CEREBRAL PALSY

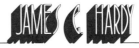

JAMES C. HARDY

University of Iowa

CEREBRAL PALSY

Prentice-Hall, Inc., Englewood Cliffs, New Jersey 07632

Library of Congress Cataloging in Publication Data

Hardy, James
  Cerebral palsy.

  (Remediation of communication disorders)
  Bibliography: p.
  Includes index.
  1. Cerebral palsy. 2. Communicative disorders.
I. Title. II. Series. [DNLM: 1. Cerebral palsy—
Therapy. 2. Cerebral palsy—In infancy and childhood. WS 342 H269c]
RC388.H37 1983   616.8'36   82-23013
ISBN 0-13-122820-X

With fond respect for and gratitude to MAC
for making life richer

Printed in the United States of America

10 9 8 7 6 5

Editorial production/supervision by Virginia Cavanagh Neri
Interior design by Maureen Olsen
Cover design by Maureen Olsen
Manufacturing buyer: Ron Chapman

ISBN 0-13-122820-X

Prentice Hall International, Inc., *London*
Prentice Hall of Australia Pty. Limited, *Sydney*
Editora Prentice-Hall do Brasil, Ltda., *Rio de Janeiro*
Prentice Hall Canada, Inc., *Toronto*
Prentice Hall of India Private Limited, *New Delhi*
Prentice Hall of Japan, Inc., *Tokyo*
Prentice Hall of Southeast Asia Pte. Ltd., *Singapore*
Whitehall Books Limited, *Wellington, New Zealand*

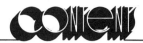

Contents

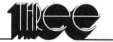

Characteristics of the problem 40

General considerations for assessment and management 74

Assessment of developmental dysarthria: The general case 100

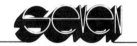

Management of developmental dysarthria: The general case 144

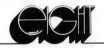

**Associated disabilities,
disorders, and
problems** 179

**The infant and
young child** 224

The severely involved:
Augmentative communication
systems 238

Appendix 255

References 267

Index 271

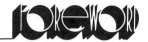

With the information explosion of recent years there has been a proliferation of knowledge in the areas of scientific and social inquiry. The specialty of communicative disorders has been no exception. While two decades ago a single textbook or "handbook" might have sufficed to provide the aspiring or practicing clinician with enlightenment on an array of communication handicaps, this is no longer possible—hence the decision to prepare a series of single-author texts.

As the title implies, the emphasis of this series, *Remediation of Communication Disorders,* is on therapy and treatment. The authors of each book were asked to provide information relative to anatomical and physiological aspects of each disorder, as well as pathology, etiology, and diagnosis to the extent that an understanding of these factors bears on management procedures. In such relatively short books this was quite a challenge: to offer guidance without writing a "cookbook"; to be selective without being parochial; to offer theory without losing sight of practice. To this challenge the series' authors have risen magnificently.

A book devoted to the subject of cerebral palsy with implications for communicative disorders has been needed for some time. James Hardy's long-time professional and personal associations with neurologically impaired persons gives him an ideal perspective as the author of such a book. Dr. Hardy has produced a work that is highly relevant for the clinical worker, and it provides a historical and research orientation that is pertinent for the scholar. What emerges between the pages of this book is a balance between theory and practice. Dr. Hardy's numerous publications and papers presented before learned societies augment his many years as a clinician and investigator. While Dr. Hardy does not shrink from stating his biases regarding management of their communication disorders, his book presents material that deals with the broad range of problems that are faced by individuals with cerebral palsy, their families, and others with whom they associate. The reader of this book will find a deep and sincere concern and understanding of the needs and rights of neurologically-impaired persons.

FREDERICK N. MARTIN
Series Editor

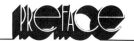

It has been my intent to write a book that deals with management of communication problems associated with cerebral palsy since the early 1970s. For over a decade prior to that time I was associated with a somewhat unique program at the University Hospital School at the University of Iowa. During that period the facility provided (1) residential education programs and related services for physically handicapped children for as many as 60 children in residence, the majority of whom had cerebral palsy, and (2) outclinic services for as many as 200 different children with cerebral palsy per year. Both groups ranged from infants to adolescents. The staff included members of the professions that were needed for ongoing services relative to cerebral palsy, and the other programs for atypical children on the University's campus were available for consultation.

The speech and hearing staff of the facility consisted of an audiologist, a teacher for the hearing-impaired, five to six clinical speech-language pathologists, and a research staff that studied (1) normal speech physiology and (2) aberrations thereof that are associated with cerebral palsy. That research program was supported in part by the Public Health Service Research Grant NB-02662 from the National Institute of Neurological Diseases and Blindness (now the National Institute of Neurological and Communicative Disorders and Stroke).

There evolved within this group of clinicians and researchers a pattern of interaction that led to consistent critiques of ideas and assumptions regarding our clinical endeavors. In addition to the involvement of the staffs of the other professions in the facility, members of the faculties of departments from throughout the University, including those of Speech Pathology and Audiology, Pediatrics, Otolaryngology, Anesthesiology, Medical Electronics, and Hydraulics Research, participated in our activities. A number of those who contributed were heavily involved with programs of the American Academy for Cerebral Palsy (now the American Academy for Cerebral Palsy and Developmental Medicine).

Those were exciting times. We were in the era of accelerated interest in conditions of cerebral palsy that is described in Chapter Two, and the exchange of ideas seemed endless.

The facilities that were available made it possible to submit a great variety of ideas to systematic observations. For example, lung function characteristics of children with cerebral palsy that could not be measured in the Speech Research Laboratory of the Hospital School were determined in the Cardiovascular Laboratory, Department of Internal Medicine, and a cinefluourographic unit in the Department of Otolaryngology that filmed articulatory movements was extensively used. Many of the pertinent clinical observations and the results of a number of the researches have not been published. These activities, however, provided the genesis of a number of the ideas discussed in Chapters Six and Seven.

It is fortunate, however, that this book was not attempted earlier. There is a tendency to take extreme positions when ideas are new and information that seems to substantiate those ideas is fresh. Many of my earlier ideas have been substantially modified by continued acquisition of information as reported in the literature, exchange of information with colleagues, the searching critiques that can be provided only by one's students, and my continued involvement with persons who have cerebral palsy. The material not only reflects those modifications, but it also attempts to present a broad perspective of clinical issues that surround this population.

As is stated or implied a number of times throughout the text, there probably is no area of speech-language pathology that is more demanding of the clinical worker. Knowledge is needed regarding speech and language development, speech physiology, neural processes of speech and language, neuromotor systems, and disorders of those systems. The heterogeneity of the communication problems of the population also requires application of information related to different types of communication handicaps, and the frequent presence of associated disabilities demands application of sound information from a number of other professions.

The attempt to integrate so much information has necessitated synthesis of a voluminous literature; what could have been lengthy discussions, with extensive documentation, have been curtailed in a number of instances. It would be unfortunate if, as a result, important considerations have been omitted. As is emphasized throughout the text, the ramifications of the clinician's endeavors require the highest degree of professional responsibility, and that responsibility cannot be met if decisions are based on ill-founded information.

To the extent that this work is found to be useful, a great number of individuals deserve my thanks. It would be impossible to list in a fair manner the many individuals who have contributed to the formulation of the ideas that are presented. Certainly, the clinical and research staffs of the program mentioned above contributed substantially by their dedicated efforts. I also am indebted to colleagues and students over the years for their willingness to share information and to critique ideas, to those individuals with cerebral palsy and their family members with whom I have worked, and to those of my current colleagues who gave so generously of their time in review of the manuscript.

JAMES C. HARDY

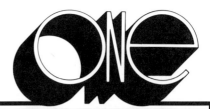

Introduction

This book deals with management of the communication disorders associated with cerebral palsy. However, the term cerebral palsy applies to a group of individuals who may have a great variety of disorders and disabilities. These other disorders and disabilities occur in different combinations and in different degrees of severity within individuals, and they may or may not have an impact on the development of communication skills. As a result, the communication disorders within the population that has cerebral palsy are extremely heterogeneous with respect to etiologies and characteristics, and it is difficult to state comprehensive, generally applicable guidelines for management of these communication disorders.

O AN ORIENTATION TO THE PROBLEM

The potential for variations of problems within a given individual who may be diagnosed as having cerebral palsy has created difficulty historically for members of all professions that have dealt with the population. Indeed, the variety of etiologies that may result in cerebral palsy and the heterogeneity of disorders and disabilities that may be associated with the condition has led to serious question that the term cerebral palsy has clinical significance. A prime basis for success in dealing with diseases and/ or disorders of humans has been the ability to identify their common elements. Whenever a homogeneous disease or disorder is identified and methods of treatment and prevention are found to be effective, the particular disease or disorder may then become subject to better understanding and, in most instances, to improved control, cure, or management. That is the prime purpose of diagnostic labels. Yet, over a century of study of the concept of cerebral palsy has shown that the label does not apply to a group with a homogeneous etiology or a common cluster of resulting disorders.

A number of definitions of cerebral palsy have attempted to encompass the heterogeneous characteristics of the individuals to whom the label has been applied. There is, however, far more general agreement about the common elements of cerebral palsy among the clinical practitioners who become involved with those to whom the label is applied than is suggested by the numerous definitions in the literature. To those practitioners, the diagnosis of cerebral palsy means that the individual has some form of dysfunction of the neuromotor systems that has resulted from a nonprogressive brain abnormality for which the onset was before, at, or shortly after the time of birth. That is also the most consistent connotation of the term throughout the historical and contemporary literature.

There are a number of etiologies that will result in early lesions or malformations of developing brain tissues. Moreover, portions of the developing brain other than those of the neuromotor systems may be involved. These factors, of course, are those that lead to the heterogeneous characteristics of persons with cerebral palsy.

Nevertheless, the term cerebral palsy will probably continue to be used as long as its definition is restricted to those common elements of (1) a developmental neuromotor disorder that is (2) the result of a nonprogressive abnormality of the developing brain. A concentration on these common elements provides a perspective that permits prediction of the unique characteristics of the cerebral palsied population, including the unique characteristics of the communication disorders of its members.

An understanding of the developmental neuromotor disorders that distinguish cerebral palsy has been slowed by a natural inclination to assume comparability between the results of brain lesions that involve the neuromotor systems of adults compared to the results of such lesions to the neuromotor systems of the developing brain. The initial belief was that there was one type of neuromotor disorder that resulted from lesions to the neuromotor systems of the immature brain. That idea, however, was dispelled rather quickly since the motor behaviors of the infants and children involved obviously differed. Also, different types of neuromotor disorders that resulted from damage to the brains of adults began to be delineated. Study of these acquired neuromotor disorders of adults showed that the different types of dysfunction might be associated with sites of damage to the brain. Thus, it became assumed that accurate delineation of types of neuromotor disorders in cerebral palsy would lead to identification of homogeneous subgroups and, hence, to better understanding of developmental neuromotor disorders. The idea of types, or subtypes, of cerebral palsy thus received emphasis, but there was the early assumption that the types of cerebral palsy should be viewed the same as types of acquired neuromotor problems of brain-damaged adults. Some of the contemporary literature that deals with cerebral palsy still contains reference to those forms of neuromotor deficits that can be differentiated in adults with acquired brain lesions.

Such attempts to compare acquired and developmental neuromotor disorders failed to recognize that an insult to the adult brain disrupts systems that have developed anatomically and that have matured physiologically. Lesions to the developing brain, however, disrupt systems whose development will be completed in the presence of the lesion. The results of these two circumstances are not likely to be directly comparable.

An understanding of the problems of persons with cerebral palsy also seems to have been obscured in another manner by the inclination to make comparisons to the results of damage to mature brains. A variety of other disorders, such as perception problems, disturbances of language function, and behavior aberrations, are known to result from damage to the brains of adults. What seemed to be comparable disorders in children began to be explained on the basis of prenatal or natal brain lesions, and, since cerebral palsy was known to result from early brain lesions, it was assumed that this variety of other specific disorders was present with great frequency in persons with cerebral palsy. As a consequence, lack of normal development of a number of behaviors and skills among the cerebral palsied population began to be attributed to alleged specific brain dysfunctions. There may be even less justification for assuming that some of these specific sequelae of damage to the mature brains of adults also can result from lesions to developing brains than there is for assuming comparable results of damage to the developing and mature neuromotor systems.

This historical inclination to attribute atypical behaviors of children to abnormalities of their brains, however, has influenced even definitions of cerebral palsy. For example, in the 1950s and 1960s the concept of the so-called brain-damaged child, or child with minimal brain dysfunction, was being accepted uncritically in this country by many professional people who worked with atypical children. Many children who behaved and learned abnormally were said to do so because of early damage to their developing brains, although the fact of brain damage could not be established for large numbers of those children. Nevertheless, some persons advocated that the child with cerebral palsy was a special case of that group of children, even though there was no evidence that all children who have cerebral palsy consistently manifest such behavior and learning problems. Such suggestions tend to divert attention from the prime distinguishing characteristic of the population—namely, the presence of a neuromotor disorder.

Discussions of the causes and characteristics of communication disorders associated with cerebral palsy routinely emphasize numerous types of bases in addition to the neuromotor disorder. Granted, these additional bases of communication handicaps may be found in selected persons with cerebral palsy, and they deserve concentrated attention by the speech-language pathologist in those cases. To set forth the premise, however, that these other bases distinguish the communication disorders associated with cerebral palsy obscures what commonality and uniqueness exists relative to these disorders.

As has been emphasized, persons with cerebral palsy manifest a high incidence of associated disabilities and disorders that may affect their development of communication skills. Mental retardation and hearing impairments are only two examples. Yet, the fact remains that the distinguishing characteristic of the population's communication disorders is a dysarthria.

Concentration on the distinguishing characteristic of the communication disorders of the cerebral palsied population—namely, a developmental dysarthria—permits a statement of manageable guidelines for remediation of these disorders. In this context, the term dysarthria implies what appears to be its current generally accepted usage: a disability in producing the speech signal due to some dysfunction of the neuromotor or neuromuscular systems or both. Thus, the assessment and management programs that are presented in detail in this book will focus primarily on the difficulties members of this population have in generating an intelligible speech signal due to their neuromotor disorder.

As mentioned, it is generally accepted that a lesion to the brain of an adult may lead to a variety of disorders. However, discussions of management of communication problems of persons who have sustained brain damage as adults frequently concentrate on one area of disability. For example, discussions of dysarthria associated with acquired neurological problems in adults may present the salient features of the speech physiology problems without emphasis on the language disorders, memory problems, or reduced intellectual function that may be concomitant problems in adults with dysarthria. It is assumed that the practicing speech-language pathologist realizes the potential presence of these other disorders and designs speech-language rehabilitation programs accordingly for appropriate cases. The same approach will be taken in this book.

The guidelines for assessment and management of the developmental dysarthrias in cerebral palsy are not identical to those for assessment and management of dysarthria that results from acquired abnormalities of adult brains. The existence of differences in the characteristics of acquired neuromotor disorders compared to developmental neuromotor disorders has already been mentioned. In addition, of course, the child with a developmental dysarthria is faced with the problem of developing speech and language with an abnormal speech-producing mechanism.

The fact that the communication disorders associated with cerebral palsy are developmental in nature adds, of course, an additional set of variables that may need the attention of the speech-language pathologist. Any of the psychological and sociological conditions that are known to contribute to problems of speech and language development also may contribute to the communication disorder of a selected child with cerebral palsy.

Again, however, viewing such variables as general contributors to the lack of development of communication skills in the population with cerebral palsy may divert attention from the usual presence of restricted function of the speech-producing musculatures. For example, there has been emphasis upon the possibility that the physical disability of children with cerebral palsy limits the extent to which they can explore their environment, and that limitation has been suggested as contributing to delay in developing language skills. However, many infants and young children who have orthopedic and/or neuromotor dysfunction of their extremities have similar limits in exploring their environment during the early ages, but they develop language and speech skills normally. Therefore, if one is to contend that experiential deprivation is a prime deterrent to development of communication skills in the cerebral palsied population, an explanation has to be given as to why children with similar physical handicaps, but with normal speech-producing mechanisms, do not as a group show delays in speech and language development. The developmental dysarthria that limits the oral interchange of infants and young children with others may be an equally crucial factor. Also, there is the strong possibility that what may be interpreted as delay in development of communication skills is primarily an inability of many of these children to express themselves due to their neuromotor impairment.

Other specific disorders have been alleged to contribute generally to abnormal development of communication skills in the population in advance of firm evidence that such problems are inevitably linked to speech and language learning problems. For example, over the last two decades interest in the role of somesthesia in motor speech behavior has accelerated. It is not the purpose here to review the theoretical formulations inherent in that research nor the conclusions that can be validly derived from it. However, the data published thus far provide only suggestive evidence that somesthetic deficits and speech production problems are related in a cause–effect manner in children with cerebral palsy. Yet, many discussions of the communication problems associated with cerebral palsy strongly emphasize the presence of the somesthetic deficits in the population as if such a cause–effect relationship can be assumed.

The responsibility of the professional person who manages any aspect of the cerebral palsied problem is too great to permit speculation and conjecture as a basis for formulating diagnostic procedures, management techniques, and prognoses. For any specific individual with cerebral palsy, a complex array of contributing factors must be considered in the management programs and statements of prognoses. This is not to say that general guidelines for assessment and predictions of outcomes of management should be based on such speculation and conjectural considerations. Rather, there is a need to be constantly realistic and objective regarding the work to be done and its potential outcome.

One disability that is very frequently associated with cerebral palsy bears directly on the activities of a speech-language pathologist who deals with this population and on the need to be objective regarding those activities. It must be accepted that a large proportion of individuals with cerebral palsy should be considered as mentally retarded. Reduced intellectual functioning, of course, has a dramatic effect on development of speech and language skills, and it may limit the degree to which effective communication ability of any type can be developed. It is difficult to face the reality of a firm, negative prognosis for a client, particularly when that client is a child within a family constellation that includes parents who, naturally enough, are inclined to hold hope for the future of their handicapped child. To perpetuate that hope falsely, however, may be a grave disservice to not only the child, but to the parents, other family members, and society in general.

That point brings me to a firm philosophy that I have developed regarding appropriate professional responsibility of the speech-language pathologist, or any practitioner in health or health-related professions. The dividends to be gained from being realistic to one's self, one's clients, and the client's family members are far greater than those achieved from being speculative, intuitive, and unjustifiably optimistic about the long-range outcome of one's professional endeavors. I have witnessed too many instances where unnecessary trauma to the stability of clients and their families has resulted from unrealistic favorable prognoses. Issuing a statement of a negative prognosis must be done with caution, and the manner in which it is done must be designed in view of a large number of variables. However, there seldom is an excuse for holding out false hope to the parents of a severely mentally retarded or severely dysarthric child who has cerebral palsy that he or she will develop reasonably good oral communication skills.

The fact that the prognosis for developing functional oral communication skills is negative in a number of children with cerebral palsy leads to another topic of professional responsibility for those who deal with this population. Frequently, that responsibility extends as much to assisting family members to adapt to the ramifications of their having a significantly handicapped child as it does to assisting the child to improve function. From the time parents recognize that their child has some type of significant abnormality, their interactions with the handicapped child, other children in the family, and each other may be altered drastically. The patterns of parent-child interaction may become counterproductive to the optimum development of their handicapped child. Any strains in a marital relationship may become exaggerated, since issues related to that child may become focal points of marital discord. Therefore, assisting families of children with cerebral palsy to become better functioning units of society may be a prime goal of the professional persons who deal with that population.

The material that follows, then, will present the position that to the extent that a unique set of guidelines can be presented to the speech-language pathologist for the cerebral palsied population, that set of guidelines is primarily related to the presence of a developmental dysarthria. Assessment and management procedures that are generally appropriate for the communication disorders of the population are those directed toward determining how neuromotor involvement interferes with speech production and how that interference can be minimized. However, the presence of an established brain abnormality that also characterizes the population predisposes this group of individuals to a wide variety of associated disabilities and disorders that may also influence their development of oral communication. Those factors contribute to the heterogeneity of the communication disorders of this population, but if the perspective is maintained that these associated disabilities and disorders are superimposed on the usual, common presence of developmental dysarthria, a reasonable orientation to evaluation and management of the communication handicaps can be maintained.

The following material also will emphasize the requirement that the speech-language pathologist must maintain objectivity in working with this population. The ramifications of the decisions that are to be made require the highest level of professional responsibility and integrity. To emphasize that point, one of the decisions that must frequently be made is whether it is realistic to expect a given child with cerebral palsy to develop functional oral communication. Although there may be alternatives, such as training the child to use some systems of nonoral communication, the basic decision of a negative prognosis for development of oral communication will have dramatic effects on the child and his or her family. On the other hand, to continue working unrealistically toward a goal of developing oral communication may have even greater adverse effects. Even though such clinical decisions may have to be based on prognostic indicators that are less than clear, they must be made, to the extent possible, from a base of realistic, objective appraisal.

Finally, because of the complexity of the factors that must be taken into consideration in the assessment and management of the communication disorders associated with cerebral palsy, the practice of speech-language pathology with this population can be one of the most challenging tasks to be faced by a professional person. Differential assessment of the many potential factors that may contribute to the communication disorders of both children and adults with cerebral palsy requires a broad knowledge of speech-language pathology. Even with that knowledge, confidence in making clinical decisions may come only after the speech-language pathologist has accumulated substantial experience in working with individuals who have cerebral palsy, their family members, and persons in other professions who have had comparable experience.

Persons with cerebral palsy present a wide array of disorders and disabilities. Definitions of cerebral palsy that have attempted to comprehensively include these disorders and disabilities divert attention from what historically has been the common element of the population to whom the label has been applied. That common element is a neuromotor disorder resulting from some nonprogressive brain abnormality that had its onset during the brain's anatomical development.

Due to the array of associated problems the communication disorders that are found among persons with cerebral palsy are also quite heterogeneous. As a consequence, it is difficult to develop a set of guidelines generally applicable to the assessment and management of these disorders. However, by recognizing the common, differentiating characteristic setting members of this group apart from other individuals, namely the developmental neuromotor disorder, it is possible to develop such guidelines. That is, assessment and management procedures that are most routinely applicable for the disorders of communication are those that concentrate on developmental dysarthria.

Those guidelines will need to be modified for each individual according to other disabilities and disorders that may be present. Unfortunately, the fact that a brain abnormality is a component of the differentiating characteristic of the condition predisposes the cerebral palsied population to a high incidence of problems for which the prognosis for dramatic improvement is poor. In addition to the neuromotor disorder, one of those frequent problems is mental retardation.

However, an appropriate orientation calls for concentration upon developmental dysarthria and the characteristics of developmental neuromotor disorders. In addition, there must be constant efforts maintained to be objective and realistic regarding professional endeavors with members of the cerebral palsied population. The ramifications of those endeavors upon the individual receiving them, his or her family members and associates, and society are too great to permit professional decisions that are based upon conjecture and speculation. Because of the complexity of the problems that are encountered and the significance of the decisions that must be made, however, work in the area of cerebral palsy can be among the most challenging and rewarding for the speech-language pathologist.

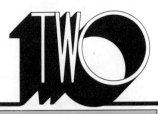

○ HISTORICAL BACKGROUND

○ PROBLEMS WITH LABELS

○ AN ERA OF ACCELERATED INTEREST

    identification of specific conditions
    phenomenon of changing signs
    the era of reflexology and systems of
    treatment

○ OTHER ASPECTS OF THE HISTORY

○ SUMMARY

The problem

Workers from a large number of professions should be available in appropriately comprehensive programs for children with cerebral palsy. From the medical profession, a neonatologist may become involved if abnormalities of the child are detected at the time of its birth. Pediatricians should usually follow the child's health status, and the services of orthopedists or specialists in physical rehabilitation, physiatrists, also may be desirable. If symptoms of the child suggest that the term cerebral palsy has been misapplied or that there also is a neurological disease present, the services of a neurologist should be available. Visual problems should be evaluated by an ophthalmologist. For the child with a hearing impairment, an otolaryngologist should be consulted to determine if the hearing problem can be improved by medical management. Since, by definition, cerebral palsy is due to a nonprogressive insult to the brain, the roles of physicians usually are to determine that cerebral palsy is, in fact, the basis of the child's abnormalities and to continue to deal with medically related problems, which includes management of neuromotor-skeletal disabilities.

Evaluating and planning management programs for specific dysfunctions usually fall to members of habilitation teams. Traditionally, physical therapists design programs to assist the child in developing or improving ambulatory skills, and occupational therapists address themselves to helping the child with what may be called functional skills (i.e., dressing, eating, toileting, and writing). Psychologists are needed who have experience in assessing both intellectual and personality problems of handicapped children. Educational consultants may be very helpful who understand the numerous handicaps that may be present and how those handicaps may affect a child's ability to master academic skills. The services of an experienced social worker may be invaluable in assisting a family to adapt to the problems that are created by having a handicapped child as one of its members.

An audiologist to assess hearing sensitivity is essential, and for those children for whom a significant hearing loss is found, the audiologist's involvement should continue. Amplification may be needed, and an appropriate educational program may call for continued involvement of the audiologist, a hearing clinician, or a teacher of the hearing impaired (or whatever may be that person's professional label) who has expertise in educational programs for children with hearing impairments.

An audiologist should carry out a routine program of hearing conservation with all children who have cerebral palsy, as is the case with other children. Also as with other children, follow-up audiological evaluations are particularly needed for those children with cerebral palsy who have shown a predisposition to otitis media and upper respiratory infections.

Since a large percentage of children with cerebral palsy have problems of oral communication, a speech-language pathologist should occupy a prime role in the habilitation of many of these children. The appropriate role of the speech-language pathologist in the habilitation team may vary as a result of a particular administrative structure or professional orientation within a particular program. Nevertheless, he or she must have an appropriate appreciation for the potential bases of communication problems associated with cerebral palsy.

In addition, the speech-language pathologist should be a member of the habilitation team on a much more meaningful level than just interacting about a given client. The orientation and goals of, and some of the information available to, the other professions must become known and understood. On a relatively superficial level, the speech-language pathologist must recognize that some techniques for determining the basis of a child's problem by another profession have limitations. For example, routine clinical evaluations by electroencephalography, or EEG, are relatively limited in specifying the location of brain pathology, particularly in children. Therefore, it is inappropriate to request an EEG from a medical colleague to determine specifically the location of an area of brain dysfunction. On a more important level, the management programs of the members of the interdisciplinary professional team may be counterproductive if they are pursued independently with equal vigor. These professional persons must interact on a level of mutual understanding and respect. If they do not, it will be difficult for them to reach optimally effective plans of habilitation.

One of the prime sources of difficulty in determining the important considerations for assessing and managing communication problems associated with cerebral palsy and, certainly, in developing an understanding of the rationales of fellow practitioners from other professions is the terminology that will be encountered. In some sciences, such as physics and mathematics, terms frequently have precise, definable referents. However, for most areas of knowledge that have an impact on an understanding of the conditions of cerebral palsy, such precision is frequently lacking.

Moreover, as increased knowledge becomes available to any professional discipline, the vernacular of that profession always increases. In disciplines other than those that deal with precisely defined entities, terms that formerly were generally understood to have one meaning come to have a more general, or altered, meaning. As these vernaculars change, ambiguity is introduced. Two different terms may come to be used that, in fact, refer to the same entity, and terms may come to have a more abstract and, hence, more ambiguous meaning that comes about from general usage.

Terminology relating to some aspects of physiology and disorders of the human has become very precise. Unfortunately, such is not the case with respect to the physiology and disorders of the brain. Even the contemporary literature that deals with neuromotor problems contains many terms that are, to say the least, ambiguous.

This problem of terminology is greatly compounded for anyone who works with individuals who have cerebral palsy. The literature and resulting ideas of a large number of professions must be synthesized. The possibility for persons misinterpreting statements from professional areas other than the one in which they have received formal training is even greater than from within their own field of endeavor. It may be impossible to estimate the preciseness of the terms used. Unfortunately, there is frequently an inclination to assume more precision than is warranted.

Also, there is the unfortunate tendency on the part of some professional people to use the vernacular of their own profession to impress rather than to communicate. The use of terms in discussions by someone from another profession with the implication that those terms reflect well-established comprehensive knowledge, when in fact there are many gaps in that knowledge, works against the goal of interdisciplinary cooperation. When members of the habilitation team are able to share points of view from their particular perspective, along with open acknowledgement of gaps in their own knowledge, they will have reached a level of professional respect and exchange of ideas that will add to the intellectual and professional challenge in serving persons who have cerebral palsy. However, it will be those who are being served who will profit optimally.

Such interdisciplinary service probably can be achieved most easily within programs specially designed for the needs of the children with multiple handicaps. Within recent decades a number of such programs have been developed within this country, some of which have been residential. With the enactment of Public Law 94–142 in 1977, many of the children who were served in those programs are now receiving professional services in their school systems. Although many large, metropolitan-based school systems have established, and will continue to establish, special programs that permit their multiply-handicapped students to receive interdisciplinary services on a day basis, achieving the desirable characteristics of the needed interdisciplinary programs for children with cerebral palsy may be difficult in many school systems. Providing related services to children receiving special education on an itinerant basis works against close interaction of the professional staff who provide those services. Yet, such interaction must be sought in order to achieve optimum programs for many children with cerebral palsy.

○ HISTORICAL BACKGROUND

It probably would be impossible to predict accurately the reactions of the early students of cerebral palsy to the tremendous specialized knowledge that now can be brought to bear on the assessment and management of the problem. Although such speculation is of little value, it is important to note some aspects of the evolution of ideas regarding cerebral palsy. A scholarly treatise of the historical observations and ideas about cerebral palsy would be inappropriate for the purposes of this book. However, a brief review of the evolution of thinking regarding cerebral palsy can highlight and, in some instances, clarify pertinent contemporary issues. (In passing, it is fascinating that some of the early statements regarding cerebral palsy closely parallel current knowledge and ideas.) Also, and perhaps most important, a historical review serves to clarify many of the ambiguities still present.

Initial identification of conditions that are now labeled *cerebral palsy* usually is attributed to W. J. Little, founder of the Royal Orthopedic Hospital, London, early in the nineteenth century. In a series of lectures published in *The Lancet* in 1843, Little described a condition he observed in infants, which he called "spastic rigidity," and he compared it to "universal spastic rigidity," a label being given to a neuromotor disorder observed in some adults after trauma or disease to their central nervous systems. Although he did offer the opinion that the condition could result from injury to the baby during birth, he stated his belief at that time that the majority of cases were associated with prematurity. He expressed the opinions that (1) for those cases, the prematurity was the result of poor health of the mother, which affected the development of the fetus, and (2) the infant, by virtue of the prematurity, was not prepared to cope with the "external agents" and was, therefore, susceptible to disability.

Almost twenty years later, Little's experiences had led him to revise his opinions considerably (Little, 1861). He described a number of events at birth, as well as whether the infant was premature or full term, that he had come to believe produced the condition, and he suggested that partial suffocation of the newborn was the principle cause of the nervous system damage that led to the spastic rigidity. He pointed out that a number of obstetricians had described "asphyxia neonatorum" as being the cause of stillbirths. However, he criticized them for failing to attend to the probability that numerous children who suffered from asphyxia neonatorum did, in fact, survive. He contended that those children had spastic rigidity and other deficits like what we now call mental retardation. Moreover, and somewhat more to the point for the present purposes, he reported that some of these children developed surprisingly good physical function and that a number of them had unimpaired intellect. Little described over fifty cases in some detail that ranged in age from fourteen months to fifteen years of age. Little's descriptions of his patients reflect reasonably well the same handicaps that are seen in persons to whom the term cerebral palsy applies today. Some of them had difficulty only with walking; others had problems not only with ambulation but also in the function of their arms and hands; some were reported to have speech problems; and the severity of their neuromotor disorders varied greatly.

The term Little's disease came to be used by many to refer to these neuromotor disorders that result from early damage to the brain. There evolved the realization, however, that Little was in error in emphasizing that these various neuromotor problems should be viewed as a common entity. Also, his later concentration on anoxia as the prime etiology was believed to be overly restrictive.[1] Therefore, even though his description of the disabilities that are frequently associated with developmental neuromotor problems due to early brain injury were comparable to those that might be used today, Little came to be viewed as having made a relatively limited contribution to knowledge of cerebral palsy due to those narrow points of view.

It is difficult to determine when the term cerebral palsy came into use. Little's publications are in English, but many of the pertinent papers of the late 1800s were published in other European languages, especially French and German. It seems, however, that by the 1890s the term cerebral palsy was in use. The translations of papers available to me suggest that Sigmund Freud contributed greatly to the use of the term as a result of his book, *Die Infantile Cerebrallahmung* (1897).[2] Freud argued that the term meant paralysis (or palsy) of childhood due to cerebral causes. Freud also argued that the term was being used at that time to apply to a number of conditions, such as epilepsy, for which it was inappropriate. Thus, attention was being diverted from the common component of the neuromotor problems just as it has been since the turn of the century. What seems to have been a very comprehensive review of the literature of the day was provided by Freud to show that even when the term is used appropriately, those children to whom it should apply have problems that differ with respect to (1) the characteristics of their neuromotor disorders, (2) the distribution of the disorders among muscle groups, and (3) the

---

[1]As reviewed in Chapter Three, anoxia of cells of the developing neuromotor systems is now known to be a prime causal factor of cerebral palsy. However, such anoxia frequently occurs prenatally. Therefore, Little's view in this regard was restrictive in that the relative lack of sophistication of the period led him to speculate that the anoxia routinely occurred at the time of birth.

[2]One translation that is available carries the title *Infantile Cerebral Paralysis* and another is entitled *Infantile Cerebral Palsy;* the texts of those two translations used the two terms consistently throughout. However, another publication in 1897 by an American physician, Sachs, refers to Freud's work as *Infantile Cerebral Palsy,* and Sachs also uses the term cerebral palsy frequently when paraphrasing, or referring to, the works of other European authors.

causes of the underlying dysfunctions of the brain. He described the presence of different types of neuromotor problems, including forms of involuntary motion disorders. He designated Little's "spastic rigidity," or what he labeled "general cerebral rigidity," as only one subtype of cerebral palsy that was, in fact, rather infrequently seen. His treatise pointed out that the variety of symptoms being observed could result from a number of etiologies and emphasized that what he was calling infantile cerebral palsy had no pathological-anatomical or etiological unity. Freud also emphasized that any unity within the group of children with cerebral palsy was to be found within subgroups, or what are now called types, of cerebral palsy.

By the turn of the century the search for the unifying variables was in full swing. Some argued that the time of the brain injury was important. That is, whether the brain was damaged before, during, or shortly after birth was said to lead to different problems, and therefore, children with cerebral palsy should be classified accordingly. Others argued that the distribution of the motor problems over the body was the unifying variable. As a consequence, homogeneity was sought, for example, within "hemiplegic forms" as compared to "diplegic forms." Some writers suggested that homogeneity could be found within the population by classifying the children with cerebral palsy on the basis of whether they showed involvement in one limb, the two limbs on one side of the body, three limbs, or all four limbs, but there came the recognition that such classifications must be combined with the type of neuromotor impairment present.

As the attempts to determine unifying characteristics of cerebral palsy continued to be made, the number of types of neuromotor disorders that were said to exist within the total population increased. This increase resulted, in large part, from observation of neuromotor disorders in brain-damaged adults. It was being learned that in a few instances the characteristics of a neuromotor disorder of such adults were somewhat predictive of the location of their brain lesions. Thus, debates as to distinctive characteristics within subtypes of cerebral palsy continued at a relatively rapid pace. These debates, as they appear in the literature, may seem to represent word games. However, to the extent that a specific label could be applied that would signify a truly unique neuromotor disorder with a common etiology, these debates held promise that significant advances could be made in the understanding of cerebral palsy.

O PROBLEMS WITH LABELS

Reference was made earlier to ambiguities in professional vernaculars that could lead to difficulty in integrating knowledge regarding cerebral palsy. Such ambiguities are present in the terms, and the entities that they represent, that have been applied to types of neuromotor disorders.[3] As better understanding of abnormal neuromotor behaviors has evolved, the terms used to denote specific types of disorders have, of course, changed. In many cases, labels that apply to types of neuromotor disorders have come to hold a generally accepted meaning that is useful but inappropriate, or questionable, in view of advancing knowledge.

The labels that have been applied to involuntary motion disorders are prime examples. There was early agreement that the neuromotor systems of some brain-damaged individuals elicited abnormal movements that were not within the individual's control. In some cases those movements could be described as rapid and jerky. In other cases the involuntary movements could be described as slow and writhing. Under the assumption that these two behaviors represented different abnormalities of the neuromotor systems, different terms were applied to each, namely (1) chorea for the rapid, jerky involuntary movements and (2) athetosis for the slow, writhing movements. It was also recognized early that the involuntary motion disorders of some brain-damaged persons appeared to be a combination of rapid, jerking movements superimposed on slow, writhing movement patterns. Thus, the term choreo-athetosis was used. Observation of individuals with developmental neuromotor problems suggested early that the bulk of what was believed to be involuntary motions could be best described as the slow and writhing type; hence, athetosis came to be viewed as a major subtype of cerebral palsy.

There were other patterns of involuntary movements that were thought to be distinctive, but the examples of chorea and athetosis serve to exemplify the point that is being made; that is, to the extent that one of these forms of involuntary motion was believed to represent a homogeneous lesion of the neuromotor systems, difficulties in the inherent conceptualizations occurred when the involuntary motions within one individual seemed to represent combinations of movement patterns that did not neatly fit within the subtypes that seemed to be identifiable. Therefore, debates ensued as to whether a given type of abnormal movement was a manifestation of one disorder or another. For those who came to believe that athetosis was the only form of involuntary motion that conceptually should exist in conditions of cerebral palsy, for example, the presence of movements other than slow writhing ones was somewhat difficult to explain.

Historically, some of the same problems were encountered in the evolution of the understanding of what is now called hypertonia. By current definition, a hypertonia is characterized by muscle tone in excess of that which is normal. Hypertonic muscle is overly resistive to stretch, and the

---

[3]Definitions of terms that are used to designate types of neuromotor disorders as they are used in reference to both acquired and developmental neuromotor disorders are provided in Appendix A.

joints of extremities for which the musculature is hypertonic are resistive
to flexion or extension. The term rigidity seems to have been the earliest
term applied to individuals whose musculatures were chronically hard to
the touch and whose attempts at movements were characterized by restricted mobility. However, as the condition of spasticity came to be recognized, the term rigidity came to be applied to a less frequently occurring
form of hypertonia. Among the children who were being identified as
having cerebral palsy, another form of hypertonia would come to be identified, which would be called tension.

The search for distinguishing, unique subtypes of neuromotor problems probably was carried too far in some cases. That is, some specific
abnormal neuromotor behaviors were identified and proposed as representing a separate, specific disability from others when, in fact, the
specific behavior was a variation of a more general disorder.

Moreover, this search for unifying, distinguishing characteristics of
neuromotor disorders presented considerable problems to the extent that
there was the inherent assumption that a specific disability represented a
homogeneous site of lesion of the neuromotor systems. In many instances, it seems that such an assumption led to a black-and-white perception of what is, in fact, a complex array of abnormal neuromotor
behaviors in a given individual. For example, cerebral palsy of the mixed
type was at one time perceived to be relatively infrequent. Although it became generally recognized that tension frequently coexisted with athetosis, there seemed to be reluctance to accept the possibility that signs
indicative of spasticity could coexist in individuals whose primary neuromotor disability was one of involuntary motion. This reluctance suggested
a lack of appreciation of the possibility that a brain lesion could affect the
function of more than one neuromotor mechanism.

○ AN ERA OF ACCELERATED INTEREST

Fewer programs were developed for habilitation of children with
cerebral palsy during the early 1900s than might have been anticipated
from the great interest in cerebral palsy up until that period. Even though
there were case reports of some persons to whom the label applied who
had developed reasonable function, many early writers expressed doubt
that the function of persons with cerebral palsy could be improved. Such
comments undoubtedly delayed general interest in organizing habilitation
programs of significant magnitude.

By the 1930s interest in atypical children began accelerating in a wide
variety of professions in this country. Study of children who were abnormal in any way began expanding, and interest increased in developing
special programs to assist those children. The potential for a rapid accel-

eration of knowledge of handicapping conditions of children was diminished, however, due to World War II. When the resources of this country could be diverted back to internal educational and sociological programs, the stage was already set for extensive study of handicapped children and development of programs to assist those children.

Although I have never seen a discussion of this point in the literature, I have formed the impression that another factor contributed to the rapid expansion of programs for cerebral palsied children and adults immediately after World War II. The need for interdisciplinary professional teams for the numerous brain-injured and physically handicapped veterans resulted in the organization of rehabilitation programs to meet those needs. Thus, society seems to have been prepared for a wide variety of activities related to better understanding, prevention, and management of the conditions of cerebral palsy.

Physicians from a variety of medical specialties who had become interested in cerebral palsy formed the American Academy for Cerebral Palsy (now the American Academy for Cerebral Palsy and Developmental Medicine) in November 1947. That organization began promoting a better understanding of cerebral palsy management programs. In 1949 what is now known as the United Cerebral Palsy Research and Educational Foundation also was founded. Along with the National Society for Crippled Children and Adults (now the National Easter Seal Society), that Foundation assisted considerably by funding public education, research, and management programs. As a result, not only did the scientific base for understanding cerebral palsy expand rapidly, but habilitation programs were organized and funded throughout this country.

Even so, many of the old issues remained. For example, in 1956 Minear published the results of a survey of members of the American Academy for Cerebral Palsy relative to the types of neuromotor problems that they believed they were observing. A summary of the results suggested that eight types of cerebral palsy were being identified. In order of highest incidence, they were: (1) spasticity, (2) athetosis, (3) rigidity, (4) ataxia, (5) tremor, (6) atonia, (7) mixed, and (8) unclassifiable. Within the subtype referred to as athetosis, four forms were recognized: (1) tension, (2) nontension, (3) dystonia, and (4) tremor. Minear's report did not elaborate to any great extent on the particular signs of each of these types of cerebral palsy. For example, no descriptions were given of the differentiating signs between what was listed as an "athetoid-tremor" and simply a "tremor."

With respect to the forms of athetosis, Minear's report referred to the fact that Phelps (1956) advocated use of eleven subclassifications of these involuntary motion disorders. Phelps had been the first president of the American Academy for Cerebral Palsy, and most reviewers of his eleven subclassifications of athetosis offered the opinion that he was probably able to identify those eleven forms of involuntary motion problems even though most other persons could not do so reliably. However, other than for a few exceptions such as Phelps' subclassifications of athetosis, most listings of types of cerebral palsy during the 1950s continued to parallel those of neuromotor disabilities for adults, such as can be seen in Minear's listing.

Some dissatisfaction with that perspective of developmental neuromotor problems, however, was beginning. The book, *The Natural History of Cerebral Palsy*, by Crothers and Paine (1959) reflected some of the change in orientation. That work reported the results of record reviews of 1,821 children who had been seen in the Children's Medical Center, Boston, Massachusetts, and for whom there had been found indications of their having cerebral palsy. Moreover, a select group of that staff systematically reexamined as many of that population as was possible. The total number of patients for whom some type of reevaluation was possible is unclear, but as many as 466 are mentioned.

The review here of some of the work of Crothers and Paine is not meant to imply that they were the only individuals who were beginning to advocate altering some of the more traditional points of view regarding cerebral palsy. They were not. They did, however, base their comments on a systematic approach to a large number of cases; moreover, they were careful to point out problems with their project and the extent to which those problems suggested caution relative to the interpretations that could be made. More important, this work represents a comprehensive transition from the more traditional to contemporary views of cerebral palsy.

Crothers and Paine concluded that the bulk of individuals with cerebral palsy can be classified within three major groups, having spasticity, involuntary motion disorders, and mixed signs. Their data, in combination with previous reports, indicated to them that cases that could be described as having rigidity and tremor are so rare that they cast doubt on validity of such classifications. Although they advocated that a few cases of ataxia might exist, they questioned that this disorder of coordination exists to the extent that previous reports indicated.

In their discussions of cases having spasticity, Crothers and Paine devoted considerable attention to the topographical distribution of abnormal neuromotor signs over musculatures of the body. On that basis, they separated hemiplegics as a subgroup differing from other cases of spasticity in a number of respects. As the term implies, signs of spasticity are to be found primarily, if not solely, on one side. If the severity of the involvement tends to differ between the two limbs of the affected side, that of the leg tends to be more severe. They also pointed out that cases of monoplegia, in which there is consistently involvement of one leg but not the arm, is a special case of the hemiplegic subgroup.

Crothers and Paine pointed out, however, that restricted mobility of the oral and facial musculatures is not commonly observed in the hemi-plegic subgroup. They also reviewed evidence, primarily from work of others, that spastic hemiplegic children frequently demonstrate bilateral somesthetic deficits. In addition, their data provided further evidence that the brain lesions that lead to spastic hemiplegia tend to occur either relatively late prenatally, at the time of birth, or after birth.

For the bulk of spastic cerebral palsied children who have obvious signs of spasticity on both sides, Crothers and Paine described two patterns of involvement. The term tetraplegia had come to be used for cases in which the neuromotor disorder is distributed over all musculatures of the body and is relatively severe throughout; the term diplegia indicates that there is relatively more severe involvement of the musculatures of the feet and legs with a diminution of the degree of involvement in the upper extrem-ities.

From the standpoint of Crothers and Paine, distribution of spastic signs in three limbs, which is referred to as triplegia, is merely one form of the diplegic situation. Triplegia is routinely characterized by relatively severe involvement of both lower extremities with a milder degree of involve-ment of the musculatures of one arm. They also believed that paraplegia, or involvement of the two legs, is a milder form of diplegia in which the neuromotor disorder does not extend up the torso to include muscula-tures of the upper extremities.

Crothers and Paine were describing what was becoming accepted as the correspondence between the topographical distribution of spasticity and the anatomical arrangement of neurons of the pyramidal motor system. As will be presented in Chapter Four, and discussed later in Chapter Six, this correspondence between neuronal arrangement and patterns of spas-ticity can be used to predict with some confidence the presence or absence of involvement of the speech-producing musculatures of persons with cer-ebral palsy whose neuromotor disorders are primarily of the spastic type.

Crothers and Paine made a strong case for not attempting to subdivide the problems of involuntary motions into a number of discrete classifica-tions. Their position was that the principle movement seen was the slow, writhing movements that had been classically labeled as athetosis. They granted that other types of movement patterns could be observed that might be described as chorea or tremor and that involuntary motions re-ferred to as ballismus, or flinging, flailing movements, could be seen occa-sionally. In fact, they reported enough variations in movement patterns that they recommended disbanding the term athetosis. They strongly urged the use of the term extrapyramidal cerebral palsy. They offered reasons for preferring that term to hyperkinesis or dyskinesis, which mean, respectively, too much movement and disorder of movement.

They reviewed a form of hypertonia, which they called *tension* accord-ing to established convention, as being frequently present in the extrapyr-

amidal type of cerebral palsy. They also discussed another phenomena
regarding the involuntary motion and tension disorders that are seen;
namely, the abnormal neuromotor signs tend to reduce or disappear
when the individual is, respectively, relaxed in a secure position or sleeping soundly.

With respect to topographical distribution of what they refer to as cerebral palsy of the extrapyramidal type, they described what had been historically described as very rare cases of involvement on one side of the
body. However, such cases are so rare that they probably are of no concern. Therefore, involuntary motion disorders can be expected to exist bilaterally, and there is some tendency for the musculatures of the upper
extremities and oral and facial structures to show more severe signs of involvement, relatively, than the lower extremities.

These authors discussed at some length the fact that the underlying
physiological signs that had come to denote both an involuntary motion
disorder and spasticity could be observed more often in an individual
than had been believed. In fact, these mixed signs were frequently prevalent, with one being relatively subtle, and they advocated that the term
mixed cerebral palsy probably should be used more frequently than had
been recognized historically.

One other type of cerebral palsy discussed by Crothers and Paine, ataxia, deserves some discussion. They pointed out that a number of cases
that were labeled as ataxic probably should have been considered as having involuntary motion. They point out, for example, that as a child with
an involuntary motion problem attempts movement, the involuntary motion does make him appear uncoordinated. However, such disordered
movements are different from the uncoordinated movements associated
with cerebellar dysfunction. Probably more important, it was pointed out
that cases of cerebral palsy of the ataxic type frequently were, in fact, children who were suffering from some type of cerebellar pathology. They
did offer the opinion that a few cases of developmental cerebellar disorders do exist.

identification of specific conditions

The heightened interest in the conditions of cerebral palsy from
the 1940s through the 1960s did greatly increase understanding of the
disabilities of individuals with developmental neuromotor problems in a
number of respects. For example, by the time of Crothers and Paine's
publication, the search for unifying characteristics within the population
having cerebral palsy had led to strong agreement that one subgroup with
involuntary motion disorders, the so-called Rh athetoid, had a cluster of
common signs. That label stemmed from the well-known effects of incompatibility of blood type between the mother and the infant, the best
known and most prevalent of which is the Rh factor.

Such incompatibility leads to a yellow substance, bilirubin, being carried in the blood that can infiltrate the nervous system of a newborn. Some clusters of neurons in the young brain are more susceptible to damage by bilirubin than others. As a consequence of the resulting pattern of brain damage, the Rh athetoid child was characterized by (1) athetosis, (2) problems of elevating the gaze of the eyes, and (3) a bilateral high frequency hearing loss. Crothers and Paine emphasized one aspect of this condition that was well-known previously but, to my knowledge, has not been integrated into the literature dealing with communication problems in cerebral palsy. Excessive bilirubin in the bloodstream can also result from liver dysfunction of newborns and, as with blood incompatibility problems, similar neural mechanisms can be damaged. Immature liver function frequently exists in premature newborns, and the infant may suffer brain damage, resulting in the above described cluster of signs. As a consequence, Crothers and Paine referred to this group of children as kernicteric rather than as Rh athetoid.

Due to sensitization of the medical profession to the kernicteric problem during this era, medication may be given to suppress the response of an Rh negative mother's blood to her baby's Rh positive blood. Steps are now taken that in many cases eliminate or reduce its severity. Blood transfusions to an affected newborn is a relatively common procedure, and it is now known that exposure of the infant to high intensities of light, particularly in the range of 420 to 470 nm (blue light), will break down the bilirubin being carried in the infant's blood. With the ramifications of kernicterus having been established, infants at risk for the condition are now identified much more frequently, and the appropriate procedures can be initiated. As a result, the incidence of the kernicteric group with cerebral palsy has been substantially reduced.

Other highly significant findings resulted from establishing habilitation programs for cerebral palsied children and, thus, longitudinally following their development. For example, some of those who were critical of the use of the term cerebral palsy as being nonmeaningful argued that as more knowledge was obtained about those to whom the term was being applied, it would be determined that many were the victims of specific disorders. As a result, it was predicted that those individuals would be excluded from the diagnostic classification of cerebral palsy. That prediction, in fact, came to fruition in a number of instances.

Large numbers of children who were labeled as having cerebral palsy were not observed systematically and longitudinally by specially trained physicians and members of habilitation teams prior to this era of accelerated interest. Even where these observations were made, they were infrequently shared nationally through publications and meetings of interested professional groups. Even for those cases that were followed over a period of years, what has now been demonstrated to be significant observations were either not made or disregarded. Unique findings and events related to a single case tended to be explained as an oddity. As highly interested, knowledgeable professional people began to share information, observations of what previously were only puzzling and seemingly unexplainable phenomena in select cases began to reveal conditions that, indeed, did not fall within the usual connotation of cerebral palsy.

One of the specific conditions that began to be identified within the population of children diagnosed as having cerebral palsy of the ataxic type was ataxia-telangiectasia, a degenerative process of cerebellar mechanisms in children with specific, identifiable signs in addition to the neuromotor disorder. Beginning in the late 1950s, numbers of children who had been diagnosed as having cerebral palsy were identified as having that condition. Evidently, the signs, and even the terminal nature, of ataxia-telangiectasia had not been shared by professional people to the point that this subgroup of children who also had a developmental neuromotor disorder were identified.

In addition, selected children who had been diagnosed as having cerebral palsy became recognized as having phenylketonuria (PKU). This now well-known genetically transmitted metabolic disorder that results in irreversible brain deterioration with resulting mental retardation and neuromotor disorders can frequently be prevented through diet control. The discovery of the prevalence of the problem in children with developmental motor disorders was one factor that led to the development of screening of infants for PKU, and through counseling of families known to have a history of the disorder, further control.

Thus, not only was one homogeneous type of cerebral palsy (the kernicterus athetoid group) identified, but other specific conditions, as exemplified by ataxia-telangiectasia and phenylketonuria, were being identified from among children who had been said to have cerebral palsy. Hence, the urging of the early investigators to continue to search for unity of conditions within those said to comprise the cerebral palsy population truly began to pay handsome dividends.

phenomenon of changing signs

In rejecting the classification of atonia, Crothers and Paine spoke to another emerging aspect of the neuromotor problems that make up cerebral palsy, namely, the phenomenon of changing neuromotor characteristics within a given individual. Some infants with cerebral palsy do manifest atonia; that type of neuromotor problem, however, changes to signs of involuntary motion or spasticity as the child's nervous system matures. It is now documented that the signs of the neuromotor disorder may change throughout the early years in a number of children with cerebral palsy.

On a superficial level, this phenomenon of changing signs can be explained rather easily. The insult to the nervous system that leads to cerebral palsy and associated problems occurs to an anatomically and physiologically developing brain. As will be reviewed later, it is well known that many structures of the central nervous system are not completely formed anatomically by the time of birth. Therefore, to the extent that there will be formation and organization of neuromotor systems after the occurrence of a lesion, the manifestations of the lesion may change in character as that formation and organization is taking place. In addition, some believe that the maturational process of neuromotor systems can be delayed by the presence of a lesion, thus extending the time over which changing signs occur.

Although the more typical change is from dramatically reduced muscle tone to either some form of involuntary motion or spasticity within the first few years of life, the evolving signs may fluctuate over some period until they stabilize to present a definable clinical picture. That is not to say, however, that changes cannot sometimes occur throughout the first decade of life. In fact, some of those who work with large numbers of cerebral palsied persons believe that the tension phenomenon that frequently accompanies involuntary motion problems sometimes gradually increases in severity up through the teen-age years.

the era of reflexology and systems of treatment

One other aspect of the report by Crothers and Paine is noteworthy for present purposes. In describing the specific signs that they believe to represent their prime subtypes of spastic and extrapyramidal cerebral palsy, they mention that in individuals with both types "release of postural and labyrinthine reflexes" could be observed. Many of those who were concentrating on the conditions of cerebral palsy were beginning to advocate that many of the abnormal patterns of muscle contraction could be explained on the basis of the exaggerated influence of reflexlike movements.

Reflexes and Cerebral Palsy. It had long been recognized that in physiologically normal newborns and infants certain stereotyped responses to specific stimuli could be observed. These responses had come to be called infantile reflexes, or primitive reflexes.

One of these responses is known as the Babinski sign; when the sole of the foot of a normal newborn is stroked by some object in a specified manner, the big toe extends upward and the other toes fan and sometimes curl. Another group of these responses can be referred to, in general, as the tonic neck reflexes. The asymmetrical type is the most frequently described, and it may be seen in normal infants at rest. The posture that signifies the reflex involves a combination of head and extremity positions. When the head is turned to one side, the arm on that side is extended, and the opposite arm is flexed so that the hand will be held up, behind the head. Moreover, the leg of the side to which the head is turned may be flexed, and the opposite leg may tend to be extended.

Perhaps the best-known infantile reflex consists of a rooting and sucking behavior. When the area of the face around the infant's lips is touched by some object, the head turns so that the mouth seeks the object (rooting), and once the object is in the mouth, the infant sucks rhythmically.

Explanations of the great variety of such behaviors that have been mentioned in the literature are numerous and, in some cases, quite elaborate. The Babinski sign, for example, has been attributed to lack of inhibition of these toe movements due to lack of neural inhibitory mechanisms having been developed at the spinal level since the lower portion of the spinal cord is not anatomically or physiologically completely formed at birth; the Babinski sign also may result from the immaturity of the pyramidal motor system at birth at the cortical level.

It has been argued that the asymmetrical tonic neck response is a phylogenetically retained behavior. Such an argument is based on the idea that reciprocal extension and flexion of the extremities in association with head movements can be observed in four-legged reptiles. As with other infantile behaviors that are said to be phylogenetically based, such arguments postulate that there remains within the human nervous system the neural organization that results in these motor behaviors. In the normally functioning human adult, however, these behaviors have come to be inhibited by neural mechanisms that complete their development after birth.

The rooting, sucking, and swallowing behavior of the newborn human represents a highly complex motor behavior that, with little doubt, has as its purpose the survival of the organism. It involves muscles of the oral cavity, neck, and torso. As the normal human nervous system matures, that behavior also becomes inhibited, and it usually cannot be readily elicited after the first year of life.

Irrespective of whether these numerous infant behaviors are due to (1) immaturity of the nervous system, (2) phylogenetically retained neuronal organizations, or (3) organized responses that are needed for survival of the human infant, the fact remains that very similar, if not identical, motor behaviors may be observed in selected brain-damaged adults. The Babinski is consistently listed as a characteristic sign of spasticity in the lower extremities of such adults. I have worked with one brain-injured adult woman for whom it would be difficult to deny the existence of a sucking reflex during the early stages of her recovery from a brain injury. The usual explanation for the return of these behaviors after brain damage is that the lesion affected the mechanisms that had come to inhibit the behaviors.

It also has long been recognized that these infantile behaviors are characteristically exaggerated in infants who have sustained some type of insult of their brains, and the behaviors may continue to be present long after they usually become inhibited in the normal young child. With respect to the asymmetrical tonic neck response, for example, most descriptions of normal infants stipulate that elicitation of this reflex is observable only through detection of increases and decreases in the muscle tone of the infant's extremities as the head is rotated passively from side to side. On the other hand, if the infant's arms and legs move into the prescribed positions when its head is passively rotated, the examiner is alerted to the possibility of a neuromotor abnormality.

It is difficult to deny that some of these behaviors are retained in individuals with cerebral palsy, and they are much more prevalent in those individuals than in those with acquired neuromotor disorders. The walking posture of many adults with cerebral palsy of the type that Crothers and Paine called extrapyramidal cerebral palsy certainly appears to be a manifestation of the asymmetrical tonic neck reflex. The head is held to one side, the arm to that side is extended stiffly, and the other arm may be held up with the elbows flexed to the extent that the hand is behind the head; moreover, the shuffling gait is characterized by the leg that is opposite to the extended arm moving with less mobility than the other.

The basis for these exaggerated and retained behaviors that result from early brain injury is that those inhibitory mechanisms that would come to inhibit the behavior in normal infants are among those that have been damaged. As a result, the uninhibited excitatory patterns of muscle activity underlying these behaviors remain unchecked as the brain matures after the lesion.

The vestibular system's excitatory influence on motor behavior is well established. Patterns of neural activity from the vestibular system in response to the head's position and movement relative to gravity enter the brain stem and, among many other destinations, impinge on cell bodies in the vestibular nuclei of the brain stem whose axons descend to influence motor activity. When you begin to pitch forward after solidly stubbing your toe, neural discharges through that vestibulospinal tract are among those that lead to rapid contraction of your muscles to create the quick reaction that is designed to prevent you from falling. Under more normal circumstances, that potentially powerful influence on musculatures assists in maintaining upright posture and otherwise assisting in motor function in relation to gravity and movement, but its potentially strong influence is kept under control by inhibitory mechanisms.

There are a number of reactions to postural change that may be seen in some brain-damaged persons that appear to be the result of inappropriate inhibition of such excitatory mechanisms. The behavior that has come to be called an extensor thrust is an example. If such a person is sitting in a chair and he or she is jostled, perhaps only slightly, the entire musculature may appear to react. The neck stiffens, the back arches, and the limbs straighten abruptly with considerable force. The person may slide from the chair if he or she is not held.

Even though these abnormal postural reactions had been observed in adults who had sustained lesions to their brains and these reactions were known to be much more prevalent in children with cerebral palsy, their potential clinical significance did not become generally recognized until this era of accelerated interest. Combined descriptions of the abnormal reflex behaviors and postural reactions in cerebral palsy began to appear, and there evolved beliefs that the motor problems of individuals with cerebral palsy could be alleviated through modification of these behaviors and reactions. Bobath and Bobath (1964), for example, were formulating a regimen of assessment and management based, in large part, on those beliefs. The Bobaths contended that the total motor behavior of the individual should be more normal if the exaggerated postural reactions and abnormal reflexes could be inhibited and if more normal postural tone and movement could be facilitated.

Mention of these behaviors as component parts of the conditions of cerebral palsy by Crothers and Paine was indicative of a growing general recognition of the importance of these behaviors in management of individuals with cerebral palsy. Despite previous advocacy of that importance, a number of influential persons dealing with cerebral palsy during that era were reluctant to accept the clinical significance of this aspect of cerebral palsy. The fact that such acceptance was being gained appears to have been a significant advance in management of the neuromotor disorders of individuals with cerebral palsy.

Systems of Treatment. The work of the Bobaths was one of many efforts to design regimens of management to assist children with cerebral palsy. By the late 1950s and 1960s the theoretical bases of these regimens were viewed as separate schools of thought, even though they frequently had much in common, and they came to be designated usually by the name of the individuals who advocated their use.

The reasons for reluctance to accept these so-called systems of therapy were numerous. However, a major one was that those who promoted a specific management system frequently advocated its use as generally applicable for all children with cerebral palsy. Many of the advocated procedures had come to be used for select cases well in advance of formulation of the systems, but those same procedures had been found to be wanting for management of other individuals. In addition, the theoretical formulations on which some of the proponents attempted to base their position were challenged. Finally, as these various systems came into use, their critics were quick to point out that no data were being generated that verified their efficacy. Thus, the proponents of a given system of treatment were viewed as overselling their case.

Nevertheless, to some professional people some of these systems seemed to have sufficient face validity to be accepted and used. As a result, these various systems began to be taught and advocated extensively.

The Bobath system of treatment became one of the more widely known. It was believed that by carefully analyzing the neuromotor patterns of a child with cerebral palsy and by manipulating that child's torso, extremities, and head, postures could be found that would optimally diminish abnormal neuromotor activity. Theoretically, as the child's nervous system adapted to the status of minimal abnormal motor activity, the child then could be taught more normal, functional motor skills.[4]

Reviews of this era of systems of treatment might lead to the conclusion that the underlying theory was rooted solely in ideas related to abnormal reflex and postural reactions. Such was not the case. Other theoretical formulations formed a basis for some of the systems, and in most cases a specific system of therapy was based on a number of theoretical contentions. For example, early considerations of the Bobaths suggested that the sequence of functional development was an important variable. That is, it was said that in order for a child's neuromotor systems to mature appropriately, it is desirable, and perhaps essential, that developmental skills (e.g., sitting, walking) be experienced in the appropriate chronological order.

That particular contention formed the primary basis of the system of therapy advocated by Fay. Fay emphasized that the phylogenetic and developmental sequence of motor activities were requisite to development of function, and he suggested that children with cerebral palsy need to be worked through that sequence in order to acquire optimal functional skills. Still another system that came to be known as the Deaver system emphasized use of mechanical devices to inhibit abnormal neuromotor patterns but to permit normal movements (e.g., leg braces).

The advocates of these systems of therapy came from a variety of professions. Karel Bobath is a physiatrist, and his wife, Berta, is a physical therapist. Martha Rood, an occupational therapist, advocated a system of treatment based primarily on somesthetic stimulation. Deaver also was a physiatrist; Temple Fay was a neurosurgeon. Winthrop Phelps, an orthopedic surgeon, made many contributions to the understanding of cerebral palsy, as exemplified by the previous reference to his classifications to athetosis; he also advocated a regimen of therapy that consisted of a variety of specific techniques.

As these systems of management became used, applications for most aspects of the habilitation process came to be recommended within the

[4]Many of the ideas that have evolved from the continuing work with the Bobath system have been incorporated into the neurodevelopmental approach to working with children who have cerebral palsy (see Chapter Nine). The theories and techniques of this approach have received greater acceptance than many of the earlier systems.

frame of reference of most of them. For examples, certain techniques that were recommended by the Bobaths became incorporated into regimens of speech work for children with cerebral palsy. Rood and those who used her system advocated specific applications to assist the speech development of such children.

Summaries of the specific characteristics of these various systems of management that were recommended during the 1950s and 1960s, can be found elsewhere (e.g., Gillette, 1969). Many professional people working with cerebral palsied individuals today were, and continue to be, trained to use those techniques. Any reader that is interested in the details of these systems is urged to refer to the basic references and associated literature that may be found in the bibliographies of summary writings.[5]

The debates that ensued during this period relative to these various systems were frequent and extensive. The proponents of the systems held strong beliefs as to their efficacy, and their critics were equally well-intentioned in pointing out problems that were inherent in the claims being made. As is usually the case when strong opinions are put forth pro and con in an area of human endeavor, concentrated observations and study were made of the phenomena at issue. The ultimate outcome when those issues relate to human problems is to the benefit of those being served, in this case children with cerebral palsy.

○ OTHER ASPECTS OF THE HISTORY

As attempts were being made to understand the manifestations of developmental neuromotor disorders and how best to manage them, there was a comparable surge of interest in other aspects of the problem. As various sectors of society saw fit to establish habilitation programs for youngsters with cerebral palsy, it became obvious that the early writers were wrong in their contention that minimal results could be expected from management. Numerous rather severely involved children demonstrated good and sometimes superior learning ability in education programs. Examples began to be cited of individuals with cerebral palsy who had reached levels of achievement that earlier would have seemed remarkable.

It was recognized that special techniques were needed for determining the learning ability of a child with cerebral palsy. The more comprehen-

---

[5]A listing of such references, along with a brief summary of some of these systems of management, may be found in an early edition of the book, *Cerebral Palsy, Its Individual and Community Problems* (Lencione, 1966). A more extensive list of these references appears in Payton et al. (1977).

sive standardized batteries of intelligence tests that were coming to be accepted for general use (Revised Stanford-Binet and Wechsler Intelligence Scales) could not be validly administered to a large proportion of individuals with cerebral palsy. As a consequence, efforts were made to devise special instruments that would reliably place children with cerebral palsy on the continuum of learning ability. As was the case with understanding the neuromotor disorders and how best to manage them, issues related to psychological assessment of learning ability were extensively debated. In addition to the effects of the physical handicaps and associated disabilities on education potential and personality development, attention was also given to family and sociological problems inherent in the cerebral palsy problem.

Martin Palmer, founder of the Institute of Logopedics, Harold Weslake of Northwestern University, and Eugene T. McDonald of Pennsylvania State University were among the speech pathologists who made significant contributions to the understanding and management of communication problems of cerebral palsied individuals. As with other disorder areas, it was being demonstrated that with assistance many individuals with cerebral palsy could improve their communication abilities.

As might have been expected from the accelerated interest in cerebral palsy, expectations for the numerous professional endeavors were high. Clinical practitioners from the variety of professions that had come to be involved with the cerebral palsy problem pursued their endeavors in the face of the insurmountable fact that a number of these children had been neurologically devastated. There frequently seemed to be the assumption that as more information was obtained about the numerous clinical problems being addressed, the obstacles to favorable prognoses could be overcome.

As the work has progressed through research and additional clinical endeavors, and as the outcomes of the earlier efforts have been observed as many of the children who received these efforts have become adults, a more realistic attitude has come to prevail. A number of children with cerebral palsy can be assisted to develop functional oral communication. Others are unable to do so, and efforts are now being devoted to help those through use of alternative means of communication. However, many questionable aspects of the history tend to linger.

The task of the speech-language pathologist responsible for providing service to those with cerebral palsy requires much more than a superficial knowledge of the physiological and sociological problems of these individuals. If that responsibility is to be fulfilled well, the speech-language pathologist must assimilate sufficient information from the many areas of knowledge that impact on the conditions of cerebral palsy so that a constant vigil of objectivity can be maintained.

It is now recognized that the problem of cerebral palsy can be managed best through comprehensive habilitation efforts of persons from a large number of professions. Moreover, these interdisciplinary efforts must be coordinated to meet the individual needs of each person.

This recognition was confirmed during the 1950s and 1960s when the interest in cerebral palsy and programs for management of the associated problems accelerated dramatically. Even though the conditions that are now called cerebral palsy were initially recognized over 100 years ago, many of the more salient issues relative to cerebral palsy were not determined until that era. There had been a search for the unifying variables that would justify considering cerebral palsy as a unique diagnostic entity, and progress was made in delineating those variables. Significant differences were determined to exist between the group of developmental neuromotor disorders that constitute the differentiating conditions of cerebral palsy and the neuromotor disorders in adults. In addition to better delineation of the problem, that determination led to the development of a number of regimens or systems of management. Even though some aspects of those systems were not generally accepted, the controversies that evolved from their being advocated resulted in still better understanding of the problem and how to deal with it.

Many of the views that were held during that era of accelerated interest must now be considered as overly optimistic relative to the outcome of management programs for numerous individuals with cerebral palsy. However, the efforts that were generated demonstrated unequivocally that many of these individuals are capable of a significantly improved life style compared to what they might achieve if such programs were not available. In addition, the work of that era identified the need to carry out professional endeavors relative to persons with cerebral palsy, their families, and society with the highest possible standards of professional responsibility and objectivity.

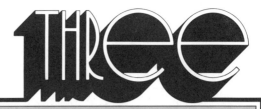

THREE

Development
of the nervous system
and etiologies

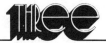

The foregoing discussion emphasized that the unique, distinguishing characteristic of persons with cerebral palsy is a developmental neuromotor disorder. As a consequence, the basis of their unique communication problems is a developmental dysarthria. Therefore, the discussion in this chapter and Chapter Four will concentrate on neuromotor disorders that result from an insult to the developing brain.

Although arguments have been made for abandoning the concept of cerebral palsy, there seems to be considerable justification for considering the group of developmental neuromotor disorders differently from disorders that result from lesions to mature neuromotor systems. The phenomenon of changing signs as a function of age in the cerebral palsied group is one such difference. Another difference is the prevalence of motor behaviors in the group with cerebral palsy that seem to be due to (1) retained and exaggerated reflexes and (2) abnormal influence of postural reactions of the neuromotor systems. Finally, it is now recognized that the types of abnormal developmental neuromotor behaviors are fewer than those observed subsequent to lesions of fully developed neuromotor systems.

Developmental neuromotor problems also differ from acquired neuromotor disorders with respect to the extreme variations that are seen in the latter relative to mixed types and topographical distribution. An adult with brain damage due to trauma, for example, may show generalized signs of some form of moderately severe hypertonicity accompanied by a violently severe tremor of one limb. The existence of mixed signs of neuromotor problems in cerebral palsy is now recognized to be relatively frequent, but they are not manifested in such obviously extreme variations. Also, although the topographical distribution of neuromotor involvement over the musculature of someone with cerebral palsy may vary, the patterns of distribution are more predictable than in acquired neuromotor disorders. These differences may be attributed to the fact that, again by definition, cerebral palsy results from a lesion to the developing nervous system. The effects of damage to the developing neuromotor systems and the subsequent maturational process of the neuromotor systems appear to bring out more homogeneous abnormal motor behaviors than is the case with lesions of the matured nervous system.

Therefore, not only may there be some virtue in retaining the term cerebral palsy to designate individuals with developmental neuromotor problems, but an understanding of cerebral palsy can be complete only if certain information regarding the development of the nervous system is at hand. The discussion in this chapter and Chapter Four also will deal with that topic.

Although the information presented in the first two chapters assumed a general knowledge of neuroanatomy and neurophysiology, the discussion to follow in this chapter and Chapter Four assumes a more detailed background. Otherwise, it will be difficult to place the concepts in an appropriate perspective. Unfortunately, readers who do not have considerable background may be inclined to take many of the statements as fact, although they deserve extensive qualification.

O DEVELOPMENT OF THE NERVOUS SYSTEM

There is no intent here to present a detailed chronology of the embryologic development of the nervous system. This discussion, rather, is designed to review only general considerations of nervous system development that are helpful in forming a frame of reference within which generalizations can be made regarding damage to the developing nervous system.

In general, structures of the nervous system develop in a phylogenetic progression, with the older portions developing first. That is, the spinal cord, the hindbrain (medulla oblongata, pons, and cerebellum), the midbrain (or mesencephalon), the basal ganglia, and cortical cells tend to develop in the order listed. However, within that general phylogenetic progression, there are numerous differences in the relative development of certain structures and pathways. For example, it has already been mentioned that the lower portion of the spinal cord is not completely formed at birth. However, that lack of complete development of the cord is somewhat relative since, at birth, many higher structures of the nervous system are much more poorly formed. In particular, cortical cells are lacking in development. With respect to neuromotor pathways that originate from clusters of cell bodies in the brain stem, the vestibulospinal neurons are among the more completely formed components of the neuromotor systems at the time of birth.

These generalizations regarding development of the nervous system provide explanations for some of the common characteristics that have been mentioned as being pertinent to neuromotor behavior of normal infants and those with cerebral palsy. Reflexes that are believed to be organized at the level of the brain stem are active; the neural networks that underly those reflexive behaviors are yet to become inhibited by the less well-developed higher mechanisms. The vestibulospinal tract is one of the more well-developed motor systems, and hence, the prevalence of postural reactions is to be expected.

This progression of development also helps explain some of the issues that have ensued. For example, it has been mentioned that the Babinski sign has been explained on the basis of the immaturity of the lower spinal cord; also, the idea that this behavior is a component of a flexor, or withdrawal, response of the leg has been advocated. Neither explanation gives the reason why that behavior seems to return subsequent to brain lesions in adults whose corticospinal tracts have been damaged. The fact that that tract is generally not well formed at birth seems a better explanation of both the Babinski sign in normal infants and its return subsequent to corticospinal tract lesions.

There is another aspect of development of the nervous system that needs to be reviewed. The specific manner in which the 100 billion or more neurons of the human nervous system come to be arranged architecturally so as to form functional neuronal assemblies is yet to be determined. However, it is reasonably clear that some neural systems have a significant predetermined specificity. That is, there is a degree of rigidity in the extent to which there can be variation in the formation of functional neuronal assemblies, or what might be thought of as neural nets, that result in the various operations of those systems. For other portions of the nervous system, however, there appears to be considerable flexibility, or plasticity, with which organization of networks for particular operations can be formed.

With respect to this latter point, there is little doubt that the organization of neural nets can be greatly influenced by repetition of transmission through the component neurons. This formation of functional neuronal nets can be thought of, in a real sense, as learning. The term plasticity of neural structures has been used by some to refer to this concept. That is, for those areas of the nervous system that possess high potential for rearrangement of functional nets as a result of learning, there is potential for different neurons to become involved in specific types of operations.

The long-range ramifications of early insult to the nervous system, therefore, may depend on the extent to which the particular system that is damaged is relatively rigid or whether it possesses considerable plasticity. Among the functional neural systems that are believed to be least plastic, the motor pathways rank quite high. As a result, it seems reasonable to assume that if some of the cells of those pathways sustain some type of insult in their course of development, there is less latitude for the remaining cells to develop the necessary networks for normal motor function.

The above descriptions are grossly oversimplified reviews of exceedingly complex concepts. However, they can be used as tentative explanations for some of the phenomena of cerebral palsy already discussed. For one example, the extent to which prenatal damage to a circumscribed area of the cortex can lead to only a specific language deficit, such as is observed in adults with aphasia, is a highly controversial topic. One of the reasons for this controversy is that there appears to be considerable plasticity of neuronal organization of those cortical cells that can become involved in language processes. There is no comparable controversy regarding restricted lesions to the neuromotor systems. As evidenced by individuals with cerebral palsy who are intellectually above average, who have no detectable problems in the use of language, and whose nervous system seems to function quite adequately except for the neuromotor problem, early neuronal damage can undoubtedly lead to neuromotor disabilities, while other functions of the individual remain relatively intact.

However, the phenomena of changing signs in young children with cerebral palsy points to the probability that some reorganization of neuromotor cells is taking place in the presence of previously damaged neurons. The relative homogeneity of developmental neuromotor problems, in contrast to the heterogeneity of neuromotor disorders acquired after the neuromotor systems have matured, may be due in part to a tendency of the young damaged neuromotor systems to become organized in relatively homogeneous manners subsequent to lesions.

○ ETIOLOGIES

Even today, specification of an etiology in a number of cases of cerebral palsy is impossible, no matter how carefully and systematically a child's gestational and birth histories are reviewed. Obviously, however, today's practitioners can be more certain of the etiology in vastly more cases than could Little, Freud, and their contemporaries.

Better understanding of the embryonic development of the nervous system has led not only to a better understanding of many of the neuroanatomical reasons for some of the characteristics of developmental neuromotor disorders, but that understanding also has assisted in better delineating etiologies that lead to cerebral palsy. The stage of development of the embryo at the time of insult has been recognized for some time as dictating the characteristics of many congenital malformations. Those portions of the nervous system and its arterial-vascular system that are in stages of rapid development are likely to be most susceptible to damage.

Destruction of cells of the nervous system may take place as a result of infections. The degree to which the brain of the fetus is susceptible to infection, however, is dictated by different variables than after birth. The maturation of the blood-brain barrier and the extent to which a specific infecting organism can cross that barrier at a given stage of development is an example. A mother's having rubella within the first trimester of her pregnancy spells dire consequences for her baby compared to her having been infected later. Although the embryonic nervous system can be affected by those general classes of infections (e.g., bacteria) that may infect other portions of the body, viral infections (as exemplified by the rubella virus) are the most common.

A number of substances are highly toxic to neurons, including many drugs and metals. However, the toxic substance that most frequently results in neuronal damage, including the nervous systems of embryos, is blood. A hemorrhage from any cause that results in blood infiltrating neuronal tissue results in destruction of neurons.

In addition, reduction in oxygen to neurons may also result in their destruction. Thus, neuronal damage can result from reduction of oxygen supply to the embryo or to portions of the embryo's brain as a result of many problems of its cerebral circulatory system. A variety of specific circulatory disorders can lead to sufficient deprivation of oxygen to cause loss of a significant number of cells.

Difficulties associated with birth have been considered, from time to time, to be responsible for a large proportion of the cases of cerebral palsy. A variety of problems that lead to difficulties of labor and of birth itself can cause nervous system damage of the newborn. However, actual mechanical injury at birth is a much less frequent cause of early brain damage than has been suggested.

As has been mentioned, at least one specific agent, namely bilirubin, has been identified as being the etiology of certain cases of cerebral palsy. As was also mentioned, certain neural structures seem predisposed to infiltration by that damaging substance, and that predisposition leads to a predictable pattern of neural destruction and resulting disabilities.

Irrespective of all of these possibilities, the two major reasons for lesions to the developing nervous system that result in cerebral palsy are now known to be hemorrhage and reduced oxygen supply. Therefore, disorders of the cerebrocirculatory system should be viewed as the most frequent etiology of neuronal damage that leads to cerebral palsy. The etiologies that lead to breakdowns in the arteriovascular system of the embryo and that result in reduced oxygen supply to its brain cells are far too numerous to even attempt to present.

Given the prenatal history, the birth history, the pattern of neuromotor involvement, and, in particular, the probable time of a precipitating episode, an etiology can frequently be determined. It must be appreciated, however, that many of the events that can lead to brain damage of the embryo are impossible to specify. In addition, case histories frequently reveal rather firm indications of the specific events that may be assumed to be the cause of selected cases, but those cases do not follow the predicted patterns that have been identified. Also, children are sometimes born for whom there is every indication that their brains will have been significantly damaged, yet they later show no obvious indications of such damage.

Differences that exist between the neuromotor disorders that constitute cerebral palsy and those that are acquired due to lesions of mature neuromotor systems are due to the former resulting from insults to developing neural systems. Just as is the case with lesions to mature brains that result in acquired neuromotor disorders, insults to developing brains that result in developmental neuromotor disorders, and hence cerebral palsy, also affect other neural systems that participate in motor function. Therefore, a variety of other disorders and disabilities may be expected in the populations that have either acquired or developmental neuromotor disorders. However, those disorders and disabilities are not likely to be comparable for the two populations since, the insults of those with developmental neuromotor disorders are to brains that are in the process of maturing.

Structures of the nervous system and the neural systems within those structures mature at different rates. The organization of some of these systems are more susceptible to modification than others due to the maturation process and as a result of neural learning. The neuromotor systems, however, are among the least susceptible to modification even during their stages of development. Therefore, relatively restricted early lesions to those systems can be expected to result in significant neuromotor disorders. Lesions to other neural systems of the developing brain, however, may not result in the variety of specific disorders that are seen in adults with acquired brain lesions.

Disorders of the cerebrocirculatory system are probably the most frequent etiologies of cerebral palsy. These disorders lead to destruction of neurons through reduced oxygen to the brain of the embryo or through hemorrhages which result in blood destroying neural tissue. Viral and other infections may destroy cerebral neurons if the circumstances are such that the infection can cross the blood-brain barrier. Mechanical injury at birth is a much less frequent cause of damage to infants' brains than might be supposed, and incompatibility of the mother's and child's blood (such as Rh incompatibility) is presently a less frequent cause due to advances in the care of the mother and her newborn.

The period of gestation over which an etiological agent destroys neural tissue is an important variable relative to the neural systems that will be affected. Hence, the time of insult is an important determinant of the type of distribution of the neuromotor disorder when that insult affects the neuromotor systems. Even though there is now a vast knowledge of potential etiologies of causes of prenatal brain damage, it is still impossible to specify the reason for the problem in a number of cases of cerebral palsy.

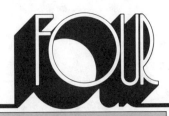

Characteristics
of the problem

Concentration will be given here to the two prime types of neuromotor disorders observed in the population with cerebral palsy, namely (1) spasticity and (2) involuntary motion and associated disorders. With respect to the second group of problems, the term dyskinesia has come to be applied within recent years, and that term will be used rather than athetosis, that has been used historically, or other terms that have been recommended such as extrapyramidal cerebral palsy.

○ NEUROMOTOR MECHANISMS AND DYSFUNCTIONS IN CEREBRAL PALSY

The neuromotor disorders associated with cerebral palsy will be discussed, for the most part, within descriptions of various components of the neuromotor systems. This approach facilitates an understanding of how the dysfunctions of various neuromotor systems are believed to contribute to the disorders of cerebral palsy, and it assists in developing a perspective that these disorders represent disruptions in the dynamics of the total of neuromotor function rather than specific dysfunctions of discrete and unrelated mechanisms.

final common pathway

The term final common pathway refers to the alpha motor neurons that provide innervation to muscle fibers. The term motor unit refers to one such alpha neuron and the muscle fibers that are innervated by its telodendria. Gradations in strength of a muscle's contraction will depend on the frequency of discharge of the motor units of the muscle and the number of those units that are recruited during the contraction.

The brain abnormalities that result in cerebral palsy are routinely above the level of the final common pathway. Dysfunctions of motor units, therefore, are not usually present in cases of cerebral palsy. Such dysfunctions are frequently referred to as lower motor neuron problems, and a review may be found in Appendix A. However, a discussion of the role of these final neurons in the chain of neuromotor activity provides a basis for understanding many of the terms and concepts related to developmental neuromotor disorders.

It is reasonably easy to conceptualize the result of the firing of one alpha motor neuron. As the action potential travels down the cell's axon
and telodendria, crosses the myoneural junction, and induces contraction
of the muscle fibers innervated by that one neuron, those fibers will contract and produce a twitch within the muscle. It also is reasonably easy to
conceptualize that the number of units that are firing and the frequency
of the firing result in gradated strength of the muscle's contraction.

It is much more difficult, however, to conceptualize the gradation of
firings of motor units among muscles that result in movement. Even for
hinge joints, such as the elbow, movement results from a finely coordinated interplay of agonist and antagonist muscles that contract, or increase in
muscle tone, and relax, or decrease in muscle tone, respectively. There
are many unresolved issues concerning how the large number of alpha
neurons that are involved in a relatively simple movement such as flexion
of the elbow are excited and inhibited so that a smooth and controlled
movement results.

There are a number of influences that contribute to the activity in the
area of the cell bodies of the lower motor neurons, and terms such as lower motor neuron pool have come to be used in reference to that neural
activity. The concept implies that in the area of the alpha cell bodies (the
anterior horn for spinal nerves and the efferent cranial nerve nuclei for
cranial nerves) there exists a pool of neural activity, and it is the characteristics of that activity that result in the patterns of alpha neuron firings
that, in turn, result in the gradations of muscle relaxation and contraction
associated with normal movements.

For many movements these patterns of neural activity are much more
complex than those associated with flexion or extension of hinged joints.
For example, the interaction among the motor units that innervate the
muscles controlling upper arm movements permits the arm to be rotated
from the shoulder in approximately 360 degrees and almost within a
plane; moreover, the arm can be extended outward from that plane in almost all possible angles. Such complexity of muscle interaction probably
reaches its ultimate in movements of the eyes and, for speech production,
the human tongue.

The patterns of neural activity within the pools of the anterior horns of
the spinal cord and the efferent cranial nerve nuclei result from neural
activity from a great variety of sources. Normal muscle function depends
on intricate interaction among (1) neural activity that comes to the neuromotor systems from a number of unspecifiable sources for initiation and
completion of movements, (2) excitatory mechanisms that either contribute to or enhance that activity, and (3) inhibitory mechanisms that serve to
regulate, diminish, or suppress the activity from those sources or from the
excitatory mechanisms. If excitatory mechanisms of the neuromotor systems are dysfunctional, the reduction of their influence to the final common pathways and the influence of the remaining inhibitory mechanisms

will result in diminished activity of those pathways. In contrast, damage to inhibitory neuromotor mechanisms will result in excessive activity to the final common pathways. The neuromotor disorders of cerebral palsy represent disruptions of this interaction of excitatory and inhibitory influences to the pools that result in patterns of activity of the final common pathways.

direct afferent influences from peripheral structures

Relatively direct transmission from receptors within the tissues of the organism influences activity in the final common pathway pool. Figure 4–1 is comparable to the usual relatively schematic diagrams that show input to the alpha motor neurons from these pathways at the level of the spinal cord. The figure also shows transmission pathways of the incoming afferent information to higher mechanisms in the nervous system. Of the receptors that respond to events in tissue, the stretch receptors, usually called muscle spindles, are the most important to this discussion.

The Gamma System. There are muscle spindles within most striated muscle. These stretch receptor mechanisms are arranged anatomically

FIGURE 4–1 Diagram of afferent information from tissues with representation of pathways to higher neural structures and transmission to area of final common pathway (alpha motor neurons). Components of the gamma system (gamma efferent neurons, muscle spindles, and spindle afferent neurons) also are shown.

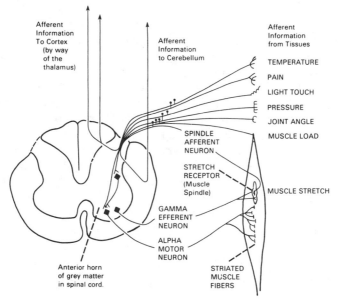

so that they respond to the muscle's being stretched. When the thresholds of the receptors are reached, action potentials are discharged along the spindle afferent fibers into the central nervous system. As Figure 4–1 shows, at the level of the spinal cord, this stretch information enters into the dorsal portion of the cord and may be transmitted directly to the anterior horn area. This incoming stretch information may have an obvious, significant influence on alpha motor activity under certain circumstances. It is, in fact, the anatomical basis of what is referred to as deep tendon reflexes. When normally innervated muscle is suddenly stretched, it may contract in opposition to that stretch as a result of (1) the stretch receptor's discharging action potentials along the spindle afferents into the central nervous system and (2) as a result, discharge of the alpha neurons to the muscle that was stretched.

The best known example of a deep tendon reflex probably is the patellar reflex, frequently referred to as the knee jerk reflex. Most persons have experienced that reflex during a physical examination. When the examinee sits on the edge of a table with the lower legs hanging free and the patellar tendon is struck just below the kneecap, the tendon is driven into an indentation under the kneecap. The muscles of the front of the thigh (e.g., the quadriceps) are thereby stretched, and they contract in a twitch-like reaction. Hence, the lower leg kicks forward. Such a deep tendon, or stretch, reflex can be elicited from any muscle group where striking a tendon, or other method, can be used to place sudden stretch on a muscle. Some physicians, for example, seem to be able to reliably elicit what is called a jaw jerk reflex. That reflex is elicited by tapping the mandible downward and observing the extent to which it jerks back to the closed position.

The muscle spindles and their associated neurons would be obstructive to movement if they responded only to mechanical stretch. That is, if strong volleys of action potentials were always distributed to the alpha motor neuron pools upon any stretch of muscle, the antagonist muscles to any movement would be resistive to stretch, and movement would be prevented. The muscle spindles, however, are not static receptors, and they play a fundamental role in normal muscle activity. These spindles have contractile components that are innervated by neurons classified as gamma efferents. Stretch on the receptor may be reduced or increased as a result of this innervation. For example, as you extend your elbow, the bicep is being lengthened throughout that movement. If the muscle spindles were static in their response to that lengthening, the movement would be resisted at some point where the thresholds of the stretch receptors were reached. However, by adjusting the contractile components of the receptors, the gamma efferents may keep their receptors close to discharge, with only some of them firing to assist in maintaining the appropriate amount of resistance to the lengthening of the bicep.

This maintenance of the proper amount of stretch on the spindle receptors might be thought of as a bias on the stretch receptor mechanism that contributes to the muscle's participating appropriately in a movement. If some weight were dropped in your hand as your elbow was straightening, the stretch receptors would be tuned to react to the stretch that would be imposed on the bicep muscle. The resulting discharge of the spindle afferents would have the effect of strengthening the contraction of the bicep so that the effect of the weight would be resisted and the planned rate of the movement would continue.

Assume, also, the case in which a volley of action potentials from some higher neuromotor system influences the motor pool in such a way as to cause the gamma efferent cells to discharge. The discharge could result in the contractile components of the muscle spindles placing enough stretch on the receptors to cause them to discharge. The resulting pattern of action potentials back into the same pool, through what is known as the gamma-alpha loop, could cause the alpha neurons to the same muscle fibers to discharge, as is the case for a stretch reflex. This gamma-alpha loop of muscle innervation is a mechanism that enables the gamma system to contribute to adjustment of rate and amount of muscle contraction as a result of influence from higher neural systems in combination with mechanical stretch.

The specific characteristics of the interaction among the gamma and alpha efferent fibers for normal movement is not totally clear. However, it is well established that relative overactivity of the gamma system is a prime component of spasticity, and the resistance (degree of muscle tone) of an antagonist muscle to being stretched is abnormally great in spasticity. Sudden stretching of the muscle will lead to an abnormally high reaction to that stretch. The knee jerk reflex, for example, will be hyperactive if spasticity is present. In addition, if the joint of a limb that has spastic involvement is suddenly flexed, firm resistance to that flexion may initially be encountered. Assume an example in which an involved arm is held by the examiner with the elbow extended, and an attempt is made to suddenly flex the arm passively. It is likely that a firm resistance will be encountered from stretch of the triceps muscle as the joint bends a few degrees. If the examiner continues to attempt to flex the joint, the resistance may recede, and it may be possible to bend the elbow completely. This is the often cited "clasp knife" phenomenon that is characteristic of spasticity. The term came to be used since this pattern of resistance to flexing a joint of a spastic limb resembles the pattern of resistance to closing the blade on a pocketknife.

The hyperactivity of the gamma system that characterizes spasticity is believed to be due to dysfunction of inhibitory influences that act on the gamma efferent cell bodies. As a result, those cells are overly active, and the stretch receptors are maintained closer to their threshold of discharge. The receptors may be so stretched by abnormal firing of the gamma efferents that they discharge continuously. The phenomenon of hyperreaction of muscle to stretch, therefore, is not totally descriptive of spasticity. Spastic muscle is rather routinely in a relatively chronic state of hypercontraction. To the extent that such constant hypertonia is present, normal movement of any type will be hindered, and it will increase in antagonists upon movement. If the constant hypertonia is severe enough, the affected structure may be maintained in an abnormal position.

Other Afferent Influences. Discussions of normal neuromotor physiology do not routinely emphasize the effects of other afferent information on the final common pathway pool. However, it does influence activity of the alpha neurons. In the abnormal state of spasticity, a typical characteristic of the gait is elevation of the heel so that the individual walks on the ball of the foot. Spraying the sole of that individual's foot with a topical anesthesia frequently results in sufficient relaxation of the calf muscles to permit a more normal gait with the heel down. When the effects of the anesthesia wear off, the abnormal posture will return. Evidently, elimination of the touch-pressure information into the overly active final common pathway pool is sufficient to reduce the contraction of the spastic muscles.

This phenomenon has led to sectioning of the dorsal root fibers to reduce the hypertonicity associated with spasticity. Some successes with that procedure were reported, but other results, such as loss of sensation in the affected limb, led to lack of the procedure's acceptance. A physical therapist who is now attempting to assist a spastic child with ambulation, however, may take great care with the fitting of shoes. If there are extreme pressure points on the surface of the child's foot as a result of a poor fit, the hypertonicity in the child's leg may be greater during ambulation than if pressure is evenly distributed.

The term tactile reflexes is frequently used in reference to such elicitation of motor activity through touch-pressure stimulation. The Babinski sign is an example, and as has been mentioned, that sign is believed to be a routine clinical indication of the presence of spasticity. In the presence of a dysfunctioning corticospinal system, the tactile stimulation sets off the motor activity of that reflex.

Hyperreflexia has come to be used in reference to some of the general clinical characteristics of spasticity. From the above descriptions of overly active deep tendon reflexes and abnormal tactile reflexes (e.g., the Babinski), it can be appreciated that the term is descriptive of many of the characteristics of spasticity. There are other justifications for its use. In reference to tactile reflexes seen in spasticity, for example, the term extended zone of stimulation may be found. That term refers to the fact that the Babinski sign may be elicited in some spastic individuals from areas other than the sole of the foot (e.g., the lower shin). Ankle clonus is another phenomena indicative of hyperreflexia. When the foot of someone with spasticity is forced upward and held, the ankle joint may be set into a reverberating, tremulous movement pattern. Through stretch of the muscles that act to depress the foot (e.g., the gastrocemious that forms the calf of the leg), those muscles contract forcefully. When, as a result of that contraction, those muscles are sufficiently shortened to lessen activity of the stretch receptors, the foot can then be pushed back into the elevated position, and the stretch reaction is repeated. Thus, a reverberating pattern of dorsal and plantar flexion is elicited.

One of the best known tactile reflexes is the gag response. The neural organization underlying the gag reflex is at the level of the brain stem. It is only one example of the fact that reflex behaviors of the cranial nerve system incorporate neuronal organizations that are much more complex (e.g., blinking of the eyes and facial grimaces to sudden, loud sounds) than for the spinal nerve mechanisms. As is well known, touch-pressure stimulation into the posterior oral pharyngeal tissues can result in a highly complex pattern of muscle activity that, with little doubt, is designed to expel the stimulating object from the gustatory tract. If the stimulation persists, this highly organized functional act can include recruitment of torso muscles to the point that the individual vomits. The gag reflex of persons with cerebral palsy who have spasticity also is frequently hyperactive.

pyramidal system

The pyramidal motor system derives its name from early identification of structures of the central nervous system by study of the intricate patterns of gray and white matter that characterize the tissue of that system. Bilateral concentrations of white matter that, in cross section, were somewhat triangular in shape were identified in the lower portion of the human brain stem. Thus, the term pyramids were given to those two bilateral structures.

It had been recognized by at least the early 1800s that the white matter of the central nervous system was composed of transmission systems. It was learned later that white matter of the central nervous system contains high concentrations of myelin sheaths of axons, and, thus, those earlier deductions regarding systems that make up white matter of the nervous system were essentially correct. When it was determined that those axons that run through the pyramids make up what now is called the corticospinal tract, and that they constitute a major motor system, the system was entitled the pyramidal system. Later, after it was learned that cranial efferent alpha neurons receive cortical innervation from the corticobulbar tract, that tract was incorporated into the concept of the pyramidal system even though its fibers do not run through the pyramids. Figure 4–2 shows a representation of the system.

A coronal section through the precentral gyrus of the cerebral hemispheres is shown above representations of horizontal sections through the brain stem and one such section of the spinal cord. The relative size of the coronal view, of course, is much reduced relative to the size of the horizontal sections.

The neurons whose cell bodies are shown to reside in the cortex of the precentral gyrus are large betz, or pyramidal, cells. The axons of these cells are shown projecting down through the cerebral hemispheres to terminate in the brain stem and spinal cord. What is now called the cortico-

FIGURE 4–2 A representation of the pyramidal system showing the topographical distribution with which neurons located within the precentral gyrus strip influence function of muscle groups. Pathways of bilateral innervation to alpha motor neurons of selected efferent cranial nerve nuclei, including the Hypoglossal nerve neuclei, and contralateral (crossed) innervation to spinal efferent (alpha) neurons are shown.

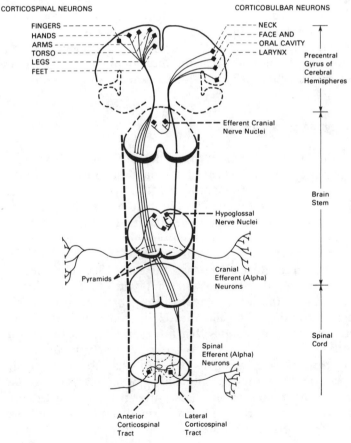

bulbar tract of the pyramidal system is represented on the right side of the drawing, and the corticospinal tract is shown on the left side. These two tracts, respectively, project their axons to the final common pathway pools of alpha neurons that are in clusters (efferent cranial nerve nuclei) in the brain stem and throughout the length of the spinal cord in the anterior horns of grey matter.

The topographical arrangement of these cells relative to the muscle groups to which they provide innervation is a most important consideration for the present discussion. As is shown, the pyramidal cells that are deep within the longitudinal fissure project their axons to the lower portions of the spinal cord to influence alpha motor neurons that innervate muscles of the feet. Progressively from the lower longitudinal fissure up and over the lateral surface of the precentral gyrus, the cell bodies provide innervation to the musculatures of the legs, torso walls, arms, and hands. The pyramidal cells over the remainder of the precentral gyrus (corticobulbar cells) influence alpha neurons that innervate muscles of the neck, face, oral cavity, and larynx.

The axons of the corticobulbar cells drop into the front of the brain stem, and they traverse internally into the tissue of the brain stem to influence either directly or indirectly the activity in the nuclei of efferent cranial nerves. Only two pairs of those cranial nerve nuclei are represented in the figure. The highest pair of the efferent cranial nerve nuclei that are shown distribute alpha neurons to some of the muscles that control eye movements, and the other pair that is shown send axons to innervate muscles of the tongue (Hypoglossal, Nerve XII).

The figure also shows that corticobulbar influence reaches the cells of the alpha neurons from the corticobulbar fibers that cross in the brain stem from the side of their origin. That innervation usually is described as being through interconnecting neurons, as is shown for one pair of the efferent cranial nerve nuclei. Due to that contralateral innervation, damage to the corticobulbar system above the level of the efferent cranial nerve nuclei will result in a motor problem on the opposite side. Therefore, when persons sustain some type of damage to the lateral area of one precentral gyrus, the muscle function of their faces and oral cavities on the opposite side may be affected.

In the great majority of such cases, however, the neuromotor problem will disappear over a period of months. What is believed to be the anatomical basis for that spontaneous recovery of function is shown in the figure. Not only do the corticobulbar fibers provide innervation to efferent cranial nerve nuclei on the opposite side of the brain stem, it is believed that they possess potential to provide innervation to those nuclei on the same side. Evidently, these ipsilateral connections serve as a backup system for unilateral damage to the corticobulbar fibers. In the presence of some type of destruction or disruption of the dominant contralateral system, the ipsilateral system does not immediately provide innervation to the efferent cranial nerves. It comes to do so, however, over time in a substantial number of cases of unilateral damage to the upper portions of the corticobulbar tract.

As is shown in Figure 4–2, the axons of the corticospinal tract enter the same general area of the brain stem from the cerebral hemispheres as do the corticobulbar fibers. They remain in the frontal portion of the brain stem, on the same side, throughout its length. After dropping through the pyramids, the bulk of the fibers cross to the opposite side and continue their downward course in the lateral area of the white matter of the spinal cord. From the point of crossing, those fibers are called the lateral corticospinal tract.

The relatively few corticospinal axons that remain on the same side drop into the front of the spinal cord, and they are called the anterior corticospinal tract. Some of those anterior corticospinal fibers cross to the opposite side of the cord before they provide innervation to the alpha motor neurons; a few of them may innervate those neurons on the same side. However, for practical purposes, the anterior corticospinal tract can be ignored. In fact, most writers take the position that the anterior corticospinal tract has little or no functional significance.

Therefore, the alpha motor neurons of the spinal peripheral nerve system do not have the backup system from higher portions of the pyramidal system on the ipsilateral side as do those neurons of the cranial nerve system. In those persons who may have a neuromotor problem on the opposite side of their faces from damage to corticobulbar neurons in one cerebral hemisphere, there will also frequently be damage to the corticospinal fibers in that hemisphere that results in dysfunction of their contralateral extremities. That dysfunction of their arm and leg musculatures cannot be expected to resolve spontaneously, as is the case with the dysfunction of their facial and oral musculatures.

This phenomenon of frequent resolution of facial and oral musculature function subsequent to unilateral corticobulbar damage is routinely described for adults who have sustained damage to their brains. I do not recall references to the possibility that these differences in unilateral and bilateral innervation of alpha neurons by the corticospinal and corticobulbar fibers respectively to be a possible explanation for the relative absence of dysarthria in cerebral palsied children with spastic hemiplegia.

There is no doubt, however, that the topographical distribution of pyramidal cells and their axons is the explanation for the distribution of spasticity in musculatures of spastic cerebral palsied children that was reviewed in Chapter Two. Figure 4–3 is designed to clarify and graphically illustrate that distribution. It can be discussed most easily by the example of a hypothetical hemorrhage in the longitudinal fissure in a case where the blood infiltrates the neural system from that area and flows upward

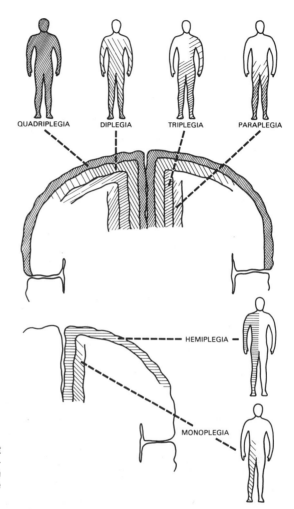

FIGURE 4–3 Patterns of insult to the pyramidal system that result in topographical distribution of neuromotor impairments in the spastic type of cerebral palsy.

and laterally over the precentral gyrus. The extent of the infiltration from the area of the hemorrhage would be predictive of the musculatures that would manifest different degrees of severity of involvement. For example, if the blood were confined to an area deep within the fissure and only on one side, a monoplegia might be expected. For another example, if that infiltration was heavily concentrated throughout both sides of the longitudinal fissure with a spreading over one precentral gyrus on one side more than the other, a triplegia might result. For a final example, the phenomenon of diplegia with lesser involvement in the upper extremities than the lower limbs can be explained on the basis that the infiltration of the blood could be expected to be less as it spread over the lateral areas of the precentral gyri on both sides than in the longitudinal fissure.

The above possible explanation for a diplegia also explains why numerous diplegic cerebral palsied children do not have dysarthria. The insult to their pyramidal systems can be conceptualized as not having spread so far over their precentral gyri as to damage their corticobulbar systems. On the other hand, the cerebral palsied children with quadriplegia routinely have dysarthria and neuromotor involvement of relatively equal severity in all four extremities. More importantly, that involvement is usually quite severe, which suggests that the quadriplegic group are victims of a general, all-encompassing insult to the pyramidal system.

These examples of pyramidal system damage also serve to help illustrate some of the comments that were made in Chapter Two relative to distribution of spasticity in cerebral palsy. That is, hemiplegia can be seen to be a more extensive form of monoplegia, and paraplegia, triplegia, and diplegia may be viewed as representing progressively more extensive involvements of the system on both sides. With the exception of some cases of quadriplegia, it can be expected that these distributions of spasticity will be characterized by the most severe involvement being in the musculatures of the lower muscle groups.

Two points in the above discussion must be emphasized. Otherwise, serious misconceptions will result.

First, although the distribution of spasticity in cerebral palsy is best illustrated by the case in which there is a hemorrhage in the longitudinal fissure, it should not be assumed that damage by blood infiltrating into the cortical tissue is the only cause of that distribution. Hemorrhages deeper within the cerebral hemispheres of the immature brain and/or reduction of oxygen to the developing pyramidal cells may, and probably more frequently do, lead to this distribution.

Second, the relation between pyramidal system damage and spasticity is so consistent that spasticity has frequently been referred to as a pyramidal disorder for both developmental and acquired neuromotor disorders. Spasticity is a usual result below a lesion to the pyramidal system no matter where that lesion is located. Yet, spasticity is not considered to be the result of damage to only that system. The pyramidal system is excitatory in function; damage to it alone, therefore, should result in a decrease of muscle tone and power of contraction. As mentioned in the earlier section on the gamma system, the hypertonicity that is characteristic of spasticity results in large part from over excitation of the gamma system. Damage to an extrapyramidal system that acts to inhibit gamma activity for normal function is therefore usually assumed to be implicated.

extrapyramidal systems

Of all concepts related to neuromotor systems and their function, the literature probably is most confusing regarding the term extrapyramidal systems. Again, history is helpful. By the beginning of this century it had been recognized that there were numerous neural systems other than the pyramidal system that directly influence motor activity. As these numerous specific neural systems began to be identified, it became difficult, from an editorial standpoint, to list the structures being discussed. As a result, the term extrapyramidal motor systems, meaning motor systems other than the pyramidal system, began to be used for editorial convenience. That use of one term to refer to a number of systems seems to have led to the erroneous conceptualization at one time that there was one extrapyramidal system. Reference to these systems in the singular may be found still in some literature.

Identification of these extrapyramidal systems resulted, in part, from recognition of a group of neuromotor disorders that were characterized by forms of involuntary motion. It had been determined that lesions among a group of nuclear masses deep within the cerebral hemispheres of adults frequently resulted in these disorders. These masses were called the basal ganglia since they are located in the base of those hemispheres, and these basal ganglia were learned to contain major components of the extrapyramidal systems.[1] Even though the character of the neuromotor disorders that became recognized as resulting from lesions to the basal ganglia varied in a number of ways, those disorders also came to be called an extrapyramidal disorder (in the singular), in contrast to spasticity that became known as a pyramidal disorder (which also seems to be inappropriate).

The involuntary motion disorders, however, not only varied in the form of the uncontrolled movements, but it became recognized that they were accompanied frequently by disorders of muscle tone. Moreover, it began to be documented that lesions to certain nuclear masses in the brain stem (e.g., red nucleus) were associated with some of the neuromotor disorders that earlier were believed to be due to lesions only to the basal ganglia. It is now known that a variety of neuromotor disorders that are acquired in adults can result from lesions to certain nuclei of the basal ganglia (caudate, putamen, and globus pallidus) and some nuclei in the

---

[1]The nuclei that were initially identified as comprising the basal ganglia are now known as the caudate, putamen, globus pallidus, and amygdaloid nuclei, and many current definitions of the basal ganglia will list those structures. However, it also became known that the amygdaloid nucleus does not have the influence on motor activity that the other three masses of neuron cell bodies do, and some authors will not list the amygdaloid as belonging to the basal ganglia. However, just as a semantic linking between the extrapyramidal systems and disorders lead to problems, such a problem exists with respect to the definition of the basal ganglia. The cluster of neuromotor problems known as Parkinson's disease were initially determined to be associated with lesions of the caudate, putamen, and globus pallidus, and Parkinson's disease became known as a basal ganglia disorder. Later, when lesions to some brain stem nuclei (red nucleus and substantia nigra) also were found to be implicated in those disorders, it was suggested by some that those brain stem nuclei be included in the definition of the basal ganglia. Usually, however, the term basal ganglia is now used in reference to the caudate, putamen, and globus pallidus.

brain stem. Despite this knowledge, the terms extrapyramidal signs and extrapyramidal disorder are still sometimes used, and they refer to neuromotor dysfunction manifested by some form of involuntary motion that is sometimes accompanied by a hypertonia.

Current neuroanatomical and neurophysiological literature frequently does not clarify the confusion. If the index of many texts of neuroanatomy are consulted for the term extrapyramidal systems, the reader will be referred to sections that list a number of neuromotor tracts that originate in the brain stem and project axons down to the motor pools of the spinal cord. Extrapyramidal influences to cranial efferent nerve nuclei are usually not discussed. However, their effects on musculatures innervated by the cranial nerves can be observed in persons who have neuromotor problems that are assumed to result from primarily extrapyramidal lesions.

It is not the intent here to offer an authoritative clarification of this confusion. Rather, an oversimplified perspective will be presented of what may be called the extrapyramidal systems. It should help form a frame of reference for understanding some of these issues. Figure 4–4 is provided to assist with that frame of reference.

Again, a coronal section through the cerebral hemispheres is shown. In contrast to the section represented in Figures 4–2 and 4–3, however, the place of this section is somewhat anterior to the precentral gyrus, or pyramidal motor strip. There is considerable evidence to support the belief that primarily inhibitory influences on motor activity project downward from that general area of the frontal lobes.[2] Moreover, this influence projects strongly at least to the caudate nucleus and putamen.

From those components of the basal ganglia, the extrapyramidal motor systems might be viewed as consisting of a second stage of vastly complex interconnections among the caudate, putamen, globus pallidus, and other nuclei that are not shown in Figure 4–4. This network involves combinations of inhibitory and excitatory interconnections that are so complex and interwoven that, on a practical, reasonably superficial level, it makes little sense to attempt to delineate them. It seems better to state simply that the combined influences of these interconnections are brought to bear on what might be viewed as a third group of mechanisms that constitute the extrapyramidal systems.

That third level of systems is composed of brain stem mechanisms whose cell bodies are located in nuclei in the brain stem and that project

---

[2]This abbreviated discussion of neuromotor mechanisms does not contain reference to the area that has come to be known as the secondary motor area. There are more and more indications that an area anterior to the precentral gyrus within the longitudinal fissure that extends slightly over the top of the frontal lobe contains neurons that participate strongly in motor activity. Although the possibility that this area of cortical neurons contributes substantially to motor function has been recognized for some time, the specific nature of that contribution still is not known.

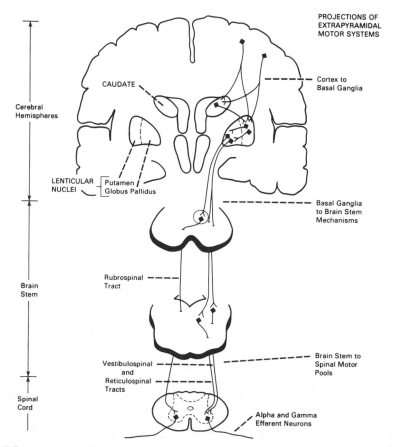

Cerebral
Hemispheres

CAUDATE

Cortex to
Basal Ganglia

LENTICULAR
NUCLEI
Putamen
Globus Pallidus

Basal Ganglia
to Brain Stem
Mechanisms

Brain
Stem

Rubrospinal
Tract

Spinal
Cord

Vestibulospinal
and
Reticulospinal
Tracts

Brain Stem to
Spinal Motor
Pools

Alpha and Gamma
Efferent Neurons

FIGURE 4–4 Representation of selected projections of extrapyramidal motor systems, show-ing pathways from (1) the cortex to basal ganglia, (2) the basal ganglia to brain stem mecha-nisms, and (3) brain stem mechanisms to spinal motor pools. A number of nuclei cells and pathways that are known to be involved in motor function in the cerebral hemispheres and brain stem (e.g., the Nucleus of Luys and the substantia nigra) are not shown. The rubro-spinal, vestibulospinal, and reticulospinal tracts are only three of at least six such brain stem projections, and no attempt has been made to accurately represent crossing of these projec-tions. Moreover, no representation has been provided to represent such projections to effer-ent cranial nerve nuclei.

their axons to the motor pools of the final common pathway. The reticu-lospinal and rubrospinal tracts are examples of these. The vestibulospinal tracts have also been included, historically, within these extrapyramidal mechanisms.

The vestibular nucleus receives information directly from the vestibu-lar mechanism, and as was mentioned in Chapter Two, the vestibulospinal tract thereby influences motor activity in relation to the posture and movement of the head in relation to gravity. The reticular formation of the brain stem has a prime function of discharging inhibitory and excitatory activity throughout the brain in association with states of attention and wakefulness; the reticulospinal tract is usually said to influence motor activity similarly. The rubrospinal tract originates in a brain stem nucleus (the red nucleus) that receives considerable information from the cerebellum; that tract is one of the pathways by which cerebellar mechanisms can influence motor function.

While it is generally assumed that pyramidal fibers primarily influence alpha neurons, some of the extrapyramidal tracts provide relatively more innervation to the gamma efferents. The vestibulospinal tract, for example, probably strongly influences gamma efferent activity to the muscles that hold us erect against gravity. It makes considerable sense as a mechanism to provide a background of muscle tone in such muscles that must fluctuate in relation to posture. As mentioned, it is believed to be damage to some extrapyramidal inhibitory system to the gamma efferents that results in the hypertonicity and overreaction to stretch of muscles that are characteristic of spasticity.

A variety of disorders of movement and muscle tone that may result from insults to the basal ganglia and associated brain stem mechanisms in adults has been mentioned. The dyskinesias of cerebral palsy, however, usually are considered to result from damage to the basal ganglia, and their prime manifestations are involuntary motions that vary from a slow and writhing type to rapid and jerky ones. However, there are other characteristics of this group of problems that have not been mentioned. For example, in some cases movements occur that are opposite to those that are being attempted. The most notable example is that the fingers of someone who has what has classically been described as athetosis tend to extend and fan as they are reaching to pick up an object prior to their closing on that object.

Also as discussed in Chapter Two, a form of hypertonia referred to as tension may be a component of dyskinesia. This hypertonia is quite different from that which is characteristic of spasticity. From the above description of spasticity, it can be appreciated that if you were to vigorously shake the hand of someone who has spastic involvement of the arm, the rapid movements would serve to increase the resistance to the movements through the resulting reaction to stretch of the muscles of the arm.

In contrast, the hypertonia (or tension component) that is frequently associated with involuntary motion tends to disappear as a result of rapid, passively induced movements. This phenomenon led to the description that the tension component observed in individuals with cerebral palsy can be "shaken away." In fact, the vigorous shaking of the limb, with the resulting diminution of the hypertonus that typically returns a few minutes after the limb is left motionless, has come to be a differentiating sign between tension and spasticity.

These dysfunctions of basal ganglia mechanisms in cerebral palsy evidently result primarily from lesions to inhibitory mechanisms. The involuntary motions, then, result from undampened waves of excitatory neural patterns flowing into the final common pathway pool. The form of hypertonicity that is called tension also results from dysfunction of some inhibitory influence, and the resulting hypertonia has the effect of restricting mobility. In many cases the tension component appears severe enough that involuntary motions of the affected structures cannot be observed. That is, the relatively constant release of excitatory neural activity may be severe enough to prevent the occurrence of the oscillating influences that result in involuntary motions.

Both the involuntary motion and tension components of the dyskinesias do tend to disappear when the individual is sleeping. Moreover, these dysfunctions may vary rather dramatically as a function of the individual's affective state. That is, they may become more severe when the person becomes excited, angry, or, in general, somewhat stimulated by the situation of the moment.

An anatomically arranged topographical distribution may exist within the vastly complex network of extrapyramidal motor systems. To the extent that this distribution manifests itself subsequent to lesions of these mechanisms, however, it certainly is not as evident in developmental disorders, as in the case of damage to the pyramidal system. The most usual distribution of the involvement over musculatures in the dyskinetic cerebral palsied group is to all musculatures.

However, as described by Crothers and Paine (1959), there are numerous cases where there is more severe involvement in the upper extremities and oral musculatures within a given dyskinetic cerebral palsied individual than for that individual's lower extremities. Such individuals may be able to ambulate reasonably well, although with a notably abnormal gait, but they may have severely restricted arm function and a severe dysarthria. For some dyskinetic cerebral palsied individuals, a dysarthria of moderate severity may be found although problems of arm and leg function are relatively mild.

cerebellar mechanisms

Views of the general roles of cerebellar mechanisms in motor activity have not changed remarkably in recent years. The cerebellum receives information from the tissues of the body (tactile and proprioceptive information), the auditory system, the visual system, and the vestibular system. In humans the cerebellum probably does not receive significant information from the olfactory system.

The cerebellum also receives information related to targets to be achieved by the neuromotor system. In this context, the term target undoubtedly encompasses both spatial and temporal characteristics of move ments that include approaches to, associated reactions with, and withdrawals from the intended accomplishments of the motor system. The usual concept of a target for the motor system might be the hitting of a tennis ball by bringing the racket face in the path of the ball. However, the target associated with the end result of motor activity might better be thought of as the comprehensive movements and postures of the head, torso, legs, and feet, in addition to those of the arm and hand, that are involved with the goal of the racket face striking the ball at the planned moment in time.

The specific neural mechanisms that provide to the cerebellum all of the characteristics of these intended targets simply are not precisely known. There is speculation, for example, that such information is derived from known connections from the precentral gyrus into the cerebellum. Irrespective of how the cerebellar mechanisms are informed of intended target specifications, it is generally agreed that all of the incoming sensory and afferent information is compared within the cerebellum to those specifications. Thus, the cerebellum acts to compare what is intended for the motor systems with what is taking place. Moreover, the cerebellum has the capability to discharge inhibitory and excitatory influences into the neuromotor systems that modify activity of the final common pathway. Those influences generally are thought to be primarily indirect through some of the so-called extrapyramidal tracts and, in some cases, it is stated that these cerebellar discharges influence activity of the gamma efferent system in addition to the alpha motor neurons. The result of these influences is believed to be minor modifications in muscle activity that correct for errors in ongoing motor activity.

In addition to this role of diminishing errors during motor acts, cerebellar mechanisms also play a substantial role in maintaining muscle tone. Coupling of these two roles within one group of neural mechanisms makes intuitive sense. That is, if the cerebellum is to be able to initiate relatively minor modifications in muscle activity, it makes sense that it also would be principally involved in regulating the general background of muscle tone on which those modifications must be made. The cerebellar influence on the gamma efferent fibers seems the most likely connections for this regulation of muscle tone.

Formulations of these roles of cerebellar mechanisms came about through, among other sources, observations of the results of cerebellar damage in adults. Such adults frequently present the clinical picture of being incoordinated, and this condition of incoordination carries the name ataxia. Ataxic movements are characterized by what can be described as undershooting and overshooting during the approach and attempts to accomplish the act, and persons with generalized ataxia appear to be intoxicated.

With respect to the effect of damage to the cerebellar mechanisms involved in regulating muscle tone, a frequent result of cerebellar damage in the adult is a generalized reduction in that tone, or hypotonia. Thus, in addition to the uncoordinated movements, individuals with ataxia frequently appear to have generalized weakness of their musculatures.

As reviewed above, cases of ataxia as a result of damage before, at, or shortly after birth seem much more rare than was previously believed. In descriptions of such rare cases, I cannot recall reading of the associated presence of hypotonia being emphasized. In addition, for the few cerebral palsied children with whom I have had contact and to whom the label of ataxia has seemed appropriate, I do not recall hypotonia as being a major problem in conjunction with the incoordination.

Neither have I read, nor have I witnessed, indications that action tremor results from cerebellar lesions to the developing nervous system. Lesions to cerebellar systems in adults often result in that condition, allegedly due to damage of an inhibitory mechanism that results in release of oscillating volleys of excitation into the motor systems when the individuals attempt movement.

Even though there are relatively few cerebral palsied children with the diagnosis of ataxia that will come to the attention of the speech-language pathologist, there are reasons for attention having been given to these cerebellar mechanisms and disorders. First, of course, the mechanisms are fundamental components of the neuromotor systems. Second, and of equal importance for the present purposes, is the fact that there is a tendency to draw an analogy between the uncoordinated movements that result from lesions to the cerebellum and the disordered movements of dyskinesia.

Such an analogy can be very misleading. Assume the example in which a teen-age cerebral palsied person with dyskinesia and a teen-age person of the same age with ataxia as the result of recent trauma are both asked to use a typewriter and both have relatively comparable severity of involvement of the upper extremities. The probabilities are very high that there will be dramatic differences in the performance of the two persons. The dyskinetic individual is likely to be much more successful in striking the keys, even though the arm and hand movements associated with the effort are obviously disordered. The individual with ataxia, on the other hand, is much more likely to be unable to strike an intended key.

For both persons, however, it should not be assumed that the gestures of the oral structures that are associated with speech production will show "incoordination" in the sense that there will be gross inconsistency in, for example, the articulatory gestures during speech production. As will be discussed later in the sections on assessment, there is considerable consistency of speech articulatory gestures for both groups.

hypotonia and cerebral palsy

A description of the condition of atonia in some cerebral palsied infants was given in Chapter Two, and the fact that signs of this neuromotor problem routinely change to some other type as the child grows older was also mentioned. In the discussion of cerebellar disorders immediately above, it was also mentioned that hypotonia was a frequent neuromotor problem that results from an acquired lesion to the cerebellum. The impression should not be gained that the hypotonia in infants with cerebral palsy is due to cerebellar problems.

Usage of terms atonia (which should mean without muscle tone) and hypotonia (or reduction of normal muscle tone) has less precise implications than many other labels of types of neuromotor disorders. Any condition that reduces the activity of the final common pathways will result in reduced muscle tonus. Therefore, for example, adults with problems of the final common pathway with resulting diminution in the activity of and/or number of alpha fibers to their musculatures may be said to have hypotonia. Their muscles will not have the normal resistance to stretch, and their general muscular activity appears to lack strength. Similar reductions in muscle tone frequently are described as being present concomitantly with other forms of neuromotor disorders in brain-damaged adults that result from lesions among the basal ganglia. Therefore, the term hypotonia is used in reference to a variety of disorders that have the common effect of reducing muscle tone.

With respect to such disorders that occur from lesions above the level of the final common pathway, the most usual assumption is that excitatory influences into the motor pool have been reduced. For hypotonia that results from cerebellar lesions, for example, it seems most reasonable to assume that reduction in excitatory influence on the gamma efferents, with a resulting decrease in the activity through the gamma-alpha loops, is a principal basis.

I have not encountered what, to me, is a totally satisfactory explanation of the anatomical basis of the now-recognized temporary hypotonia in cerebral palsied infants. It evidently results from relatively generalized dysfunction of excitatory mechanisms in the brain. If the change in the form of the neuromotor disorder were routinely from the hypotonia to spasticity, it could be stated with some confidence that the pyramidal system had been the system that sustained the principal damage. That would make considerable sense, in that "pure lesions" of the pyramidal systems are believed to result in conditions of reduced muscle tone. However, the hypotonia in cerebral palsied infants may change to signs of spasticity or dyskinesia or both.

The term atonia probably should not be applied to most such weakened infants with cerebral palsy since some muscle tone is present. However, muscle tone in some of these infants is so lacking that their torso, limbs, and head literally "flop around" as they are handled. Their muscle mass is pliable to the touch and seemingly without tone. In severe cases there is minimal capability of movement.

As the improved movement capability begins to be observed as a result of increases in muscle tone, that tone comes to be abnormally great and/or involuntary movements come to be present. The continued maturation of the neuromotor systems subsequent to the lesion that produced the initial hypotonia is a generally accepted explanation for such changes.

○ ABNORMAL REFLEX BEHAVIORS AND REACTIONS

The material in Chapter Two emphasized the growing recognition in the 1950s and 1960s of the significance of abnormal motor patterns in cerebral palsy that were referred to as reflexes. As mentioned there, some of the systems of management of cerebral palsy that were being advocated and used relied heavily on evaluation and modification of these motor patterns.

Current recognition of the potential clinical significance of these abnormal reflex behaviors in conditions of cerebral palsy is reflected throughout the literature by extensive lists and discussions of them. These presentations frequently imply that the behaviors represent specific, well-defined phenomena that can be reliably identified. However, a comprehensive review of the descriptions of these entitled behaviors suggests that different labels are frequently applied to similar behaviors.

Not only are many of these behaviors difficult to identify reliably, there is a more basic problem of specifying the extent to which some can be said to be reflexes. Defining what constitutes a reflex is certainly more than a trivial consideration. Review of a number of relevant issues should be helpful.

There is no doubt that a number of specific reactions of the human organism can be designated as reflexes. That is, they are manifested by consistent stereotyped responses to specific types of stimuli. The reaction of the sphincter muscles of the iris of the eye to intensity of light (pupillary reflex) is an example. In the normally functioning individual, the areas of the pupils of the eyes that are exposed will be increased or reduced as a function of the intensity of light entering the eyes; the response is so consistent that deviation of the normal reaction indicates some type of dysfunction of selected neural mechanisms that are known to result in the reflex. Moreover, this reflex cannot be modified by learning, and there are relatively few neural operations other than the afferent, interconnecting, and efferent neural mechanisms that are involved in the response. The pupillary reflex, then, can be thought of as being relatively hardwired within the nervous system. Responses and activities of the organism that are mediated primarily by the autonomic nervous system frequently have this type of neural organization as their bases.

Many of the neural organizations that result in reflex behaviors that may have diagnostic and management significance for conditions of cerebral palsy, however, are subject to strong influence by other neural mechanisms. Those influences serve to exaggerate, diminish, or produce variations in the response within one individual from time to time. In addition, the variations in the lesions to the developing neuromotor systems, the differences in maturational organization of the neuromotor systems in the presence of those lesions, and the differing organizations of those systems that result from neural learning will produce dramatic variations in many of these behaviors among cerebral palsied individuals. Implications that they may be consistently and readily identified provide little preparation for the variations seen within individuals and the dramatic variations that may be observed among individuals.

The examples of both normal and abnormal neuromotor behaviors that are called reflexes and that have already been reviewed in this book attest to the heterogenity of these behaviors. These responses result, as has also been discussed, from a comparable variety of afferent, interconnecting, and efferent mechanisms.

A point of clarification may be needed at this juncture. The orientations that emphasize the significance of reflex behaviors in cerebral palsy that are being discussed do not routinely encompass the manifestations of hyperreflexia that characterize spasticity. Rather, these orientations speak to the significance of abnormal activity of more elaborately organized neural influences to the final common pathway. Examples of such behaviors that have already been mentioned in Chapter Two are retained and exaggerated primitive reflexes (e.g., the asymmetrical tonic neck reflex) and overly dominant postural reactions (an extreme form of which may be an extensor thrust).

Since these behaviors result from the dynamics of organization with less direct connections to the final common pathway, their influence cannot be expected to be as consistent as for those reflexes that have more direct connections. Even where there is a strong tendency for some of these behaviors to dominate the motor behavior of an individual, the variations in the influence of excitatory and inhibitory mechanisms that result in discharge of the alpha neurons may vary dramatically from moment to moment; hence, so will the manifestations of these behaviors.

Some of the criticisms that have been leveled against the orientation that abnormal reflexes are a clinically significant aspect of cerebral palsy have been (1) implications that their influence on motor function is highly predictable and consistent, and (2) the inherent problems in conceptualizing that such a variety of behaviors can be subsumed under the connotation of the single term reflex. Recognition of this latter factor seems to have led to some of these behaviors being referred to as responses or reactions rather than reflexes. The most prevailing obstacle to acceptance of what may be an appropriate orientation to the significance of these behaviors are extreme positions in that regard; these positions postulate that such behaviors are the most significant aspect of the problem and that analysis and management of developmental neuromotor disorders should be based almost solely on identification and modification of such behaviors.

The professional person who must address these issues may be better prepared to deal with them by understanding the bases of these reflex behaviors. Viewing them as an array of discrete behaviors tends to lead to the probable misconception that they may be unrelated within a given individual with cerebral palsy. Approaching these issues from an understanding of the interactions of the neural mechanisms that elicit these behaviors may be more helpful, and a perspective that many are interrelated or are variations of a common phenomenon may be possible.

As mentioned in Chapter Three, there is no doubt that there exists within the nervous systems of newborn infants a variety of neural organizations whose neuronal arrangements are predetermined. Their function is not dependent on learning. Many of the resulting behaviors are readily elicited in human newborns and throughout the early months of life. The sucking reflex of the newborn mentioned in Chapter Two and the flexion of the infant's leg to withdraw its foot from a noxious stimulus are examples. In addition, the motor activity of the young infant tends to be dominated by those neuromotor systems that are more completely developed; as mentioned in earlier chapters, the vestibular motor systems that eventually come to influence muscular activity as a function of the relation of the head to gravity and body posture are relatively well formed and are strongly influential in the infant's motor behavior. During the early stages of life a number of the motor behaviors mediated by these predetermined neural organizations and well-formed neuromotor systems may be relatively consistently elicited by specific stimuli, and the resulting motor patterns may be relatively stereotyped.

As the total nervous system matures, however, developing inhibitory systems come to suppress the activity of many of these neural organizations and early dominant excitatory motor mechanisms. Moreover, the totality of the developing neuromotor systems comes to influence motor function through maturation, and concomitant modifications will also develop within the neuromotor systems as a result of neural learning. Therefore, in the normally functioning adult, some of these early motor behaviors may be nonexistent; some may continue to have a strong but not a dominating influence; others remain as a part of normal motor function that closely resembles their initial forms. The sucking reflex is an example of a behavior that diminishes completely; reactions of limb and torso muscles to changes in posture are among those that continue to reflect influence of the vestibular neuromotor systems on motor activity; and actions of the posterior oral and pharyngeal musculatures during swallowing resemble early motor behaviors.

Infantile motor behaviors

The review in Chapter Two of the growing recognition of the potential significance of reflex behaviors in cerebral palsy mentioned that a portion of the motor behaviors of infants seems to result from (1) immaturity of neuromotor mechanisms, (2) manifestations of phylogenetically retained neuronal organizations, and/or (3) organized responses that are needed for survival of the human infant. Examples were reviewed, namely, the Babinski response, the asymmetrical tonic neck response, and the sucking reflex. Some of the more frequently mentioned additional examples are reviewed here.

Stimulation of the ball of the foot of an infant within the first few months of life may lead to all toes curling, and an object placed across the palm of the infant's hand in a specified manner will lead to the fingers curling and sometimes grasping the object. These grasping behaviors have been said to be examples of reflex organizations that are phylogenetically retained in the human nervous system. That is, they are said to represent remnants of stereotyped responses that can be seen in paws of monkeys in response to such stimuli.

In contrast, when the lateral plantar surface of the young infant's foot is stroked upward toward the ball of the foot, the big toe may curl upward, and the other toes may curl downward. This Babinski response, as already mentioned, is a normal reaction in very young infants, but its presence later is said to be a classic sign of spasticity. As already reviewed, its basis is thought to be quite different than the grasp response of the foot and toes.

The Moro reflex may be elicited relatively consistently in very young normal infants. When (1) the infant's head is supported slightly above a table while it is lying on its back and the head is suddenly released, (2) the upper portion of the infant's body is raised slightly off the table by pulling it upward with the arms and releasing them, or (3) the table on which the infant is lying supine is slapped to create a loud sound, the infant's arms will extend slightly upward in an abducted posture and then adduct as if the baby were attempting to wrap its arms around something. The legs may also move in a similar action. A number of authors indicate that influence of the Moro can be seen in the response to any sudden movement of the infant in space. The Moro is usually thought to be the result of stimulation of the vestibular system.

Within the first month of life, supporting the baby in an upright position so that its feet are touching the surface under it can result in a number of behaviors that involve the legs and trunk. The baby may lift itself from a squatting position to stand, and if its body is tilted forward, it may make steplike movements. These behaviors are relatively complex, and they seem to result from early-formed neuromotor organizations within the brain stem and spinal cord that respond to tactile and proprioceptive stimuli in combination with vestibular responses.

With respect to the sucking reflex, a variety of behaviors of the young infant that involve the oral and pharyngeal musculatures are also associated with ingestion, including lip closure around an object, sucking actions through tongue valving within the oral cavity, and swallowing. In addition, the baby's head may turn and move toward an object that touches its face in the area of its mouth. Some writers describe certain aspects of these behaviors (e.g., specific movement of the lips) as separate reflexes. Others include all of these behaviors under the label of a rooting and sucking reflex. Holding to this latter view permits appreciation of the elaborate nature of early-formed organizations within the infant's nervous system.

Descriptions of early motor behaviors also usually include a review of reactions of limb and torso musculatures to the position of the head to the body. They may be detected in normal infants by changes in muscle tone as a function of changes in head position. The asymmetric tonic neck response is one that may be observed in early normal infancy as subtly affecting muscle tone, as described in Chapter Two. The symmetrical tonic neck response is another of these behaviors. When the head is moved backwards, the extensor muscle tone of the arms increases as does the tone of the flexors of the legs; when the head is moved forward and down, these differences in tone reverse; there may be extension and flexion of the torso with those respective head positions.

The labyrinthine reflexes interact with the tonic neck reflexes as a function of the head's relation to gravity; one of their manifestations is that the tone of those muscles that extend the back and neck increases when the infant is lying on its back. Normal infants begin to develop a variety of postural reactions that become more sophisticated as motor skills are developed, and they persist in normal individuals as body and limb reactions to maintain balance.

The neuronal organizations that mediate these infantile motor behaviors and postural reactions reside for the most part at the level of the brain stem, and it is their interaction with the other existing motor mechanisms that brings about the sum of the motor behavior of which their manifestations are components. That is, these organizations cannot be viewed as discrete, separate mechanisms that operate independently. The intensity of the stimulus that elicits these behaviors will do so in relation to the intensity of the stimuli that may elicit others. Moreover, the influence of those stimuli may be enhanced or reduced by the developing inhibitory or excitatory neural patterns that eventually affect the activity of these organizations in the mature nervous system.[3]

It has been suggested that the activity of some of these lower organizations is a precursor of normal movement, and that possibility can be argued on a logical basis. Whether that is so or not is a moot point in regard to the effects of damage to the developing neuromotor mechanisms that normally come to inhibit and modify their activity. As mentioned in Chapter Two, the walking posture of many persons with the dyskinetic form of cerebral palsy very closely resembles that which would be dictated by descriptions of the extreme manifestation of asymmetrical tonic neck response. The reactions of the musculatures of numerous children with cerebral palsy to sudden changes in their postures leaves no doubt that abnormal, exaggerated reactions to those changes suddenly dominate their neuromotor systems.

significance for diagnosis and management of cerebral palsy

As has been mentioned, the exaggerated forms of some of these infantile motor behaviors are known to be indicative of damage to the developing neuromotor systems. An infant whose limbs assume the positions of the asymmetrical tonic neck reflex when its head is rotated from side to side is suspect of having cerebral palsy. Retention of the infantile reflexes (e.g., the sucking reflex) past the age when they usually become inhibited is also suggestive of a problem. Lack of emergence of those reflexes (e.g., the stepping reflex) is another diagnostic sign.

Alterations in the normal sequence of these infantile behaviors may result from existence of some of the forms of neuromotor disorders that have been discussed in this chapter. A significant hypotonia will serve to diminish them, and a hypertonia may serve to obscure their presence.

Rarely does some deviation in one, or a very few, of these behaviors prove to be a firm diagnostic sign of a significant neuromotor disorder. Rather, it will be a cluster of such deviations, and especially with accompanying signs of a neuromotor disorder, that will confirm the presence of such a problem.

There also seems to be a growing acceptance on the part of those who work with conditions of cerebral palsy that these abnormal reflex behaviors and postural reactions have significance for management. To the ex-

[3]The entirety of the material presented by Payton et al. (1977), may assist in understanding these points. For example, a perspective of the potential interaction of the classically described labyrinthine and tonic neck reflexes may be obtained. For another example, descriptions of how manifestations of the tonic neck reflexes vary as a function of posture may be found.

tent that these behaviors and reactions strongly influence motor behavior of selected infants, children, and adults with cerebral palsy, it seems reasonable that if activities can be designed, or the person can be handled in a manner that alleviates their influence, the chances will be enhanced that the person will be able to develop improved motor function.

In particular, there appears to be growing support for use of such management procedures with the very young cerebral palsied child. This support is based on the belief that early management, which includes procedures designed (1) to reduce the influence of these behaviors and reactions that are exaggerated and (2) to increase the influence of those that are diminished, may well provide one of the better approaches to management of developmental neuromotor disorders. This view seems reasonable if it is assumed that the possibility for modifying and developing neural patterns is greatest with the very young brain.

A number of movement patterns of the oral musculatures that are associated with mastication and deglutition of individuals with cerebral palsy have now been indicated as retention of reflex behaviors. It is known that the tongue movements associated with sucking and swallowing in infants are different from those used later for chewing and swallowing. Also, what appear to be the more infantile tongue movements can be observed in the oral behavior of some older cerebral palsied children. However, as with the case of head, body, and limb movements, there are now descriptions of a number of specific movements of the oral structures of children with cerebral palsy that are said to be manifestations of specific reflexes.

There will be additional comments regarding management that emphasize these behaviors in Chapters Five and Nine. However, from my point of view, the exceedingly strong emphasis that has been placed on abnormal reflex behaviors has led, in some cases, to an inappropriate frame of reference for the speech-language pathologist. Excessive concentration on this aspect of the problem diverts attention from more clinically relevant considerations for many speech-handicapped cerebral palsied speakers.

Many discussions of these abnormal reflex behaviors are presented in such a manner that it is easy to assume that an ability to recognize each specifically described behavior and to design management programs accordingly is essential to planning habilitation programs for the speech production deficits found in the cerebral palsied population. Certainly, an understanding of these abnormal behaviors is important. For the bulk of children with cerebral palsy who are capable of developing intelligible speech, however, concentration on dysfunction of the speech producing musculatures may be far more important. To the extent that this assertion is valid, it is possible to approach assessment and management of the specific characteristics of the dysarthric problem of individuals with cerebral palsy in a way that will lead to improved speech-production capability

without relying solely on analyzing and attempting to manage these abnormal reflex behaviors and reactions.

○ OTHER CHARACTERISTICS

The disorders of the motor systems that are described above are
the more important signs that are used currently to distinguish among the
types of cerebral palsy. Other such signs also may be used. For the
speech-language pathologist, however, the above descriptions should be
of assistance in understanding a number of the neuromotor aberrations
that are observed. There also are other characteristics that deserve review.

Individual differences

The point has been made that the neuromotor disorders in the
cerebral palsied population are relatively homogeneous compared to
those seen in adults with acquired neuromotor disorders. There are, however, individual differences among the movement patterns of those with
cerebral palsy that can be legitimately classified as having a common type
of problem. Some children with cerebral palsy of the dyskinetic type do
demonstrate the described reverse breathing pattern later. However,
some do not. For another example, even though there may be present a
generalized restriction of the mobility of the speech articulators in a given
individual with cerebral palsy, the tongue may be better controlled and
show more mobility than, for example, the lips. As will be emphasized later, one of the tasks of the speech-language pathologist is to determine
these relative patterns of immobility among the lips, tongue, jaw, and velopharyngeal port mechanism.

Even though known characteristics of developmental neuromotor disorders may assist in identifying and explaining physiological aberrations
of cerebral palsied individuals, it should not be assumed that such general
characteristics of the speech-producing musculatures are prime contributors to a speech deficit in the individual case. Whether or not, for example, a respiratory physiology problem of a dyskinetic child contributes to
the child's speech production deficit may depend upon a number of factors that are unique to that child. An uncritical assumption that it does
may obscure other physiological contributors that are of far more significance.

variations in signs and mixed signs

Discussions of the abnormalities of reflexes and postural reactions
also frequently imply that these behaviors can be consistently elicited in an
individual with cerebral palsy. As has been emphasized, nothing could be

further from fact. Even those manifestations of the various so-called signs of types of neuromotor disorders in the cerebral palsied population may vary dramatically from moment to moment. For example, in attempts to demonstrate classical signs of spasticity to a group of medical students, a physician may be forcefully driven to explain such variations within individuals. He might begin by describing ankle clonus and then proceed to grasp the child's lower leg in one hand, its foot in the other, and force the foot upward. No indications of clonus may result. This can happen even though twenty minutes earlier in an examining room the same physician had been able to elicit a sustained clonus with the same patient in the same ankle joint. Later in the same demonstration with the students, the physician may attempt to repeat the demonstration with success. Such variations in the abnormal neuromotor behaviors probably reflects changing patterns of inhibitory and excitatory activity within the various motor pools of the neuromotor systems. Therefore, in contrast to the impression that these behaviors can be consistently demonstrated, they are, in fact, subject to change.

Such changes also bear upon the comments made earlier relative to mixed types of cerebral palsy. The growing recognition that such mixed signs are relatively prevalent was due, in large part, to the ability to detect subtle indications of various signs. It became recognized, for example, that relatively weak, yet undeniably present, signs of hyperreflexia could be observed at times in persons who otherwise showed obvious, quite remarkable, signs of dyskinesia with what had seemed to be an accompanying tension component. Determination that a mild hyperreflexia was sometimes demonstrable might explain why that individual's tension could not be "shaken away" consistently.

Irrespective of their bases, the potentially subtle, fluctuating indications of these mixed signs probably have very little significance for the speech-language pathologist. Rather, in most cases, these subtle variations should be viewed as manifestations of the fact that function of the nervous system is dynamic and that caution should be exercised in assuming that its dysfunction will conform to predictable signs in a black-and-white manner.

fluctuations in severity of dysfunction

There are fluctuations in the severity of neuromotor dysfunctions associated with cerebral palsy that are quite significant to the speech-language pathologist. The generalized increases in muscle tone that may result from an individual's suddenly reacting to postural insecurity may bring about an intermittent deterioration in what is otherwise a reasonably adequate ability to produce speech. Such increases in dysfunction may appear to spread into muscle groups that otherwise show little or no signs of involvement of the neuromotor disorder. Thus, a child with a spastic diplegia who has very mild dysarthria may momentarily lose the ability to communicate orally as he or she is lifted in a manner that brings about such a postural reaction.

Another stimulus for increased muscular dysfunction may be a maximum effort on the part of the individual. The discussion of respiratory function for speech production in Chapter Six reviews the effects on the normal system when a speaker attempts to talk at the lowest levels of his or her vital capacity. Muscles throughout the torso and neck that usually are not involved in the speech-producing process may be brought into the attempt to maintain a speech-generating air stream when maximum contraction of the thoracic cage is required to do so. Such recruitment of associated muscle groups into acts that require extreme effort may, in fact, be detrimental to accomplishing the act in normal individuals.

In persons with cerebral palsy this recruitment of associated muscle groups is often referred to as "overflow." Such overflow may spread not only into associated muscle groups but also into musculatures not in any way associated with the act. In addition, the severity of the neuromotor dysfunction usually increases significantly, particularly where hypertonia is present. This overflow may be elicited quite easily in individuals with cerebral palsy. Such overflow throughout the speech-producing musculatures can, as might be anticipated, result in a temporary deterioration in speech-producing ability.

A third relatively common source of increased severity of dysfunction was mentioned in the earlier discussions of dyskinesias, namely, that the signs may vary as a function of the affective state of the individual, particularly for those who manifest tension. For a number of individuals with cerebral palsy who have dyskinesia, these fluctuations in severity can dramatically alter their ability to produce speech. Such persons' speech may usually be readily intelligible, but it may become unintelligible when they are upset, apprehensive, or excited. This source of increased severity of the neuromotor disorder may even manifest itself in speaking situations where the individual is uncomfortable for any reason.

○ SIGNIFICANCE OF THE CHARACTERISTICS

An earlier comment stated that the speech-language pathologist who deals with the cerebral palsied population must be well versed in all aspects of speech-language pathology. Also, it was stated that these endeavors can be among the most challenging to persons of that profession. A comprehensive understanding of the potential significance of the characteristics of the neuromotor disorders to speech physiology aberrations is, in and of itself, a challenge. Logical conclusions in that regard may be misleading in many cases.

During the era of accelerated interest in the conditions of cerebral palsy that was described in Chapter Two, attention was frequently given to the phenomenon of reversed breathing that could be observed in a number of children with dyskinesia. The behavior was not easily explained on the basis of earlier knowledge, and it reflected a physiological respiratory problem that appeared to contribute to a speech-production deficit.

The behavior was characterized by what appeared to be the reverse of the contraction-expansion patterns of the abdomen and thorax observed in normal persons during breathing. That is, during inspiration the abdomen was seen to expand dramatically, and the thorax appeared to contract. During expiration, the abdomen contracted, and the thorax appeared to expand.

Such observations may be explained on a logical basis from knowledge of the above-mentioned topographical distribution of the dyskinesias. That is, dyskinetic cerebral palsied persons sometimes show more severe involvement of their upper extremities and, hence, upper torso, than of their legs and, hence, abdominal wall muscles.

To the extent that a dyskinetic child has relatively more involvement of the upper torso than the lower torso wall musculatures, more flexibility would be expected in the expansion-contraction capability of the abdomen than of the thorax. Inhalation and exhalation would then be accomplished most easily by action of the diaphragm in combination with the abdominal wall muscles. Most normal persons can accomplish such "belly breathing" with relative ease by maintaining a relatively rigid position of the thorax during respiratory maneuvers, and the above described reciprocal, seemingly out-of-phase, contraction-expansion patterns of the thorax and abdomen will be observed. As will be discussed later, this type of breathing behavior probably does not contribute as significantly as has been assumed to the speech-production deficits of the dyskinetic speakers who use it.

The last topic to be presented in the above discussion of characteristics of neuromotor disorders was the fluctuating nature of the tension form of the hypertonias. An example of the problems that this phenomena can create for the speech-language pathologist not only demonstrates the need to understand the characteristics of the problem, but it also serves to verify the contention relative to the challenges that this area poses.

Some years ago I had occasion to work with a young woman who was attending the University of Iowa with a career goal of becoming a social service worker. She had a relatively mild, generalized dyskinesia. Her gait was only somewhat slow, her writing was readily legible, and she was maintaining a better than B average in her course work. She was an exceedingly gracious individual who appeared to have a very insightful understanding of human behavior.

Based upon the above description it might be assumed that this young woman possessed all of the characteristics necessary to achieve her career goals. The one exception was her speech, which was usually of slow rate but was quite adequate and only somewhat distracting to the listener. However, when she used the telephone her prosody diminished, her speaking rate slowed still further, and her articulation became imprecise. In questioning her about circumstances in which there was a comparable deterioration in her ability to speak well, she related other occasions in which she had refrained from speaking, if possible, because of this problem. She could recall, for example, avoiding oral recitations in school. However, at the age of twenty, speaking over the telephone remained the prime, and almost sole, problem situation.

After considerable counseling, it was possible to convince this young woman that the problem probably was due to heightened anxieties that remained regarding use of the telephone and a resulting increase in her mild hypertonia. She eventually was able to control her reactions to the point where she could at least converse comfortably over the telephone, even though at the time of my last contact with her, her speech in that circumstance was not as good as it routinely was.

I can recall full well one of the students of the Department of Speech Pathology and Audiology who drew an assignment to work with this young woman who said, "We are treating her like she is a stutterer." Indeed, the management of this problem was quite analogous to that which many people might use with stutterers who have significant difficulties with specific speaking situations. Of course, a prime difference is that in this case the reactions to the speaking situation led to a demonstrable, generalized restriction in the mobility of the person's vocal tract. Even so, effective management of the problem necessitated not only an understanding of the fluctuating nature of the tension but also of variables inherent in the principles of clinical practice of a totally different area of speech-language pathology.

As should become clear in the discussions to follow, a comparable understanding of the areas of speech physiology, speech and language development, and so on, including a thorough understanding of the effects of velopharyngeal incompetence on speech production, are required to work in the area of cerebral palsy. Indeed, that work is exceedingly challenging.

A review of the neuroanatomical components of the motor systems along with a discussion of their dysfunction in spasticity and dyskinesia places the speech-language pathologist in a position to appreciate the important characteristics of most cases of developmental dysarthria. In addition, such a review provides an understanding of less frequently occurring forms of developmental neuromotor disorders, and it assists in interpreting much of the literature that deals with those disorders.

One of the major differences between acquired and developmental neuromotor disorders is the prevalence of abnormal reflex behaviors and postural reactions in the developmental group. Numerous infantile motor behaviors in combination with patterns of development of the neuromotor system are the basis for these behaviors and reactions when there is early damage to the developing neuromotor systems. These abnormal reflex behaviors and postural reactions are used in many instances as signs that indicate cerebral palsy is present in infants and very young children. In addition, they have been used as the foundation of approaches to management of the cerebral palsied problem. However, the speech-language pathologist is well advised to consider these behaviors and reactions as only components of the total problem of cerebral palsy, and overemphasis upon them may lead to overlooking more important characteristics of developmental dysarthria.

Other important characteristics of cerebral palsy are some of the individual differences that may be observed in the neuromotor disorders of selected individuals within diagnostic types and the variations in signs from the usually expected patterns of neuromotor involvement. In some individuals with cerebral palsy, fluctuations in the severity of the neuromotor problem are to be expected.

These characteristics are of crucial significance to the speech-language pathologist who works with individuals who have cerebral palsy. It is these characteristics that form the unique differentiating communication problems of that population.

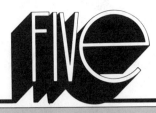

○ THE REALITY OF THE PROBLEM

○ NEUROMOTOR NETS FOR SPEECH PRODUCTION

○ THE SPEECH-PRODUCING MECHANISM AS AN AERODYNAMIC-MECHANICAL SYSTEM

○ FUNCTIONAL OVERLAY AND PHYSIOLOGICAL LIMITS

○ REFLEX BEHAVIORS AND POSTURAL REACTIONS

○ POSITIONING

○ ASSESSMENT AND MANAGEMENT AS A FUNCTION OF AGE

○ INTERDISCIPLINARY ASSESSMENT AND MANAGEMENT

○ SUMMARY

General considerations for assessment and management

Assessment procedures have the prime purposes of (1) providing indications of the bases of the problem, (2) giving the speech-language pathologist indications of the degree to which the client will be able to develop or improve his or her communication skills and (3) providing guidelines for the management procedures that will bring that prognosis to fruition. No matter how carefully and comprehensively the assessment procedures are carried out, prognostic indicators are, in many instances, obscure. That is particularly true when dealing with very young children who have cerebral palsy. Even when those indicators appear relatively clear, continuous reappraisal of the initial impressions of the prognosis is necessary as management proceeds.

○ THE REALITY OF THE PROBLEM

There may be a strong tendency to err in the direction of overly optimistic prognoses by speech-language pathologists for children with cerebral palsy. It is a natural tendency for a professional person to identify to a certain degree with a child and to share the hopes of that child's parents for a favorable outcome of professional management, and there certainly should be an attitude of guarded optimism underlying professional endeavors. However, in a number of cases an orientation that a child with cerebral palsy will make substantial improvement in developing oral communication skills if enough continued effort is put forth may result in a gross misservice to all who are concerned. As mentioned in Chapter One, the responsibilities of those professional people who work with the cerebral palsied population are too great to justify other than being realistic to one's self, the client, and that client's family members.

There is some latitude within the neuromotor systems for change as a result of learning. Otherwise, the known effects of various types of motor training could not be realized. It is intriguing to speculate about the events that transpire within the nervous system as improvement in some disordered movement pattern takes place as a result of a management regimen. However, statements made in the literature to explain such improvement are misleading if they result in an assumption that normal motor function can be achieved in the great majority of cases of cerebral palsy. As has been mentioned, neuronal transmission through the neuromotor systems probably has less latitude for change as a result of learning than many of the other neurological systems. Irrespective of the physiological bases of improvement of neuromotor performance as a result of learning, there will be a limit to that improvement.

A fundamental orientation underlying the suggestions for assessment and management given in the remaining chapters of this book is that dysarthric speakers must be assisted to produce the best speech of which they are capable within the limits of their disordered speech-physiology mechanism. This orientation is in contrast to an assumption that, through management procedures, the basic physiological capability of a dysarthric speaker can be improved dramatically. That frequently will not be the case. It may be possible to extend those limits somewhat with appropriate management, but it is much more likely that optimum improvement can be achieved by assisting most of these speakers to produce speech within the limits of their mechanisms.

Later discussions regarding respiratory function problems associated with cerebral palsy, their effect upon speech production, and how those effects can be minimized serve as an example of this present orientation, and there is an analogy to expectations for esophageal speakers. It is clear that those speakers have a limit to the amount of air they can inject into the esophagus and then use to drive the vocal tract. Management routinely does not include procedures designed to dramatically increase that amount of air. Rather, it is assumed that the esophageal speaker must function to the best of his or her ability within the physiological limitation by speaking in short phrases. In lieu of substantial evidence that the speech-producing function of respiratory muscles of speakers who have cerebral palsy can be dramatically improved, it may be far better for those speakers who present a significant problem of respiratory function to concentrate on producing the best speech possible within the limits of his or her respiratory system than to engage in a regimen of respiratory exercises with the assumption that his or her respiratory function for speech production will be improved.

The reality of a neuromotor disorder also must be recognized relative to involvement of other speech-producing musculatures. In the earlier discussion of the final common pathway, the complexity in movements of the human tongue during speech production was emphasized. The musculature of the tongue, however, is a relatively small group of muscles compared to the totality of the muscles involved in speech production. The neuromotor activity that underlies the total speech-physiology process requires synchronous patterns of muscle activity associated with respiration, phonation, and articulation. These patterns consist of sometimes subtle but significant adjustments in muscle tension that are at least as rapid as changes in the acoustic speech signal and that are requisites to normal speech production.

The phenomenon of perceived speech stress serves to exemplify the point. Differences in stress, or syllabic emphasis, are characterized by rapid fluctuations in fundamental frequency of the vocal tone, vocal intensity levels, and timing of phonatory and articulatory movements. Changes in subglottal air pressure also are associated with different fundamental frequencies and intensities of the vocal tone. Although those differences in subglottal air pressure may be due as much to changes in interaction of the vocal folds with the speech airstream as they are due to pulsatile activity of respiratory muscles, it is likely that such respiratory activity plays a role in production of some stress differences. Stress patterns, then, which are a component of perceptually normal speech, depend on subtle, rapid, and synchronous changes of tension in a variety of muscles of the total speech-producing system.

The presence of a neuromotor disorder will negate such rapid, subtle muscle activity. Therefore, to anticipate that a speaker with cerebral palsy who has generalized involvement of the speech-producing musculatures will be able to produce speech that sounds normal is unrealistic in many cases. The more usual realistic goal for such speakers is for them to be able to produce speech with optimum intelligibility within the limits of their specific speech-physiology problems. Even the goal of routinely being intelligible is unrealistic for some.

The fact of a physiological limitation to improved performance also must be recognized with respect to disabilities other than the neuromotor disorder. It is tempting to speculate, for example, that a given cerebral palsied child may have an aphasic-like problem in addition to the neuromotor disability, and considerable attention may be devoted to that possibility. Numerous other examples of disabilities that have been alleged to be the result of brain abnormality in children have been assumed also to be present in selected children with cerebral palsy, and many times statements regarding these disabilities imply that if they are appropriately recognized and managed, significant improvement will be realized.

A great deal of professional attention to children with abnormal brains can result in some improved performance in a number of skills, even for those who have been rather grossly devastated neurologically. However, to anticipate dramatic improvement, and especially normality, may be very unrealistic. To the extent that disabilities other than the neuromotor problem are present, and to the extent that those disabilities are also due to the abnormality of the developing brain, the reality of the neurological limitations increases the probability of a poor prognosis.

It is my contention that, as has been implied in the earlier portions of this book, preoccupation with the complex array of potential contributors to communication problems associated with cerebral palsy has led, in many instances, to diversion of appropriate attention from the more salient clinical features of the problem. Determining (1) the speech-physiology deficits that are present in a specific speaker with cerebral palsy and (2) the extent to which such a speaker can modify his or her speech-producing behaviors in order to speak with optimum intelligibility within the limits imposed by those deficits may pay greater dividends. By concentrating on that aspect of the problem, the speech-language pathologist frequently can assist individuals with cerebral palsy to make dramatic improvement in their communication skills. In numerous cases that improvement will be sufficient to demonstrate that consideration of factors other than the dysarthric component of the problem is unwarranted.

In addressing the principal task of determining the speech-physiology limitations of speakers who have cerebral palsy, there may be the inclination to attribute all deleterious speech motor behaviors to abnormal neuromotor patterns. Such speakers, however, may adopt a number of counterproductive motor behaviors in attempting to learn to produce speech in the presence of selected speech physiology deficits. As might be anticipated, such learned behaviors that contribute to the speech deficit are usually relatively easy to modify compared to those that represent the limits imposed on the speech-producing musculatures by the neuromotor disorder.

The emphasis in this book on the dysarthric aspects of the communication problems of speakers with cerebral palsy should not obscure the fact that any of the variables that cause or maintain communication problems in physically normal children may lead to, and maintain, such problems in children with cerebral palsy. Therefore, even though the probabilities are extremely high that a communication problem of someone who has cerebral palsy will have a neuromotor problem as its prime basis, the speech-language pathologist should be constantly alert to the possibility of other bases.

Because individuals with cerebral palsy are routinely physically handicapped to some degree, they are also surrounded by a cluster of associated psychological-social problems that require attention in a speech habilitation program. In general, these problems may be viewed as a natural outgrowth of a child's or adult's being significantly handicapped. They range from attitudes the cerebral palsied individual develops to those that evolve with the individual's parents, other family members, and associates. It should not be assumed that such problems are unique to those with cerebral palsy. Rather, they frequently appear to represent attitudes and reactions of individuals who have problems in adjusting to, and or competing in, society for a wide variety of causes.

The following discussion of assessment and management procedures relative to communication disorders associated with cerebral palsy will concentrate on the dysarthric aspect of those disorders. The presence of other contributory disabilities, disorders, and their implications as well as associated attitudinal and adjustment problems on the part of the individual, family members, and associates also will be reviewed. Finally, a position will be maintained that all persons involved with an individual who has cerebral palsy, including the professional persons working with the individual, the family members of the individual, and that individual, will best be served in most cases by an objective, realistic approach to the management program and its potential outcome.

○ NEUROMOTOR NETS FOR SPEECH PRODUCTION

Considerable attention was given to relatively specific irregularities of motor patterns of articulatory, laryngeal, and respiratory function of cerebral palsied speakers during the era of accelerated interest in cerebral palsy. Problems in repetitively moving the tongue up to and down from the alveolar ridge and lateralizing the tongue from one corner of the mouth to the other were examples. The general idea had evolved that a single such irregularity was likely to be a contributor to a clinically significant speech-production problem. Moreover, the recommended evaluation regimens emphasized the need to identify those specific irregularities, and in many instances, management procedures entailed training the child with cerebral palsy to improve those specific irregularities.

The staff of speech-language pathologists with whom I was associated and their work, as described in the Preface, began to cast doubt on the relationship between many of these irregularities of the speech-producing musculatures during nonspeech acts and irregularities of motor behaviors associated with speech production. There were instances in which it was observed that a cerebral palsied youngster, for example, could not elevate the tip of the tongue to touch the alveolar ridge because of restricted mobility of the tongue and problems of jaw movement. Yet, that same child could produce acoustically acceptable lingua-alveolar consonants, and cinefluorography confirmed relatively rapid, mobile action of the anterior portion of the tongue to accomplish the needed lingua-alveolar contacts. Some of the early research efforts (e.g., Hixon and Hardy, 1964) showed that the relationship between restricted mobility of articulatory structures during nonspeech movements and the severity of speech-physiology problems of children with cerebral palsy was not sufficiently strong to use nonspeech movements as firm predictors of speech-physiology problems. Thus, the concept evolved that the neuromotor nets associated with speech production are dissimilar for speech and nonspeech acts. These nets are, moreover, sufficiently different that irregularities in motor performance during acts other than speech production may hold limited significance for the speech-language pathologist who is assessing and managing a developmental dysarthria.

The historical concentration on motor behaviors of relatively specific, isolated muscle groups (e.g., mobility of the lips) had also led to the orientation that significant speech physiology problems could best be understood by conceptually segmenting structures of the vocal tract. It seemed to be assumed, for example, that a problem of tongue function should be given attention in a management program, irrespective of mobility problems of other muscle groups associated with speech production.

The results of a number of unpublished researches began to cast doubt on such an orientation. There were strong indications that the manner in which the respiratory, laryngeal, and articulatory systems interact with the speech airstream may be of more significance than the function of one of those systems. A model for clinical work began to be developed that was based on the ideas that (1) the speech-producing mechanism should be viewed as an aerodynamic-mechanical acoustic generator in which the respiratory system supplies the aerodynamic energy on which various valves (the laryngeal and articulatory structures) interact to produce the acoustic speech signal and that (2) the dysarthric problem should be conceptualized as a disruption in the interaction of those valves with the airstream. This model emphasizes the importance of viewing the speech-producing system in its entirety in assessing and managing the dysarthric problem.

The previously mentioned publication by Hixon and Hardy (1964) resulted from one of the earlier attempts to address systematically the issue of the relationship between irregularities in nonspeech movements of the articulatory structures and the severity of the speech-production problems in the cerebral palsied population. The rates with which a group of dysarthric cerebral palsied children could (1) perform reciprocal movements with their tongues, lips, and jaws and (2) produce trains of consonant-vowel syllables were determined. The strength of correlations between those rates and the severity of judged speech defectiveness showed that the latter were much more strongly related to the severity of speech problems than the former. Moreover, a review of what was then contemporary thinking regarding organization of the neuromotor systems by Paillard (1960) was used to support one of the resulting conclusions, namely, that the neuromotor nets that result in speech production are probably uniquely organized for that activity.

Paillard had pointed out that the anatomy of the human pyramidal system provides a neurophysiological capability for performance of extremely complex, rapid, and precise movements with the hands and oral structures. As can be seen in Figure 4–2, a much larger proportion of the pyramidal cells influence the final common pathways of motor units that innervate hand, facial, and oral musculatures than other muscle groups. Paillard also pointed to phylogenetic differences among species in this regard. For example, relatively more pyramidal fibers contribute to the functioning of a monkey's forepaws than to that of its oral structures.

Paillard also reviewed the belief that this relatively large proportion of neurons that influences the activity of specific muscle groups forms the neuroanatomical basis for development of exceedingly complex and precise movements, which he referred to as "skilled movements." The concept of skilled movements now seems generally accepted as a manifestation of organizations within the neuromotor systems that are dissimilar to those organizations resulting in other types of movements of the same musculatures. In some cases these skilled movements are defined on the basis of their speed, complexity, and other criteria. However, the basic contention is that there exists within the neuromotor systems the potential for developing elaborate networks that result in rapid, complex movements involving numerous muscles that come to be "automatic" in the execution. One frame of reference regarding these so-called skilled movements says that their execution results from excitation of neuronal nets that have become organized in a manner that results in the ongoing movements from plans that have been laid down in the nervous system. Moreover, the usual conceptualization of skilled movements also includes the idea that in spite of their speed, precision, and complexity, they may be executed with little or no conscious attention.

The patterns of limb and torso movements that result in walking, for example, also are routinely accomplished without concentration. Those who emphasize the automatic nature of skilled movements might be in a better position if they would recognize that the types of acts to which they are referring may be distinguished more by their complexities and rates of associated motor activity than by the extent to which the relatively vague concept of "attention" is involved.

Nevertheless, this concept of skilled movements has come to be applied to speech production and to patterns of hand and finger movements. Moreover, it has come to include the idea that the neuromotor systems become organized to achieve an end result, irrespective of the manner in which specific muscle groups participate. An often-cited example is handwriting, which is comparable and distinctive to individuals whether they are writing, for example, their signatures on a blackboard with chalk or on a piece of paper with a pencil. In writing on a blackboard, muscles that control the shoulder, elbow joint, wrist, and fingers are involved. Using a pencil to write on paper involves fewer muscles, but the resulting configurations of marks on the paper are quite comparable to those made by the chalk on the blackboard. Similarly, the perceptual characteristics of a person's speech are comparable, irrespective of head position or other contingencies (e.g., holding a pipe between the teeth) that require modification in the speech producing movements.

A comprehensive model of neuromotor processes associated with speech production also must include innervation of muscle groups associated with respiration and phonation. The earlier description of the physiological correlates of stress attests to the need for concomitant synchrony of phonatory and articulatory movements. Even though action of respiratory muscles for stress differences is equivocal, there is evidence to suggest that the respiratory system strives to maintain specific magnitudes of air pressures within the vocal tract during speech. Therefore, the activity of the respiratory system must be included in considering the total neuromotor nets for speech production.

The uniqueness and inherent complexity of the neuromotor organization for speech production can be emphasized even more by pointing out that the transmission time of action potentials along the axons of the alpha motor neurons of the brain stem to muscles that control respiration, phonation, and articulation vary as a function of those axons' length. Therefore, the neuromotor organizations that result in speech production include patterns of excitation of the final common pathways that vary temporally, but all of the synchronous movements that are needed for speech production are accomplished with appropriate timing. It seems likely that the neuromotor processes for speech production involve elaborate networks that innervate the motor units of the entirety of the speech-producing musculatures whose cell bodies are located throughout the lower portion of the brain stem in a number of efferent cranial nerve nuclei.

There is evidence from a number of sources that the neuromotor systems do come to be organized dissimilarly for different acts of at least the oral structures. For example, in patients who are undergoing brain surgery, electrical stimulation of the cortex in the area of origin of the corticobulbar tract may result in prolonged phonations; in other instances swallowing behavior may be elicited. Thus, it would appear that appropriate excitation of cortical mechanisms will, in some instances, excite the neuronal organization that results in phonatory activity; in other instances, the neuromotor net that has become organized to produce swallowing behavior may be excited.

Earlier material also stressed the need to understand that the input to the final common pathway motor pools may be from a variety of different sources for different acts. Elicitation of a gag response does not provide input to the efferent cranial nerve system comparable to that which results in velopharyngeal port closure during speech production, and there should be no puzzlement as to why a child with cerebral palsy may have a gag reflex that includes extensive palatal movement but whose palate moves minimally during speech. Yet, observation of the extent of palatal movement during the gag response has been used, historically, as a predictor of that movement during speech production. There also have been suggestions that repeated elicitation of such movement by the tactile stimulation of the oral pharyngeal area should be incorporated into a regimen of muscle training to promote palatal movement in order to improve speech production.

It has been amply demonstrated that palatal immobility during speech production, with resulting velopharyngeal incompetence, is frequently found in many individuals who have dysarthria as a result of a lesion to the neuromotor systems above the level of the brain stem. Those same individuals frequently have extensive palatal movement and velopharyngeal closure during a gag response. That response may be hyperactive in cases of spasticity to the point that vomiting may occur from rather mild stimulation, and the zone in the oral cavity from which the response can be stimulated is frequently extended. Therefore, the presence of palatal movement during the reflex gag really gives no indication of palatal movement during speech production.

I also question the possibility that routine elicitation of a gag response can be used to improve velopharyngeal competence during speech production, on the basis of points that have just been covered. For the neuromotor disorders of cerebral palsy, the abnormal neural patterns to the final common pathway pool that result from incompetence during speech production are from sources other than the relatively direct interlinkage between the afferent and efferent branches of the cranial nerve system involved with the gag reflex. Therefore, eliciting a gag response is unlikely to affect the neuromotor patterns that are responsible for the incompetence.

A number of examples with comparable implications for management of dysarthria associated with cerebral palsy could be cited. A substantial discussion will be devoted later to only one of those examples: dysfunctions of respiratory musculatures that may contribute to a speech problem of a cerebral palsied speaker. Also, an individual with celebral palsy may exhibit extreme excursions of the chest wall and inhalation of a large quantity of air during yawning. Such an extensive respiratory maneuver may be impossible for that person to accomplish otherwise. I have witnessed some speech-language pathologists whose management regimen was based on the assumption that inducing yawns in such persons will improve control of their respiratory systems. Requiring a child with cerebral palsy to breathe into a bag held over the nose and mouth will soon result in replacement of the oxygen in the bag by the child's expired carbon dioxide, and yawning occasionally may be induced.[1]

---

[1]This procedure also was used under the assumption that one of the underlying bases of the involuntary motion disorder frequently seen in cerebral palsy is a chronic reduction in optimal levels of carbon dioxide in the blood stream. This belief was never verified experimentally; nevertheless, some individuals did use such procedures under the assumption that not only would carbon dioxide levels be increased and result in reduction of involuntary motion, but also, as mentioned, the inhalation ability to those children would improve. These two purposes, in fact, would achieve opposite results. The mild hypoventilation probably would serve to increase carbon dioxide levels, but improvement in inspiratory ability would serve to increase ventilation of oxygen when the child was not ventilating into some kind of closed container, resulting in reduced carbon dioxide levels.

From my point of view, inducing yawning with the rationale that it improves respiratory function for speech production differs very little from repeatedly eliciting a gag reflex of a dysarthric child in the belief that it will improve the child's velopharyngeal function during speech production. Some speech-language pathologists today reject such suggestions, particularly with respect to the rather extreme example of inducing yawning. Those same clinical practitioners, however, may be inclined to use isolated, nonspeech movements of the tongue, lips, and jaw as a part of the assessment and management regimens with cerebral palsied speakers. The yawning act is initially stimulated from chemoreceptors within the respiratory system, and the neuronal patterns to the final common pathway pools of alpha neurons that results in the yawn probably comes principally from the autonomic nervous system. As mentioned earlier, transmission to the final common pathway pools for the gag response comes through relatively direct interconnections between tactile receptors in the oral pharyngeal area. For nonspeech acts of the tongue, lips, and jaw, input to the final common pathway pools is probably impossible to specify precisely; nevertheless, it seems illogical to contend that such input is from the same neural mechanisms as those that emit speech-producing movements.

I seriously question the efficacy of any clinical technique that assumes abnormal movements can be improved by repetition of similar movements of the same musculatures that result from a different source of innervation to the final common pathway pool. Phrases such as "transfer of vegetative movements" to movements during speech production have been used to imply or state that such techniques have a place in the clinical regimen. I know of no evidence to support the validity of such claims. However, my general position in that regard applies to more than just the use of reflexes to induce movements that allegedly can be transferred to some other type of functional act, and I will return to that topic later.

There may be some value in determining the effects of neuromotor involvement during nonspeech movements of the speech articulators. Even so, for the speech-language pathologist to utilize nonspeech movements for assessment or management purposes with the idea that such activities are predictive of significant speech physiology problems or that their repetition will directly improve the speech physiology capability of their client is, to me, based upon untenable assumptions regarding organization of the neuromotor systems for speech production.

The most efficient general guideline to bring about any possible improvement in neuromotor function for speech production, therefore, would seem to be through use of activities associated with some form of speech production. Such activities are those that are most likely to involve the total neuromotor net for speech production.

○ THE SPEECH-PRODUCING MECHANISM AS AN
AERODYNAMIC-MECHANICAL SYSTEM

When the speech-producing mechanism is conceptualized as an aerodynamic-mechanical acoustic generator, the respiratory system may be viewed as providing the power source for the speech signal, namely an expiratory airstream with certain characteristics. Those characteristics probably are dictated by requirements for certain magnitudes of air pressures at specified locations along the vocal tract. Those locations can be viewed, in general, as being below the vocal folds for phonatory activities and in the oral-pharyngeal cavity for production of voiceless consonants. When the relationships between the magnitude of subglottal air pressure and vocal fold tension are appropriate, for example, phonation results from the vocal folds being set into vibration; for phonation to be maintained, there must be retention of appropriate tension of the vocal folds and a specified magnitude of mean subglottal air pressure. As another example, for production of the turbulence associated with continuant consonants, the appropriate articulatory structures are positioned to present a resistance to the airstream; the noises that either constitute or are components of those consonants are produced by forcing air through those restrictions; in order for that forcing to take place, certain magnitudes of air pressure within the oral-pharnygeal cavity must be generated and maintained. For a final example, the plosive phase of stop consonants results from the articulators occluding (or creating an infinite resistance to) the airstream; that occlusion creates air pressure behind the occlusion, and that magnitude of air pressure can be thought of as a potential aerodynamic energy source. When the occlusion is opened, the release of that energy, in a burst of airflow, creates the plosive phase of aspirated stop consonants. Thus, the mechanical valves that interact with the speech-generating airstream can be viewed as the vocal folds, the various configurations of the tongue in its relationship to other oral structures, postures of the lips in conjunction with each other and the teeth, and finally, the soft palate in conjunction with pharyngeal wall movements that close the velopharyngeal port.

The function of the velopharyngeal port within the concept of the speech-producing system as an aerodynamic mechanical sound generator deserves special consideration. Its function emphasizes the dichotomy between the aerodynamic-mechanical and the acoustic aspects of speech production. Closure of the velopharyngeal port results in an aerodynamically efficient generator within the oral cavity; that is, as air pressure is generated within the oral-pharyngeal cavity air cannot leak through the nasal cavities. When the velopharyngeal port is open, such a leak of air reduces the efficiency with which noises can be generated in the oral cavity.

Of course, velopharyngeal port opening is associated with the production of nasal consonants. Egress of air from the oral cavity is blocked, and there is airflow through the nasal cavity. However, it is the change in the acoustic characteristics of the vocal tract that results in the phenomenon of nasal resonance. That is, the masses of air in both the nasal and oral-pharyngeal cavities are set into vibration. The resulting resonance of these two acoustically coupled masses of air usually results in the perception of what we refer to as nasality. The frame of reference that calls for viewing the speech-producing mechanism as an aerodynamic-mechanical system does not take into consideration such changes in the resonance characteristics of the vocal tract that result from the velopharyngeal port being either open or closed.

Similarly, the model of the speech-producing mechanism as an aerodynamic-mechanical generator essentially ignores the changes in the resonance characteristics of the vocal tract that result in different vowel productions. Those characteristics are determined by the changes in sizes of air masses within the pharynx and mouth that result from changing positions of the tongue. The resulting amplifications and attenuations of frequencies of the phonatory acoustic spectrum result in the acoustic differences among vowels.

During vowel productions the major resistance to the speech airstream is at the level of the glottis, and it is important to recognize that it is the major resistance to the speech airstream against which the respiratory system must work to perform its function as a power source. That is, it can be assumed that the vibrating vocal folds present the major resistance to the speech airstream during vowel productions. As long as the respiratory system is creating an appropriate subglottal air pressure to maintain the folds in a vibratory mode, it can essentially ignore lesser restrictions to airflow through the oral cavity until those restrictions become greater than that presented by the vocal folds.

These comments should not be construed to imply that the ability or inability of an individual with cerebral palsy to produce vowels should be disregarded. To the contrary, attention to the adequacy of vowel productions probably has not received enough attention. The points being made here, however, are (1) that clinically significant aspects of dysarthria can usually best be analyzed and managed by giving attention to the aerodynamic-mechanical interactions of the entire speech-producing mechanism and (2) that there is a very important differentiation to be made between those interactions and the changes in the dimensions of the vocal tract that lead to differences in its resonance characteristics. However, for the immediate purposes, those changes in the dimensions of the vocal tract that lead to different resonance characteristics are being ignored.

A final point should be made regarding the aerodynamics of speech production. Airflow through the glottis is interrupted during the adduction phase of phonation; during the implosion phase of stop consonants the expiratory airstream also is momentarily blocked. However, such blockages are so transient that they are ignored for the present purposes. For those purposes, it is desirable to view the respiratory system as having to make relatively continual adjustments to reduction in internal volume while simultaneously maintaining the appropriate air pressures within the vocal tract.

As a first example of how viewing the speech-producing system as an aerodynamic-mechanical system makes it possible to understand many of the potential effects of restricted mobility of the various structures involved in speech production, consider the function of the tongue musculatures in the production of /s/. In the usual normal circumstance an aperture is formed by a groove in the tongue against the alveolar ridge, and that aperture is relatively small. As a specified amount of air pressure is developed behind that aperture, the rate of airflow being forced through the aperture is rapid enough to create the turbulence to produce /s/ as that airstream is disrupted by some structure such as the edge of the teeth.

If restricted mobility of the tongue results in the aperture's being larger, and if the respiratory system generates an airstream of comparable force, as was the case for the normally narrow aperture, characteristics of the aerodynamics through the aperture will be altered. With the same airflow, the larger opening will cause a drop in the air pressure behind the aperture. Even so, the loss of air volume will be greater through the larger opening; finally, the velocity of particles of air will be slower. A reasonable analogy can be made by thinking of the effects of adjusting the nozzle of a garden hose. When the nozzle is adjusted to produce a concentrated jet of water through a narrow opening, the water pressure within the hose is substantial, and the velocity of the particles of water through the nozzle is great enough that the jet carries for a considerable distance. When the nozzle is opened maximally, there is an increase in the volume of water flowing from the hose, but the water pressure within the hose is less, and the speed of the water particles also is less.

For the speech-producing system, it is the velocity of air particles that creates the turbulence needed for production of fricatives and sibilants. If the opening is abnormally large during production of such consonants, the respiratory system must generate an airstream of greater force if the needed air turbulence is to be created. For stop consonants, the inefficiency of articulatory function due to neuromotor involvement may result in slower movement toward occlusion of the airstream, and the precision of that occlusion may be less. The respiratory system, again, must compensate for the increased loss in internal volume. The greater respiratory effort may result in the production of the sound, but it also results in an even greater volume of air flowing through the system to produce the sound.

Thus, because of the inefficiency of articulatory valving of the airstream, which is a component of most cases of dysarthria, a greater work load is placed on the respiratory system for speech production. The extent of that increased demand on the respiratory system will vary, of course, with the manner and place of articulation of various speech sounds and the extent of reduced mobility of the articulatory structures associated with their production.

However, restricted function of one articulatory structure, the velopharyngeal port, will result in reduced aerodynamic efficiency of the speech-producing system in general. The presence of velopharyngeal incompetency results in leak of the expiratory airstream through the open velopharyngeal port as the respiratory system generates the needed intraoral air pressures. In that circumstance, the total aperture through which the airstream will flow is a sum of the areas of the velopharyngeal port opening and the oral aperture, (e.g., the groove of the tongue against the alveolar ridge for /s/). Such an additional area through which air will escape increases even more the force with which the respiratory system must generate a speech-producing airstream. That is, if the /s/ is to be produced, the respiratory system must accommodate for a more rapid loss of internal air volume as it attempts to generate the intravocal tract air pressure needed to drive air with the needed particle velocity through the tongue–alveolar ridge aperture.

Velopharyngeal incompetence, however, is likely to be more dehabilitating than inefficiency of oral structures. Air will follow the path of least resistance. When the aperture of the velopharyngeal port is larger than the articulatory aperture in the oral cavity, a relatively large volume of air will leak through the nasal cavity. It may, therefore, be impossible to generate sufficient intraoral air pressure to force air at the needed particle velocity through the oral aperture for continuant consonants or to create the needed potential aerodynamic energy for plosion of stop consonants.

Even though speakers with cleft palates in general, have anatomically and physiologically normal respiratory systems, many of them cannot use their respiratory systems with sufficient force to overcome the leakage of air from the oral cavity through the velopharyngeal port. As a consequence, they frequently have severe difficulties in producing consonants that require generation of relatively high magnitudes of intraoral air pressures. That is so even though speakers with cleft palates usually are considered to have normally mobile tongue function in addition to normal respiratory systems. For cerebral palsied speakers who have combinations of restricted mobility of tongue, lip, and jaw function and velopharyngeal incompetence, their ability to use the respiratory system to compensate for inefficient valves of the speech airstream is also usually compounded by restricted function of their respiratory musculatures.

In order to complete the perspective of the speech-producing mechanism as an aerodynamic-mechanical system, it is necessary to consider the case where there is normal mobility of the laryngeal and articulatory structures in the presence of restricted function of the respiratory musculatures. There is substantial evidence to support the contention that normal speech production, at conversational levels of vocal intensity, minimally taxes the potential of the respiratory system as an aerodynamic power source. That is, the normal respiratory system possesses the potential to generate within the vocal tract air pressures that greatly exceed requirements for driving that tract. Moreover, the physiologically normal respiratory system can generate the needed pressures throughout most lung volume levels.

The literature that has dealt with the contribution of respiratory function problems to the speech-production deficits of the cerebral palsied population tends to imply that such problems may be a sole physiological basis of a speech-production deficit. Such implications may seem reasonable in view of the various behaviors of selected cerebral palsied speakers as they attempt to make themselves understood. Some seem to exert extreme physical effort near the end of phrases as if they are "running out of air." They may be able to produce no more than a few syllables on one expiration. There may be notable inspirations between each short utterance and other behaviors suggestive of significant difficulty in using the respiratory system for speech generation.

In contrast, various diseases and injuries have left many persons with significant dysfunction of their respiratory musculatures, but they can produce speech quite normally for conversational purposes. More important for the present purposes, there are numerous normally speaking individuals with cerebral palsy who have neuromotor involvement of their respiratory musculatures. As will be reviewed in Chapter Six, there will be no involvement of laryngeal and articulatory muscle groups of paraplegic persons, and some diplegic individuals also have normally functioning laryngeal and articulatory mechanisms. Such individuals typically have normal speech production skills at conversational levels of intensity, but the nature of their respiratory dysfunction is comparable to that of cerebral palsied dysarthric speakers whose respiratory function problems appear to contribute to the speech-production difficulty.

Therefore, it seems reasonable to assume that respiratory dysfunction resulting from a developmental neuromotor disorder will contribute to a clinically significant speech production problem only in the presence of restricted mobility of laryngeal and articulatory musculatures. That is, the inefficient valving of the speech airstream that results from that restricted mobility and the associated increase in demand for respiratory function for driving the vocal tract will exceed the capability of the involved respiratory musculatures. In the presence of normal articulatory and laryngeal function, however, a respiratory function problem is unlikely to lead to a clinically significant speech problem.

The earlier discussion of neuromotor nets associated with speech production suggested exercising caution in assuming that relatively specific irregularities of motor patterns of oral, laryngeal, and respiratory function of speakers with cerebral palsy could be used with confidence to identify significant speech physiology deficits. The potential effects of dysfunction of one muscle group of the speech-producing mechanism on the aerodynamic requirements of the total speech system also supports the notion that limited information regarding the significance of a specific speech physiology deviation can be obtained by observing the function of isolated speech-producing structures. Therefore, the most desirable approach to assessment and management of dysarthria associated with cerebral palsy would appear to be through integration of the results of a number of observations that provide a general overview of the operation of the entire speech-producing mechanism. Otherwise, the significant problems of the interdynamics of the various structures and muscle groups may be overlooked or inappropriate conclusions may be drawn regarding the effects of isolated physiological problems.

O FUNCTIONAL OVERLAY AND PHYSIOLOGICAL LIMITS

It should not be assumed that the speech-motor behaviors presented by the speaker with cerebral palsy represent the direct manifestation of the neuromotor disorder nor the current physiological limits of his or her speech-producing musculatures. Such an individual will be attempting to learn, or will have learned, to produce speech not only in the presence of those limits, but with musculatures that do not have normal mobility. This situation usually leads to numerous inappropriate or deleterious speech-producing behaviors.

Identifying and modifying such behaviors are likely to be the more productive of the efforts to assist children with cerebral palsy in improving their speech production skills. That is, it may be much easier to change these motor behaviors than to extend the current limits of the system. For example, because of hypertonicity of the lower lip, a slight overbite, and some restricted mobility of the jaw, a speaker with cerebral palsy may have learned to produce lingua-dental approximations for bilabial consonants; yet, when instructed to do so, that speaker may be able to produce bilabial consonants with relative ease. For another example, the discussion to follow will point out that the manner in which many individuals with cerebral palsy have come to use their involved respiratory systems for speech production is inappropriate for the requirements of their speech-producing mechanism; moreover, it may be within their immediate capability to modify the use to improve their speech. It may take substantial work to incorporate such readily possible changes into habitual speaking behavior, but there may be early evidence that such a goal is realistic.

Some deleterious speech behaviors may be found that seem to be present due to the interaction of muscle groups of the involved speech-producing system. For example, as will be reviewed in detail later, habitually producing voiced for voiceless consonants may be the result of the individual's having adopted that behavior in order to valve the speech airstream more efficiently. Yet, when that individual produces speech samples that are, and in ways that are, minimally taxing to the respiratory system while making desirable changes in use of the respiratory system, he or she may use voiceless consonants with little or no difficulty.

I tend to refer to deleterious speech-producing behaviors that are readily within the capability of the dysarthric speaker to modify as components of *functional overlay* to the dysarthria. The term is a misnomer since it implies, within the vernacular of the profession of speech-language pathology, that these behaviors have no anatomical or physiological problems as their bases. Obviously, as defined, they have usually come to be used because of such problems.

The following discussions will review a number of these components of functional overlay that seem to represent (1) the most easily achieved approximations of the desired motor behaviors, (2) attempts to compensate for the presence of restricted or limited function of the speech musculatures, and (3) mislearning of motor patterns that may have been precipitated because of such restrictions and limits. In contrast, there will be mentioned numerous other examples of such behaviors that the person seems unable to modify irrespective of how he or she attempts to do so.

A principal goal of the assessment process is to determine the extent to which functional overlay is present and the circumstances in which it can be modified most easily. Although the speaker may not be able to incorporate such modifications into his or her habitual speaking behavior, the presence of these functional components indicates a favorable prognosis for those aspects of the deviant speech signal they produce.

A more negative prognosis is indicated for those deviant aspects of the speech signal that are manifestations of limits of the function of the speech musculatures. It may be unrealistic to anticipate that such behaviors can be changed.

A conclusion that a given speech musculature is being used to its limits should not be drawn too quickly. As some of the functional components of the problem are diminished, a greater capability for function of the remainder of the speech musculatures may become apparent. As a consequence, the assessment process must be continuous throughout the management program, and the therapeutic activities must be changed as a result of revised impressions.

○ REFLEX BEHAVIORS AND POSTURAL REACTIONS

Early impressions also may need revision if there are positive results from management of reflex behaviors and postural reactions. The discussions in Chapters Two and Four reviewed an evolution of thinking relative to manifestations of the uninhibited or exaggerated reflexes and reactions present in a number of individuals with cerebral palsy. The discussion of the so-called systems of treatment in Chapter Two briefly reviewed a few of the approaches to management of cerebral palsy that were based on that evolution of ideas, and some of the difficulties with those systems of treatment were pointed out. Later material suggested that there is currently more general acceptance of management programs that are contemporary outgrowths of that era. It follows that characteristics of the speech production problem as initially seen will change in cases where management programs successfully reduce the influence of these reflex behaviors and postural reactions on the speech physiology mechanism. Speech-language pathologists may wish to obtain special training in current approaches to this type of management, particularly if they work with infants and very young children who have cerebral palsy.

It would be unfortunate if the special training, the literature emphasizing this approach to management of cerebral palsy, or contact with professional people who strongly advocate such approaches were to lead the speech-language pathologist to deemphasize the understanding in management of aberrations of speech physiology as seen in individuals with cerebral palsy. An understanding of these reflex behaviors and postural reactions should be used as a tool in the assessment and management of the speech problems of this population in a manner comparable to the way information from the profession of psychology is used to understand the effects of intellectual and personality characteristics in assessing and managing the types of communication problems.

Speech-language pathologists should not independently design and carry out programs of management of general neuromuscular-skeletal dysfunction. Physical therapists and occupational therapists should have primary roles in such programs.

Despite more general acceptance of this type of approach to management of cerebral palsy, there continues to be a lack of common agreement in that regard and objective evidence as to the effectiveness of such programs. Some of these orientations have not stood the test of time. Others remain as viable orientations in the minds of some individuals.

Whether the orientation toward management calls for the use of therapy techniques to inhibit abnormal reflex behaviors, use of braces to maintain appropriate alignment of the lower extremities, or combinations of these and other approaches to neuromuscular-skeletal management, the principals of assessment and management of the speech physiology deficit will be comparable. The realistic goal of such programs is reduction of the influence of reflex behaviors and postural reactions.

More attention will be given to management of these behaviors and reactions in the discussion of the very young child with cerebral palsy in

Chapter Nine. Even for infants and very young children, however, it is unrealistic to anticipate that in many cases the influence of these abnormal neuromotor behaviors will be eliminated by such management regimen. Again, the realistic goal will be reduction of that influence.

○ POSITIONING

The earlier discussions of postural reactions in cerebral palsy have used the behavior known as an extensor thrust as an extreme example. However, abnormal postural reactions in this population may take the form of increases in the severity and distribution of the type of the neuromotor disorder that usually dominates the individual's motor dysfunction. For example, a young spastic diplegic child, or a child with dyskinesia, may show considerable movement capability of the upper extremities and a dysarthria of relatively mild severity when he or she is sitting in a chair designed to provide optimum support of the legs, back, and head. If that same child, however, is lifted from the chair by an adult who holds the child under the armpits so that the head is not supported and the extremities swing freely, the child may show an immediate increase in generalized hypertonia. The legs may extend and assume a scissorlike position, the torso may stiffen, the arms may flex, and there may be signs of generalized muscle contraction throughout the neck, oral, and facial musculatures. Moreover, this generalized increase in hypertonia may persist, with its dramatic adverse effects on functioning, as long as the child is held in the posture described. Milder reactions to posture and increases in both hypertonia and involuntary motion may be seen when cerebral palsied individuals are sitting in conventional chairs or wheelchairs.

There is an element to management programs for cerebral palsy that is designed to reduce these manifestations and that now has considerable general acceptance. It is usually referred to as positioning. Positioning procedures are not comparable to the various paradigms of management of reflex behaviors and postural reactions that have been previously discussed. For example, they do not incorporate any teaching of new movement patterns. Positioning is related to such systems of management only in that it is designed to provide the individual with spatial security while being in a position that promotes optimum functioning with the limits of his or her physical capability. The procedures consist of use of a wide variety of devices in which the individual with cerebral palsy may lie, sit, or stand. A number of such devices are available commercially, but many interdisciplinary teams who recommend use of these devices believe that they must be tailor-made for each individual. Some of the commercially available devices are designed to permit a range of adjustments. Even so, there is a frequent belief that such adjustments do not meet the precise needs of many individuals. As a consequence, positioning devices may be constructed according to precise specifications, and modifications may be made on a trial-and-error basis as they are used.

A frequent positioning device is modification of a wheelchair, usually constructed with plywood and some type of foam pads. More recently, a variety of plastic materials that can be molded into the desired configurations are being used. Either such pads or the molded plastics are usually covered with some type of washable upholstery material. The positioning device is constructed so as to provide maximum support, with the back and seat contoured specifically for the individual. Wedges may be mounted to a high back so that the individual's head is held in a normal, upright position; a removable wedge may be attached to the seat to maintain the thighs in a slightly spread position; and the lower legs and feet may be positioned in contoured cushions mounted to a foot board. Straps or vests may be added to hold the individual's torso or limbs where indicated, as, for example, when there is a tendency for an extensor thrust to occur.

The goals for such positioning usually extend beyond providing the individual with a sense of optimum security and placing him or her in a position that diminishes reflexlike behaviors. The individual usually is positioned in a posture that is optimally conducive for eating and other activities that require the use of the upper extremities. Special lap boards may be constructed to assist with such activities, including schoolwork. The need to avoid muscular-skeletal deformities also is taken into consideration.

The variety of devices that may be constructed range from wheelchair adaptations to standing tables, chairs, and infant seats. The design of these devices requires input by physical therapists, occupational therapists, and, on occasions where health management is of concern, medical personnel. The speech-language pathologist should actively participate to determine the effects of the positioning on the individual's speech production capability, and input is particularly needed when a system of nonoral communication is appropriate, as will be discussed in Chapter Ten.

○ ASSESSMENT AND MANAGEMENT AS A FUNCTION OF AGE

There seems to be a wide-spread belief that professional attention should be given to the needs of the child with cerebral palsy at the earliest possible age in order to begin assessment and to assist parents to cope with their situation. Not only does that belief seem to be accepted today, but it may be that abnormal neuromotor behaviors of cerebral palsy are most subject to change at a very early age. It would appear, then, that management programs should begin as soon as the diagnosis of cerebral palsy is made.

In addition, an overview of current beliefs and practices concerning management of communication disorders associated with cerebral palsy suggests that very general goals are appropriate for different age groups of those with cerebral palsy, an associated developmental dysarthria, and the capability of developing intelligible oral communication. From infancy through the very young years, concentration should be on (1) those general aspects of the neuromotor disorder that seem subject to modification and (2) motivating the child to use and develop speech-production skills within the limits of his or her speech-producing mechanism. A prime goal through the elementary school years usually will be to concentrate on relatively specific changes in speech-producing behaviors that contribute optimally to intelligibility. Programs during adolescence and throughout adulthood may be devoted primarily to maintenance of the speech-production skills that have been developed.

It should not be inferred that these programs should involve working only on articulation skills. Rather, the emphasis should be on optimal development and use of speech-producing skills, taking into account function of the entirety of the speech-producing system. Even though the emphasis here is on the speech physiology problems of this population, these programs must also include the broad range of psychological and sociological variables that influence children's development of communication. Within these general frames of reference, a few specific concepts related to management as a function of the client's age are offered.

Hixon and Hardy (1964) suggested that their findings indicated the desirability of motivating the child with cerebral palsy to produce speech at the earliest age possible. The rationale was that early speech production would facilitate the organization of the neuromotor systems for speech generation. The implication was not intended that normal neuromotor function for speech production can be achieved in the presence of a lesion of the neuromotor systems. The suggestion is in line, however, with current thinking that establishing more normal motor patterns is most possible at very early ages.

As has been mentioned, there seems to be increasing support for the belief that modification of some undesirable neuromotor behaviors is best accomplished at very early ages. Also, it cannot be denied that the sooner the child with cerebral palsy can be motivated to begin producing speech, the sooner his or her efforts can be evaluated and modified. To the extent that the organization of the neuromotor systems can be influenced by such early learning, motivating the cerebral palsied infant and very young child to engage in as much speech-producing activity as possible should do more to facilitate the eventual optimal use of the child's speech-producing musculatures than professional attention during later years.

As will be discussed in Chapter Nine, working with the cerebral palsied infant and very young child can be very demanding. In view of some of the specific behaviors that need to be evaluated and modified, many cerebral palsied children, even through the early elementary years, will have limited ability to understand and concentrate on the desired activities. Any reward system that is used to shape the behaviors deemed desirable will have to be applied very consistently.

Therapeutic activities that involve "playing games" or "fun" learning paradigms that are appropriate for relatively young children are relatively easy to design and carry out without strongly emphasizing the specific goals to be achieved by those programs. Children with developmental dysarthria, however, should understand, within the limits of their maturity, what is to be gained from the therapeutic activities. Activities can be designed so that they are highly motivating, and much may be accomplished in therapeutic sessions. However, those accomplishments are likely to be for naught if a ten-year-old cerebral palsied child does not understand, for example, the reason for maintaining a slow speech rate at all times. Optimum progress will depend on the consistent use of the best speech-producing behaviors possible for the speaker, and an intellectual understanding of the problem should assist the speaker in maintaining that consistency.

Finally, I have formed a strong impression that the longer the deviant neuromotor patterns that constitute developmental dysarthria persist, the more difficult they will be to change. As a result, the prognosis for improving the dysarthria of an adult with cerebral palsy may be much poorer than for improving that of a child with a comparable pattern of speech physiology problems. To the extent that these impressions are valid, early, consistent, and prolonged professional attention is needed if many speakers with developmental dysarthria are to develop and maintain optimal speech-producing skills.

○ INTERDISCIPLINARY ASSESSMENT AND MANAGEMENT

A number of comments have been made regarding the need for appropriate interaction among the personnel from the various professions that deal with the problems associated with cerebral palsy. In particular, the discussion to come of associated disabilities, disorders, and problems in Chapter Eight should reinforce the necessity of such interaction. As already indicated, that interaction must involve more than simply sharing reports and recommendations. Ideally, it should include a mutual sharing of impressions relative to assessment findings, planning for management, and understanding of each profession's orientation toward the problem.

The administrative structure of some programs permits the professional persons of the habilitation team to work in the same facility and, perhaps, to perform evaluations and conduct the management programs simultaneously as a common staff. This is an ideal situation. However, there must still be a mutual respect among the professional persons. The skills and knowledges of each profession suffer from limitations. Open sharing of these limitations with a critical evaluation of all assumptions and conclusions will enhance the possibility that the most relevant clinical problems will be identified and that the most appropriate management program will be designed.

For work settings in which frequent interprofessional contact is not possible, such mutual sharing of impressions and planning may be more difficult. Yet, it is imperative that attempts be made to accomplish the needed interactions.

The speech-language pathologist should be able to depend on workers from other professions to provide information and impressions that are crucial to interpretation of the assessment and to planning the management program for the communication problems of a child with cerebral palsy. In some instances the information and impressions may seem to be erroneous, and the degree of mutual interprofessional respect may be tested as a result. Nevertheless, open and frank resolutions of the issues should be attempted. If program planning is at issue, an arbitrator with the professional knowledge to make judgments regarding the issue probably should be consulted.

Great care should be taken in the manner with which clients and their parents should be made aware of any interdisciplinary issues. No greater disservice can be given than to undermine their confidence in another professional person who also is providing services. That is particularly so when there are no other alternatives available. The speech-language pathologist should maintain the same professional ethics in interacting with those in other professions as he or she does with other speech-language pathologists.

SUMMARY

There are a number of general considerations that apply to both assessment and management of the speech production problems of persons with cerebral palsy. Above all, objectivity must be maintained throughout the entire clinical process.

The reality of the neuromotor problem suggests an orientation of assisting the speaker with cerebral palsy who has neuromotor involvement of the speech-producing musculatures to produce the best speech possible within the physiological limits of his or her speech mechanism. There may be some instances in which those limits may be extended, but is unrealistic to expect great gains in that regard for most cases.

Concentration should be upon activity of the speech-producing musculatures for speech production. To assume that activity of these musculatures during non-speech-producing acts represents neuromotor activity comparable for speech production overlooks the neuromotor systems' unique organization for the speech-production process. Observation of the speech-producing structures during nonspeech-producing activities may give an indication of the presence of neuromotor involvement, but it should not be assumed that the degree of restricted mobility that is observed is comparable to that during speech-production. Similarly, use of nonspeech-producing activities as a part of the management process also overlooks the fact that the neuromotor organization for speech production is not only unique to that process, but that organization involves synchronous innervation of the speech-producing musculatures, including those associated with not only articulation but also with respiration and phonation.

The major clinically significant aspects of the dysarthric program can be viewed as a disruption of the components of the speech-producing system as an aerodynamic-mechanical sound generator. That perspective facilitates understanding and analysis of how restricted mobility of specific speech-producing musculatures and structures interact with the other musculatures and structures of the system. Moreover, that perspective recognizes that function of the speech-producing system must be considered in the assessment and management process.

Since speakers with developmental dysarthria attempt to learn speech-production skills in the presence of physiological problems, they tend to develop deleterious speech-producing behaviors that are not due to the physiological limits of their speech-producing mechanism. These behaviors may be relatively easy to modify in the management program, and that improvement may result in substantial improvement in their speech. Those inappropriate speech-producing behaviors that are imposed by the neuromotor disorder are likely to be more difficult to modify.

Attention to the abnormal reflex behaviors and postural reactions that are frequently a part of the cerebral palsied problem deserve attention in the programs of the speech-language pathologist. Indeed, if programs that are designed on the basis of management of those behaviors and reactions are successful in improving the speech-producing capability of a child with cerebral palsy, initial impressions relative to that child's prognosis may have to be revised. However, the speech-language pathologist should not devote his or her attention to management of these behaviors and reactions to the exclusion of a thorough analysis of and concentration on the speech-physiology problem.

The need to provide postural support devices is becoming increasingly recognized as a needed part of the management of a number of persons with cerebral palsy. Such positioning devices provide postural security and reduce the negative influence of postural reactions upon function. They should be designed so as to place the individual in optimal functional positions. The contribution of the speech-language pathologist to both the assessment and management of the cerebral palsied problem should take into account the need for and the potential benefits to be derived from such positioning.

It now seems possible to outline general goals for the clinical process with speakers who have developmental dysarthria that vary as a function of those speakers' ages. Finally, in order to bring results of any aspect of the assessment and management process to an optimum conclusion, interdisciplinary efforts of the highest quality and professional integrity are required.

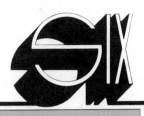

SIX

Assessment of developmental dysarthria: The general case

Procedures will be described in detail for assessment of speech physiology aberrations and the speech-production problems created by those aberrations associated with developmental dysarthria. No single aspect of the management process of these speech-production problems is more important than that assessment. The findings will not only serve as a guide to planning management goals, but they will point to relatively specific therapeutic activities that may most efficiently lead to achieving those goals.

The general case to which these assessment procedures are applicable are speakers with developmental dysarthria who have the intellectual capability and maturity to cooperate in the assessment process. The presence of any of the associated disabilities, disorders, and problems that are described in Chapter Nine may necessitate modifications of the procedures to be used and the impressions that will be formed.

○ INVOLVEMENT OF THE SPEECH-PRODUCING MUSCULATURES

The literature routinely reviews the characteristics of neuromotor disorders in cerebral palsy as they are seen in the limbs, and these manifestations, in general, form the basis of differential diagnoses. There are limits, however, to which generalizations made from these characteristics in the extremities apply to those in the speech-producing musculatures. Therefore, a discussion of the manner in which developmental neuromotor disorders are manifest throughout the speech-producing musculatures of persons with cerebral palsy will be helpful. It is possible to predict to general cases that will encompass the bulk of the cerebral palsied population by considering these manifestations within each of the two major subtypes of cerebral palsy, spasticity and dyskinesia.

These discussions, by necessity, cannot review many subtle variations of the neuromotor involvement of the speech-producing musculatures. However, the more frequently seen significant exceptions to those usual expectations that do have significance to the speech-language pathologist will be summarized.

spasticity

The severity of involvement among the articulatory masculatures within one person who predominantly has spasticity may vary substantially. For example, the velopharyngeal port may not narrow appreciably, much less close, during an individual's attempts to produce speech. In that same individual, tongue function during speech production may appear to be relatively better. At one time, I considered the possibility that these variations in function of the oral structures could be explained on the basis of differing degrees of abnormal neural input into the final common pathway pools of selected cranial efferent nerves. However, that consideration was not productive.

The extent to which muscle spindles (stretch receptors) exist throughout all of the speech-producing musculatures is uncertain at this time. They have been demonstrated to be present in certain muscle groups associated with respiration, the tongue, and the larynx. The fact that some physicians rely on an abnormally hyperactive jaw jerk reflex as a manifestation of spasticity indicates hyperreflexia of jaw musculatures may be present in cases of spasticity. As mentioned, the gag reflex of cerebral-palsied persons with spasticity frequently can be described as hyperactive. Therefore, it probably is reasonable to assume that the concept of hyperreflexia can be generalized to a number of muscle groups innervated by the cranial efferent nerves, and, to the extent that this is so, it must be assumed that increased hypertonia results from rapid and extensive movement of the oral structures.

The distribution of spasticity will be discussed within the context of the conventional labels of monoplegia, hemiplegia, paraplegia, triplegia, diplegia, and quadriplegia (or tetraplegia). The artificiality of these classifications was introduced in Chapter Two and addressed in Chapter Four. That is, for one example, diplegia can be conceptualized as a more severe form of paraplegia in which there has been a more extensive spread of the lesion throughout the pyramidal system. Nevertheless, these classifications have come to have considerable meaning clinically, and they may be used to predict generally the distribution of the neuromotor impairment throughout the speech-producing musculatures.

Spastic Hemiplegia and Monoplegia. Even though it is not typical of the group, some children who are given the diagnosis of cerebral palsy of the spastic hemiplegic type may manifest a dysarthria. There may be a number of reasons for these cases. The diagnosis may be inappropriate, and the child, in fact, may manifest demonstrable bilateral neuromotor involvement. Damage to the individual's central nervous system may have occurred substantially after the time of birth, and as a consequence, the case may not be representative of the typical patterns of developmental neuromotor problems. On the other hand, such a case may be one of the infrequently seen variations in the usual distribution of involvement associated with developmental spastic hemiplegia.

However, members of this group frequently have developmental communication problems. Most of these appear to be problems in learning to produce the speech signal. The prevalence of somesthesia in the spastic hemiplegic group may contribute to these speech-learning problems, as discussed in Chapter Eight. Mental retardation, which also is prevalent in this subgroup, may contribute.

The speech-language pathologist is even less likely to encounter a case of spastic monoplegia with dysarthria. The probability is very low that damage could be sustained to the developing pyramidal motor system so as to affect mobility of the musculatures of one foot, one leg, and the speech-producing musculatures and leave the other muscle groups spared.

Nevertheless, the speech-language pathologist may receive referrals from other professional persons implying that the communication problems of spastic hemiplegic and monoplegic children have dysarthria as their bases. In fact, parents may have been told that the developmental speech problem of their hemiplegic or monoplegic child is due to their child's having "cerebral palsy." The introductory comments in the preceding chapter mentioned that variables leading to communication deficits in children who do not have neuromotor disorders may impact on the development of the communication skills of children who do have such disorders, and a number of the cases, particularly those with monoplegia, exemplify that point.

Spastic Paraplegia. Again as reviewed in earlier discussions, the distribution of spasticity in paraplegic cases by definition involves primarily the musculatures of the lower extremities. In many cases, the involvement may extend into the torso wall musculatures, but a criterion for this classification is that the function of the upper extremities is unaffected.

To the extent that torso wall muscles are involved, there will be dysfunction of certain expiratory acts, since the abdominal wall muscles serve an expiratory function. If the restriction of muscle function extends into the thoracic wall muscles, expiratory function may be further affected and inspiratory function may also be reduced. This is so since the internal intercostal muscles act to reduce the dimensions of the thoracic cage and thereby contribute to expiratory effort, and the external intercostal muscles act to elevate and expand the thoracic cage for inspiratory efforts.

For the reasons given in the preceding chapter, these patterns of respiratory dysfunction in the spastic paraplegic cerebral palsied group should not be expected to result in significant problems of speech production. Even those whose pattern of involvement extends into the thoracic wall musculatures are not likely to have a dysarthria. They may have difficulty in using loud vocal intensities, and they may have some problems playing wind musical instruments well. However, in the absence of involvement of the articulatory and/or laryngeal musculatures, this group can be expected to develop communication skills normally if mental retardation, hearing impairment, or other contributing factors to a communication problem are not present.

Spastic Diplegia (and Triplegia). Spastic diplegia implies neuromotor involvement of musculatures of all four extremities, but of lesser severity in the upper than the lower extremities, and it can be expected that the entirety of the torso wall musculatures will be involved to some extent. Since the neuromotor involvement of the upper-body wall muscles usually will be less severe than those of the lower torso wall, this group will show the same relative deficits of inspiratory and expiratory function as the more severe and extensive cases of paraplegia. The extent of those deficits, however, should be relatively more severe.

There will be considerable variation, however, with respect to involvement of musculatures of the oral structures within the spastic diplegic group. For a few, the nueromotor disorder seems nonexistent, literally, from above the level of the shoulders. In this subgroup, as with cases of more extensive distribution of involvement with spastic paraplegia, dysarthria may not be present. Such individuals may show, in fact, gross impairment of arm and hand function, yet there may be little or no dysfunction of their neck musculatures, and restriction of the mobility of their oral structures cannot be detected. These children may develop normal speech-production skills for conversational levels of vocal intensity, especially if there are no other developmental disabilities or other factors that would contribute to development of a communication problem.

Others of the spastic diplegic group may show no restricted function of the oral structures, and they may develop good articulatory skills. Yet, they have pronounced dysprosody. There may be a tendency to attribute that speaking behavior to restricted function of the intrinsic laryngeal muscles. For reasons to be explained shortly, this seems to be unlikely. Reduced flexibility of laryngeal function due to hypertonicity of the neck musculatures in combination with the expected problems of respiratory flexibility may be an explanation.

For the diplegic group whose neuromotor involvement extends into the oral structures, a developmental dysarthria can, naturally enough, be expected. By definition, the involvement will be relatively less severe than that of the lower extremities. However, the resulting developmental dysarthria will not necessarily be mild. The involvement of oral musculatures may be fairly severe, but even in cases where the restricted mobility of the articulatory structures appears relatively mild, the resulting reduction and efficiency of utilization of the speech airstream may cause a relatively severe speech-production problem because of the reduced respiratory function typical of spastic diplegia.

I have been impressed by there being relatively few spastic diplegic persons who appear to have significant dysfunction of the intrinsic laryngeal musculatures. To the extent that the commonly held view regarding correspondence between distribution of spasticity in cerebral palsy and arrangement of the pyramidal system is valid, and that pattern is characterized by diminution of severity of damage to the pyramidal system from those neurons that influence activity of the lower extremity muscles up through the laryngeal musculatures, it would be predicted that intrinsic laryngeal muscles would be the least involved of all musculatures.

Numerous spastic diplegic individuals who have dysarthria, however, manifest speech behaviors suggestive of laryngeal dysfunction. They may, for example, tend to use voiced consonants for voiceless cognates. However, as has been stated and as will be explained later, this behavior may be due to problems other than laryngeal adduction and abduction. Reduced stress contrasts and intonation patterns also are typical. These characteristics also may not be due to dysfunction of intrinsic laryngeal musculatures in the great majority of cases. The following discussion on laryngeal function will point out that the combined attributes of stress and intonation patterns depend on more than intrinsic laryngeal muscle function. Also, involvement of the extrinsic neck musculatures may have a deleterious effect on intrinsic laryngeal activity through restriction of movements of the laryngeal cartilaginous complex. Therefore, there are a number of alternatives to the belief that these deviant speech characteristics are due to neuromotor involvement of the intrinsic laryngeal musculature.

The material in Chapter Four pointed out that triplegia probably represents a form of diplegia in which the damage to the pyramidal system has been more extensive on one side than the other. My experience suggests that dysarthria is not routinely seen in this group.

Spastic Quadriplegia (or Tetraplegia). Either quadriplegia or tetraplegia is used in reference to those with cerebral palsy who have equal degrees of spasticity in all four extremities. Both terms mean involvement of all four limbs, but quadriplegia now seems to be more commonly used. The neuromotor disorder is often quite severe, which suggests a relatively complete lesion over the bulk of the pyramidal fibers bilaterally. This possibility seems very likely in most of these cases, since they frequently have comparably significant involvement of the muscles of the oral cavity, and their speech-producing behaviors are also suggestive of notable laryngeal dysfunction.

Some cases of spastic quadriplegia, however, may have relatively milder involvement of their oral musculatures than of their extremities. Such a distribution suggests a less complete problem of the corticobulbar fibers. As can be appreciated, however, it is difficult to judge with confidence that the involvement of the upper extremities is exactly comparable to that of the lower extremities. Therefore, a number of cerebral palsied individuals who are labeled quadriplegic may in fact have a severe diplegia. Hence, the pattern of lesser involvement to those musculatures that are provided innervation by the corticobulbar system would be anticipated.

dyskinesia

As reviewed earlier, the form of involuntary movements that constitute dyskinesia may vary considerably in rate and character, but the form most usually seen is that of slow, writhing movements that have classically been called athetosis. Such involuntary motions sometimes can be observed in the lower facial muscles and tongue. The undulating movements characteristic of the extremities, however, can usually be seen in the lower facial muscles and tongue only when they are at rest or during nonspeech movements. For example, the tongue may show the slow, writhing movements of athetosis when it appears to be resting as the mouth is held open, and such movements may become exaggerated during attempts to protrude the tongue. However, during speech production, the same individual's tongue may move in a consistent pattern as one mass with little or no independent flexibility of the tongue tip from its body.

The most usual manifestations of facial and oral musculature involvement in dyskinesia during speech production are (1) a tendency toward overly extensive movement in selected instances and/or (2) generally restricted movement. As an example of the former, the dyskinetic individual's jaw may open abnormally wide when he or she starts to speak. Lack of involuntary movements in the speech-producing musculatures are exemplified also by behaviors of the jaw; that is, involuntary opening and closing movements are not typically seen.

Neither are involuntary movements typical in respiratory maneuvers. If the dyskinetic person is sitting or lying securely, and there are no involuntary motions present in the extremities, particularly the upper extremities, that person routinely will perform inspiratory and expiratory efforts in a smooth, uninterrupted manner. If notable involuntary movements of the upper extremities occur during those efforts, however, momentary accelerations or decelerations of the respiratory airstream may be observed, evidently resulting from impingement of these movements on the thoracic structure. The prime manifestation of the respiratory dysfunction associated with dyskinesia is restriction of function.

The tendency for (1) articulatory gestures to be characterized by relatively inflexible, stereotyped movement patterns and (2) respiratory maneuvers to be characterized by restricted function suggests that a form of hypertonia is present in those musculatures. However, it is of minimal import to the speech-language pathologist to know why these differences exist in manifestations of dyskinesia in the musculatures of the oral and respiratory musculatures. To anticipate that such differences exist, however, is important. Also, since the manifestations of dyskinesia typically seem to be restricted mobility in the speech-producing musculatures, there will not be dramatic differences in the movement patterns of the musculatures between dyskinetic persons who show signs of the tension disorder and those who do not.

Fluctuations in Severity. Earlier discussions pointed out that the severity of the neuromotor disorders associated with dyskinesia frequently fluctuate as a function of the affective state of the individual. Although the extent of involuntary motions in the limbs can be clearly seen to increase as a result of such individuals' becoming excited, the effect of such an increase in severity on their speech-producing musculatures usually is more extensive immobility. A boy with dyskinesia who is using a typewriter to complete a spelling assignment may show a dramatic increase in the interference of intended typing movements by relatively violent involuntary motions of his arm when he suddenly seems to remember how to spell a difficult word; if the child is responding to the spelling test orally, his seemingly sudden recollection of how to spell the word may result in a generalized increase in the overall severity of his dysarthria with a resulting deterioration of speaking ability. The young woman whose situation was described at the end of Chapter Four and who had relatively mild dyskinesia with a relatively selective problem of speech production when talking on the telephone also exemplifies this general reduction in the speech physiology capability of many dyskinetic individuals under conditions of stress.

Topographical Distribution. It is usually assumed that dyskinetic involvement is generalized over all muscle groups. During the era of accelerated interest in conditions of cerebral palsy when dyskinesia was routinely referred to as athetosis, this assumption was characterized by the frequent statement, "a severe athetoid is a severe athetoid." As the statement implied, some degree of dysarthria can be expected as a result of involvement of articulatory and respiratory musculatures. As in individuals with spastic diplegia, however, function of intrinsic laryngeal musculatures seems to be reasonably good in many individuals with dyskinesia.

As was mentioned in some of the earlier material, however, a number of persons with dyskinesia show relatively more severe involvement of the upper extremities, including thoracic wall musculatures and facial and oral musculatures, than they do in their lower extremities. In Chapter Four this pattern of involvement was offered as an explanation to what has been referred to as "the reversed breathing patterns" of some dyskinetic individuals. That is, they seem to compensate for the relatively re-stricted mobility of the thoracic cage by extensive movement of the diaphragm; as a result the abdomen expands extensively on inspiration while the circumference of the thorax remains unchanged. Indeed, in some cases this characteristic seems to be so extensive that the thorax ap-pears to contract on inspiration. On expiration, the abdomen contracts, driving the diaphragm into the thoracic cavity, and the thorax may seem to expand during expiration as a result. This extensive, compensatory use of the diaphragm also may lead to a structural characteristic of the thorac-ic cage that at one time drew much attention to selected dyskinetic chil-dren, namely a "flaring" of the lower rib cage. Rather than the usual tapering of the lower thoracic cage, the lower ribs in such cases seemed actually to flare, or bulge, outward from the configuration of the upper ribs. Again, these characteristics of the so-called reverse breathing pattern are probably insignificant in and of themselves to a speech-breathing physiology problem; rather, they should be considered significant only to the extent that they reflect a respiratory function problem in combination with reduced efficiency of other speech-producing structures.

The difference between the severity of dyskinetic involvement in upper musculatures as compared to lower muscle groups can be quite dramatic. A few cases of dyskinesia may be observed in which the involvement of the oral musculatures is extremely severe; yet there may be very mild in-volvement of all four extremities.

As with spasticity, and despite the usual assumption of generalized in-volvement associated with dyskinesia, the severity of involvement of se-lected speech musculatures may show considerable disparity within an individual. That is, the tongue may function relatively better than the lips or vice versa.

other types of neuromotor disorders

As mentioned in Chapter Four, hypotonia in cerebral palsy is seen as a generalized weakness primarily in infants, and the manifestations of the neuromotor disorder typically change to some other form with in-creasing age. At the time the hypotonia is the prevalent problem, howev-er, the reduced muscle tone, as demonstrated in the disability of limb, tor-so, and neck function, is more severe, relatively, than for the oral structures. That is, although the severely hypotonic infant may show es-sentially no movement capability of its limbs, there typically will be some movement capability of the tongue. However, there will also typically be oral function difficulties, and feeding such infants may be a significant problem. The point being made is that some capability for movement of the oral structures routinely seems present.

Despite a growing belief that ataxia is rarely seen as a true developmen-tal neuromotor disorder, an occasional child may be seen who certainly appears to be accurately diagnosed as having ataxic cerebral palsy. If the problem is ataxia, the speech gestures will not be characterized by the same patterns of uncoordinated movements as are manifest in limb movements. Rather, speech-producing gestures, again, seem impaired by restricted mobility, and they are typically imprecise and abnormally slow. Assessment procedures usually give the impression that these characteristics are generalized throughout the speech-producing system.

○ ASSESSMENT PROCEDURES

It is impossible to observe directly many of the physiological events that produce certain aspects of the speech signal. Also, there are limitations to the conclusions that can be drawn as to the physiological events that produce certain characteristics of the speech signal. Nevertheless, assessment of the speech physiology deficits of a cerebral palsied speaker must entail (1) to the extent possible, observations of the physiological events that generate speech during a wide variety of speech-producing activities,[1] (2) careful attention to the characteristics of the speech

[1]The assessment procedures described in detail in the text do not require instrumentation for observation of speech physiology events and related behaviors. Numerous uses of instrumentation will permit measurements of such events that may give more precision to the assessment. Unfortunately, needed descriptions of the use of such instrumentation as is currently available and that has practical clinical utility with the cerebral palsied population is, in general, lacking. However, a number of descriptions of the application of instrumental techniques for use with cerebral palsied speakers are available. Some of these descriptions resulted from work that assisted in formulating the approaches to assessment and management discussed in the text.

Methods for determining the partitions of the lung volume are described by Hardy (1964) and Hardy and Edmonds (1968). Procedures for obtaining the maximum expiratory pressure-producing capability of the respiratory system as a function of the lung volume are described by Hardy (1967); this reference also presents methods for using cinefluorographic films of the articulatory structures to determine patterns of velopharyngeal function. That latter procedure also may be used to observe and document patterns of jaw, tongue, and lip movements (Kent and Netsell, 1978). A method for determining the area of the velopharyngeal port during speech production by simultaneously measuring nasal airflow rates and intraoral air pressures is also given by Netsell (1969). A procedure for measuring the volumes of air expired during speech production may be found in Hardy and Arkebauer (1966). Much of the technology that may be used to study normal speech physiology (e.g., Hixon, 1972, and Hixon et al., 1976) has limited application for use with speakers who have cerebral palsy. Many of the procedures associated with this technology require physical performance in cooperating for the procedure that is not within the capability of most individuals with cerebral palsy.

Some of the instrumentation described in the literature requires equipment and technological assistance that are not available to many speech-language pathologists. Even when such equipment is available, considerable experience may be needed before it can be used with confidence with the cerebral palsied population. As emphasized in the text, such instrumentation frequently is not needed for sound clinical judgments.

signal during such activities, and (3) an integration of those observations and characteristics within a frame of reference of the available knowledge regarding the speech physiology process.

A major portion of the following discussion of assessment procedures will be organized within the topic headings of respiratory system, laryngeal system, velopharyngeal port mechanism, and lips, tongue, and jaw. This editorial organization is not meant to contradict the point of view that the interdynamics of the entire speech physiology process must be considered in assessment of dysarthria. Rather, such discussions are needed in order to review the characteristics of the speech physiology mechanism that must be taken into consideration in the use of the prime assessment tool, namely, an analysis of the speech-producing behaviors.

Another qualification in regard to the immediately following material needs emphasis. There will be numerous statements relative to the effects of the interaction of various speech-producing musculatures when differing degrees of function are present within an individual speaker with cerebral palsy. These effects, of editorial necessity, are presented in a context that suggests that they will be relatively constant within a speaker. The fluctuations in the severity of the neuromotor disorder within an individual will intermittently alter the relationships to be presented. An important example is the case in which there is relatively severe dysfunction of the respiratory musculatures compared to the articulatory and laryngeal musculatures. For many of the spastic diplegic individuals who show this pattern of neuromotor involvement, it will be stated that the respiratory dysfunction will contribute minimally to the speech production problem in the presence of the mildly involved articulatory and laryngeal musculatures. This will be true when the individuals are functioning in the absence of those intermittent increases in the severity of their neuromotor problem. However, when their musculatures become dominated by a strong postural reaction, the spread of increased muscle tone throughout the speech-producing musculatures may dramatically alter the pattern of the speech physiology aberrations. It would be impractical to repeat a description of such intermittent changes on the speech physiology problems in each of the applicable instances that follow. Therefore, it should be taken for granted that for selected speakers with cerebral palsy, intermittent changes in the severity of their neuromotor problem will alter the character of the speech physiology problems are described.

The speech-language pathologist who has experience in working with developmental dysarthria will probably select from among these extensive assessment procedures. The discussions of these procedures, the rationales for their use, and the information to be derived may serve as a review of guiding principles for assessment of developmental dysarthria rather than as a dictum for routine, necessary procedures for all cases.

The last section of this chapter that deals with speech testing provides the crucial portions of the assessment process. The procedures called for in that section should be completed initially in the assessment session. The immediately following discussion of specific aberrations of the speech producing mechanism will serve to assist in interpreting the results of those procedures.

respiratory system

As it became obvious that respiratory function problems contribute to the speech-production difficulties of cerebral palsied speakers, terms such as poor "breath support" and "breath control" for speech, began to be used. Certain characteristics of respiratory function of the population drew considerable attention. The previously described "reverse breathing pattern" of selected children with dyskinesia and the fact that many children with cerebral palsy have reduced vital capacities compared to their physiologically normal peers are examples.

However, an adequate definition of some of these terms and an explanation of how these specific characteristics contributed to a speech production problem was lacking. The research program mentioned in the preface addressed some of these issues. As the work continued, a number of the findings began to be applied to clinical work.

A review of some aspects of respiratory physiology will be helpful to understanding those applications. The reader who is not comfortably knowledgeable in that area is encouraged to refer to a comprehensive review of speech breathing physiology (e.g., Hixon, 1973). Only those aspects of normal respiratory function that are essential to the present discussion will be reviewed here.

The left side of Figure 6–1 presents one of those aspects, namely, a graphic display of the partitions of volume of the human respiratory system. That display can be understood best by imagining an individual who is breathing into an apparatus that displays the volume of air being inspired and expired on some type of paperwriter. During inspiration the writing pen moves upward, and during expiration it moves downward.

The total lung capacity (TLC) of the respiratory system is defined by the volume of gas contained within the pulmonary cavities after a maximum inspiratory effort. For purposes of measurement and identification of mechanical properties of the system, that TLC can be conceptualized as divisible into a number of subvolumes, or partitions of the lung volume. These various partitions are not mutually exclusive, and only selected partitions are shown in Figure 6–1. Most of the partitions shown are measured from the lung volume level labeled as resting respiratory level (RRL). The respiratory system is an elastic-mechanical mechanism, and the RRL is the internal volume when there are neither inspiratory forces acting to expand that internal volume nor expiratory forces operating to reduce that volume. When the internal volume is larger or smaller than

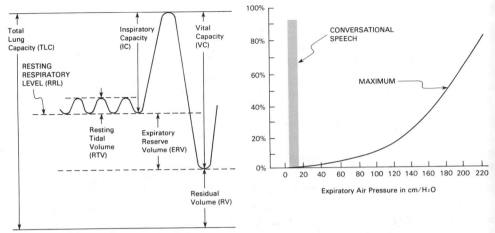

FIGURE 6–1 A graphic display of the total lung capacity (TLC) of the human respiratory system, showing the resting respiratory level (RRL), or that volume of air in the lungs when the system is at rest. The resting tidal volume (RTV) is the volume of gas exchanged during rest breathing; the inspiratory capacity (IC) is the volume of gas that can be inhaled in excess of the RRL on maximum inspiration; the expiratory reserve volume (ERV) is the volume that can be expired from the RRL; the volume of air that remains in the lungs is the residual volume (RV). The vital capacity (VC) is the gas that can be expired after the lungs are completely inflated. To the right is a graph of the maximum expiratory air pressures that might be generated by a healthy young adult male at percentage levels of his VC and the range of air pressures that would be generated in the vocal tract for conversational speech.

RRL, the elasticity of the respiratory system creates a force to return that volume to RRL.

Exchange of gas in and out of the respiratory system for rest breathing results, in general, from inspiratory muscles acting to expand the internal volume to more than RRL; then relaxation of respiratory muscles results in the elastic recoil of the system, creating expiration and returning the volume of the system to RRL. Resting tidal volume (RTV) is defined as the volume of gas exchanged during rest breathing; this volume will be dictated primarily by oxygen needs of the organism.

As can be seen in Figure 6–1, a maximum inspiratory effort from the RRL results in inhalation of a relatively large volume of air, which is referred to as the inspiratory capacity (IC). A maximum expiratory effort after a maximum inspiratory effort will result in expiration of a volume of air referred to as the vital capacity (VC). As shown, such a maximum expiratory effort results in exhalation of more air than was inhaled during the inspiratory capacity effort. That is, the internal volume of the respiratory system can be reduced from the RRL by using expiratory musculatures to exert greater force than that of the elastic recoil of the system. The amount of air that can be expired below the RRL is defined as the expiratory reserve volume (ERV). The VC, then, is the sum of the IC and ERV.

However, even when a maximal attempt is made to exhale all of the air in the lungs, there will remain a given volume of air internally. That volume, shown in Figure 6–1, is referred to as the residual volume (RV).

The right side of Figure 6–1 shows the magnitude of expiratory air pressure that can be generated by the respiratory system at different lung volume levels. That is, the pressure-volume curve labeled *maximum* gives approximate values of the air pressure that a healthy young adult male might generate at different levels of his vital capacity if he blew into a closed tube with maximum force at different levels of his vital capacity.

As can be seen, the respiratory system is capable of generating much greater expiratory air pressures at higher lung volume levels than at lower levels. At relatively high lung volume levels, the elastic recoil of the system assists in generating expiratory air pressures. That assistance is progressively less at lower levels of the IC; at lung volume levels below that of the RRL, that elastic recoil actually resists the generation of expiratory air pressures. At 0 percent of the VC, the individual cannot overcome the elastic recoil of the system with the expiratory musculature and reduce more the size of the respiratory system, even though a substantial volume of gas (RV) remains in the respiratory system.

To maintain a given magnitude of expiratory air pressure for speech production throughout the vital capacity, inspiratory and expiratory muscles must interact. At high lung volume levels, the inspiratory muscles may act to check the elastic recoil of the system so that the air pressures in the vocal tract will not be too great. At mid-lung volume levels, both the inspiratory and expiratory may act simultaneously to control those pressures. At lower levels, expiratory muscles must work not only to generate the needed air pressures, but they must also work against the system's elastic return to RRL.

The pressure volume graph also shows the range of average air pressures in the vocal tract (5 to 15 cm/H_2O) associated with speech production at conversational levels of intensity. Since the demand for intravocal tract air pressures is relatively minimal compared to the capability of the respiratory system to generate such pressures, the normal speaker can generate speech, for practical purposes, throughout the entirety of his or her vital capacity.

However, the expiratory musculature must overcome the relatively strong elastic recoil at extremely low levels of the VC, and considerable expiratory effort is required to drive the vocal tract at those low levels. If you exhaust your respiratory system to a volume level where you feel it is almost impossible to expire more air, and you then attempt to speak, you will readily perceive the effects of reaching your limit in overcoming the elastic recoil of your respiratory system. The muscular effort associated with speech generation will be extreme; you literally have to exert perceptible force with your torso muscles to drive the vocal tract; you will be inclined to inspire air so that you can drive your vocal tract more easily and extend the length of utterances; your speech will sound "strained"; there will be a reduction in stress contrasts.

These effects of trying to drive your vocal tract from lung volume levels that tax your respiratory system probably result, at least in part, from recruitment of all possible associated muscles, including those of the neck, into the effort. (As discussed in Chapter Five, such "recruitment" of associated muscle groups in acts of maximal effort is frequently seen and easily elicited in persons with cerebral palsy, and the term overflow has been used to designate motor behaviors that seem explainable on that basis.)

Measurement of air pressures in the vocal tract during speech production will show peaks, or pulses, of those pressures in association with restrictions presented to the air stream by the adductions of the vocal folds and various articulatory structures. As has been mentioned, it is unclear whether the respiratory system functions to provide such pulses of aerodynamic energy that may be associated with some unit of speech such as a syllable. There is some suggestive evidence that it does, but it is also possible that many of the peaks of air pressure within the vocal tract during the utterances result from intermittent resistances to the airstream. The most reasonable statement at this time seems to be that pulsatile contractions of respiratory muscles probably are associated with very strongly stressed units of the speech signal.

FIGURE 6–2 A graphic display of the total lung capacity (TLC) of the respiratory system with relative alterations in selected partitions of that capacity from normal that tend to be found in cerebral palsied individuals with (1) spastic paraplegia, mild spastic diplegia, and mild dyskinesia, (2) moderate spastic diplegia and dyskinesia, and (3) spastic quadriplegia, severe spastic diplegia, and severe dyskinesia.

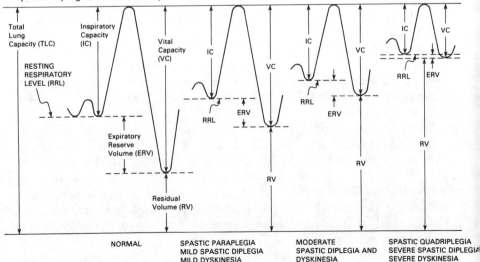

Respiratory Function Problems. Figure 6–2 shows the effects of the previously described patterns of respiratory musculature involvement on the partitions of the lung volume of individuals with cerebral palsy. Considerable variation, of course, can be expected in the patterns of the subgroups indicated.

The RTV can be varied while maintaining the same volume of gas exchange by increasing rate and decreasing the volume of each breath cycle or vice versa. The RTVs of speakers with cerebral palsy are, in general, comparable to those of physiologically normal persons of matched physical size, but their RVs tend to be greater.[2]

The reduced ability of all of the spastic subgroups to expire below their RRLs probably results, in large part, from the involvement of their abdominal wall muscles. Even mild paraplegic individuals may show some reduction in their ability to expire below RRL if their involvement extends into their abdominal wall muscles. The capability to reduce the lung volume below RRL becomes progressively less for those in which involvement of torso wall muscles extends up into the thoracic wall musculatures. This progression in reduced expiratory capability for the more extensive cases of paraplegia and diplegia probably results from dysfunction of not only the abdominal wall muscles but also the involvement of those thoracic wall muscles that also have expiratory function. In cases where all torso wall muscles are moderately to severely involved, little or no capability to expire below RRL exists.

A progressive disability to perform inspiratory efforts also is shown for the three spastic subgroups. In the case of paraplegia, the slight reduction in inspiratory capability might be explained on the basis of the diaphragm having to work against a relatively immobile abdominal mass that is being held in place by the involved abdominal walls. With the more extensive in-

[2]This statement is based on relatively few data. In order to measure the residual volume (RV) of an individual, a relatively complicated gas-mixing technique is used. The measurement, in fact, is made of a person's functional residual capacity (FRC), which is not shown in Figure 6–1. That partition of the lung volume is the sum of the expiratory reserve volume (ERV) and residual volume (RV). The individual whose FRC is being measured breathes in a closed apparatus containing known amounts of an inert gas and oxygen. The person rest breathes for the amount of time necessary to thoroughly mix the gases in the apparatus with those in the lungs. The percentage of the volume of the inert gas is then calculated, and from that calculation the person's FRC can be determined. The person's RV can then be estimated by subtracting the ERV from the calculated FRC. Rest breathing in a closed respiratory apparatus for the time necessary to complete such a gas-mixing technique is relatively difficult, and only few data of this type exist with cerebral palsied speakers. The data that do exist indicate, as shown in Figure 6–1 that the RVs of cerebral palsied individuals will be increased, compared to matched physiologically normal individuals, by the amount of reduction in their VCs. This alteration in the mechanics of the respiratory systems of cerebral palsied individuals appears to be one of those abberations of function of a mechanism that is involved in producing speech that may have little or no direct significance for the speech pathologist.

volvement up the torso wall as in the extreme case of quadriplegia, the ability of the individual to inspire becomes progressively more limited. This increasing limitation can be explained on the basis of the increased immobility of those thoracic muscles that have inspiratory capability as well as decreased capability of the diaphragm to flatten against a relatively rigid abdominal mass.

In regard to the diaphragm, I am of the opinion that the function of that large, powerful inspiratory muscle is spared, relatively, in cerebral palsied persons compared to their torso wall muscles. Whether or not the diaphragm is involved, its function will be reduced by the extent to which there is involvement of torso wall muscles. That is, if the abdominal wall muscles are resistive to stretch and firmly hold the abdominal contents, the diaphragm will be limited in its ability to flatten and thus increase the internal dimensions of the thoracic cage for inspiration.

For dyskinetic speakers who have relatively comparable severity of involvement throughout their torso wall muscles, alterations in the partitions of the lung volume can be expected to be progressively affected as a function of the severity of that involvement, in the same manner as the continuum of dysfunction across the groups with spastic paraplegia, diplegia, and quadriplegia. That is, for the milder dyskinetic individuals, the function of the abdominal wall muscles and both the inspiratory and expiratory musculatures of the thoracic wall will be affected to some extent, and there will be diminution in their expiratory ability with only some reduction in inspiratory ability. For the moderately involved dyskinetic person, the expiratory musculatures of both the abdominal and thoracic walls will be more severely affected; there will be some dysfunction of the inspiratory thoracic wall musculature; and with the diaphragm functioning relatively well, these speakers will show a severe reduction in their ability to perform ERV efforts and only some reduction in performance of IC efforts. The very severely involved dyskinetic person will show dramatic reduction in performance of an IC effort with little or no ability to perform an ERV effort for the same reasons as in cases of spastic quadriplegia.

The previously offered explanation of the so-called reverse breathing pattern of some dyskinetic cerebral palsied individuals was based on the assumption of relatively more severe involvement of the thoracic wall muscles than of the abdominal wall muscles. That explanation would seem even more reasonable if their diaphragms functioned reasonably well. Since the thoracic wall muscles, as a group, have both inspiratory and expiratory function, there would be a trade-off, with the abdominal muscles being less severely involved for expiration. If that is so, alterations in partitions of the lung volume of those with the reverse breathing pattern would be similar to those dyskinetic persons whose severity of involvement is comparable throughout the abdominal and thoracic muscles.

To the extent that the ability of a person with cerebral palsy to perform ERV and IC efforts is limited, his or her vital capacity also will be reduced by the sum of those limitations. As is shown in Figure 6–2, and in view of the alterations in the partitions of the lung volumes of cerebral palsied persons just discussed, it can be expected that, compared to normal persons, those persons will have reductions in their vital capacities.[3]

In most cases, there is no cause-effect relationship between only these reductions in vital capacity of cerebral palsied speakers and their speech production deficits. The extent of such a relationship will depend as much on the function of the speaker's laryngeal and articulatory structures as on the respiratory dysfunction. Since more air per unit of speech, such as a syllable, may be expired in the presence of neuromotor involvement of the speech articulators, a reduced vital capacity may present a limitation to the speech production process.

If a normal speaker repeats a train of the CV syllable /bɑ/ at a conversational level of intensity, he or she will expire approximately 30 cubic centimeters (cc) of air per syllable. If the CV syllable contains a voiceless stop (e.g., /pɑ/), more air per syllable will be expired. Still larger expired volumes per syllable are associated with production of voiceless continuants. The consonant /h/ requires more volume flow than any other speech sound. Dysarthric cerebral palsied individuals may expire three to four times as much air per syllable as the normal speakers, with the amount dependent on the characteristics of the restricted function of the speakers' laryngeal and articulatory structures.

Assume the example in which a physiologically normal ten-year-old child has a vital capacity of 2.4 liters, or 2400 cc of air, and that she routinely expires an average of 40 cc of air per syllable as she speaks. Assume further a child with spastic diplegia of moderate severity who has a comparable body size and total lung capacity; such a child might have a vital capacity of two-thirds her normal counterpart, or 1600 cc. Although the normal child could produce utterances of up to sixty syllables in length if she spoke over the entirety of the vital capacity, the cerebral palsied youngster could produce only sixteen syllables over her entire vital capacity if she averages 100 cc of expired air per syllable.

That reduction in potential length of an utterance, however, does not

---

[3]There is some evidence that the oxygen requirements of selected individuals with cerebral palsy may be somewhat higher than for normal persons that are matched by appropriate variables. For those selected individuals, the volume of gas exchanged during rest breathing may be somewhat greater, and their tidal breathing during exercise will be larger than for matched normal persons. The most reasonable explanation of such a finding seems to be that the muscular activity that results from the hypertonicity and/or involuntary motions associated with cerebral palsy requires the increased oxygen consumption. Therefore, the possibility that a selected person with cerebral palsy might routinely rest breathe at a slightly more rapid rate and/or greater tidal volume probably is of no import to that person's speech physiology problem.

explain why numerous cerebral palsied speakers seem to be limited to a very few syllables on one expiration. Thus, reduction in vital capacity is not the only significant aspect of the speech breathing problems of cerebral palsied speakers.

A far more crucial problem may be the ability to generate the positive expiratory air pressures needed to drive the vocal tract. As might be expected from the earlier discussion, the ability of cerebral palsied persons to produce expiratory air pressures is, in general, reduced. The amount of the reduction will, of course, depend on the specific pattern and severity of respiratory musculature involvement.

The left portion of Figure 6–3 shows the pressure-volume relationships of the above mentioned normal and cerebral palsied children. The magnitude of air pressure needed to drive the normal vocal tract is also shown in Figure 6–3, as it was in Figure 6–1.

In viewing the relationships shown in Figure 6–3, keep in mind that a speaker cannot be expected to drive the vocal tract at a lung volume level below that where the ability of the respiratory system to generate expiratory air pressures is less than the pressure that is required. Therefore, the cerebral palsied child would be unable to drive his or her vocal tract below approximately the 50 percent level of the vital capacity, and he or she would be limited to producing phrases to about eight syllables in length on one expiration. However, when speech is produced at the lower levels of the vital capacity where the magnitude of air pressure needed to drive

FIGURE 6–3 A graphic display of the vital capacities of a normal child and a spastic diplegic child who are of comparable physical size. This figure shows the maximum expiratory air pressures that they can produce at levels of their vital capacities along with the range of air pressures that might be generated within the children's vocal tracts for speech production. Also shown is the volume of air that might be exchanged as the children inhale maximally and produce a train of consonant-vowel syllables for as long as possible on one expiration. The drawing shows that the children will terminate that speech effort at a level of their vital capacities where their respiratory systems cannot generate the air pressures needed within their vocal tracts to produce speech.

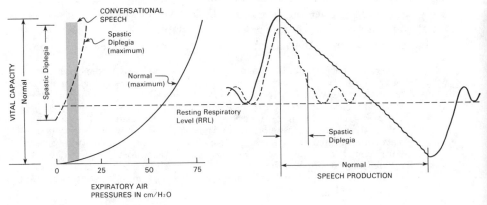

the vocal tract is only slightly less than those that can be generated by the respiratory system, the cerebral palsied speaker will be exerting considerable effort to generate a speech airstream. The effects may be comparable to the normal speaker who attempts to produce speech near the lower limits of the vital capacity, as described earlier. For practical purposes, then, the cerebral palsied child being described in this example might be limited to production of only three to four syllables on one expiration.

These relationships between the effects of dysfunction of the respiratory mechanics of dysarthric cerebral palsied individuals and the inefficient valving of the speech airstream due to the restricted mobility of their laryngeal and articulatory structures are further illustrated in the righthand portion of Figure 6–3. A tracing of the volume flow during speech production is shown for both the normal and spastic diplegic child.

Those tracings are for a train of CV syllables that each might produce under instructions such as, "Take as deep a breath as you can, and say puh-puh-puh-puh for as long as you can without taking a breath." Note that the slope of the resulting trace will be steeper for the child with cerebral palsy than for the normal child, a result of the former expiring more air per unit of speech than the latter. Also note, as would be predicted from the above discussion, that the spastic diplegic child terminates the speech effort relatively high in the vital capacity. In fact, the trace shows that the child expired air after terminating the speech effort at the lung volume level where the needed air pressure in the vocal tract equaled the respiratory system's capability to generate expiratory air pressure. At lower lung volume levels, the cerebral palsied youngster could generate the minimal expiratory pressures needed to expire air through an open vocal tract, but could not generate the magnitudes of such pressure needed to drive the vocal tract. Such tracings are generally typical for cerebral palsied speakers who have dysarthria.

Examples of different variations in the extent of neuromotor involvement of various muscle groups demonstrate how respiratory dysfunction and mobility problems of laryngeal and articulatory structures interact. For one example, a severely involved respiratory system in combination with severe restriction of movement of the articulators might result in a situation in which the speaker could be expected to produce only one syllable per expiration, and such extremely severe cases are seen. For another example, a cerebral palsied speaker who has relatively mild involvement of the respiratory muscles but with some articulatory involvement including the velopharyngeal port may be incapable of generating the intraoral air pressures needed for consonant production. For a final example, the spastic diplegic individual in which the respiratory system is significantly involved with little or no dysfunction of the laryngeal and articulatory structures may be capable of essentially normal speech for conversational purposes.

Assessment of Respiratory Function for Speech. Speech-language pathologists do not routinely have available the type of instrumentation that is needed to measure the characteristics of respiratory function that were just reviewed. Therefore, in the usual clinical situation it will be impossible to quantify the severity of respiratory function problems of a given cerebral palsied speaker. However, the severity of such problems is not the crucial determination to be made. Some deviation from normal respiratory function is to be expected as a component of developmental dysarthria. The critical assessment task is to determine the extent to which a respiratory function problem contributes to the speech-production deficit and the limitations that the problem presents to the speaker in improving his or her speech.

The person's usual speaking behavior will give some indications of problems of driving the vocal tract with the respiratory system. Short utterances with inhalations between each, the appearance of using considerable generalized effort for speech production, and slowing of speech and sounding "strained" at the end of phrases are such indications. A set of selected speech activities may clarify the limits with which the respiratory system can drive the vocal tract. These activities should be designed to assess (1) any differences that might exist in the manner with which the speaker routinely uses his or her respiratory system for speech compared to the capability of that system to drive the vocal tract and (2) the extent to which the individual's respiratory system can drive that tract under optimum conditions of laryngeal and articulatory valving of the speech airstream. At least four types of activities may be used for these purposes: (1) counting, or other activity as will be described later, (2) producing a train of CV syllables in which the consonant is voiceless, (3) repeating another CV train in which the consonant is the voiced cognate of the consonant used in (2), and (4) prolonging of a neutral vowel. Each of these four types of activities entail different types of valving of the speech airstream.

The first activity should contain a variety of phonetic contexts. The speaker should be likely to produce it spontaneously, and it should require more than one inspiration for completion. Its purpose, of course, is to obtain a speech sample in which the speaker is using the respiratory system as he or she routinely does while speaking.

The results of the speech testing that are described later should be used in selecting the voiceless-voiced consonant pair and the vowel for the CV syllable trains. The consonant pair should be those that the speaker produced most accurately and with what appeared to be the greatest ease. Typically, these consonants will be a pair of stops. The vowel that is to be coupled with the consonant pair should be chosen on the basis that it, too, is the one that is produced most accurately when combined with those consonants.

For the vowel prolongation, a neutral vowel should be used, under the assumption that its production places the least physiological stress on the speaker's articulatory system. The results of the speech testing may demonstrate, however, that some other vowel should be used.

These four activities should be presented twice. The first should be with instructions that are designed to elicit a prolonged effort but without reference to the speaker's respiratory behavior. "Count for me until I tell you to stop," or "Sing the sound /ɑ/ over and over until I tell you to stop," are examples.

Instructions designed to elicit behavior that is used routinely for speech production should be given first throughout the evaluation process. Otherwise, as the speaker concentrates on the speech-production process during the assessment session, he or she is likely to produce speech in ways that will obscure the manner in which the speech-producing system is routinely used.

Since activities to assist in the assessment of routine use of the laryngeal system will also be presented, the second set of activities for assessment of respiratory function should be deferred until later. When these activities are repeated, the instructions should be changed in order to motivate the speaker to produce them at higher than usual levels of the lung volume. "Take a deep breath and count as long as you can on one breath," is an example.

Comparisons should then be made between the durations of these activities and the number of syllables produced on one expiration for the three activities in which syllable productions are involved. Changes in the quality of production and the steadiness of pitch and loudness throughout each act also should be noted. Even though the literature has mentioned a problem of "breath control" as being one of the speech physiology problems associated with cerebral palsy, it will typically be found that trains of CV syllables and vowel prolongations are produced with relatively constant fundamental frequency and intensity. This would not occur if there was a problem in controlling the force of the speech-generating airstream. Selected speakers, particularly the more severely involved, may have a very restricted range of lung volume levels over which they can generate utterances of steady pitch and loudness, even when they are optimally secure. This should be the range of lung volume levels over which it is assumed that their respiratory systems can optimally drive the vocal tract.

It will be rather routinely found that the ease and durations with which dysarthric speakers can produce these four types of activities will be, from the best to the poorest, prolongation of the vowel, repetition of the voiced CV syllable train, repetition of the voiceless CV syllable train, and the more routine type of speech production. If the speaker's larynx functions reasonably well during prolongations of vowels, it may be assumed that sustaining vowels is an activity in which the speech airstream is most efficiently valved. The valving of the speech airstream usually is more efficient for voiced than for voiceless consonants, and, during a speech act in which there is a variety of phonetic contexts, the physiological demands upon the involved speech-producing system may be greatest, as will be discussed later.

These same activities will usually be spoken for longer durations on one expiration and with better quality after the speaker follows the instruction to inhale deeply prior to each. Thus, an indication will have been obtained as to the degree to which the speaker's respiratory system is capable of driving the vocal tract under varying conditions of valving of the speech airstream and levels of lung volume.

Respiratory dysfunction may contribute to restrictions of ranges of pitch and loudness due to the increased subglottal air pressures that are associated with rises in fundamental frequency and increases in the intensity of the vocal tone. As mentioned in Chapter Five, the frequently observed substitution of voiced consonants for their voiceless cognates may have been adopted to conserve respiratory effort.

The information to be gained from these observations is (1) the extent to which the speaker's respiratory system is taxed by the speech production process and (2) the extent to which the speaker can modify his or her respiratory system to better drive the vocal tract. In general, then, these observations should be made with the idea that they will provide an indication of the physiological limitation imposed by the respiratory system on the speaker's ability to improve his or her speech.

laryngeal system

Function of the laryngeal mechanism for speech production is directly dependent on an appropriate interaction with the speech-generating airstream. The phonatory wave form possesses three characteristics that are requisite to perceptually normal speech production: (1) the fundamental frequency, which is determined by the rate at which the vocal folds vibrate, (2) the intensity of the wave form, which is determined, in large part, by the magnitude and pattern of the vibrations, and (3) the perceptual quality of the vocal tone, which is determined primarily by the pattern of vocal vibration.[4]

With respect to changes in fundamental frequency, the important determinants are the length of the vocal folds, their thickness or mass, the tension with which they are held in the expiratory airstream, and the force of that airstream against their inferior surfaces as reflected by subglottal air pressure. Increases in the fundamental frequency of vibration, which are reflected perceptually by rises in pitch, are associated with combinations

---

[4]The term vocal quality in this context does not refer to perceived differences due to changes of the resonance characteristics in the vocal tract. The phenomenon of hypernasality is due to such changes.

of increased vocal fold length, increased vocal fold tension, thinning of the cross-sectional mass of the vocal folds, a simpler mode of vibration, and greater subglottal air pressure. The associated laryngeal adjustments are, of course, dependent on intrinsic laryngeal activity, but the appropriate magnitudes of subglottal air pressure must be present.

The changes in phonatory activity that are components of vocal intensity differences may be more dependent on variations in the subglottal air pressure. The vocal folds, however, are held in the adducted position for a greater proportion of the phonatory cycle as vocal intensity increases, and the open phase is characterized by more extensive and complex movement of the folds. Since greater subglottal air pressures are also associated with increases in vocal intensity, it would appear that the intrinsic laryngeal muscles hold the folds together with greater tension, and they are literally blown apart with greater force for high levels of intensity. The changes in the open and closed phases of the phonatory cycle creates more harmonics in the vocal tone and, hence, greater intensity; the alteration of the duty cycle also is due to intrinsic muscular adjustments.

It is somewhat easier to attribute the quality of the vocal tone primarily to action of the intrinsic laryngeal musculature. Even so, the specific physiological events that lead to the abnormal phonation described as harsh and strained are not known. It can be said with some confidence that a breathy voice is due to inadequate vocal fold tension and/or adduction. However, it seems reasonable that an inappropriate relationship between tension of the vocal folds and the speech airstream could lead to a deviation in even that quality of the voice.

The complexity of the interaction of all of these parameters of laryngeal function is compounded by the requirement of abduction for voiceless consonants. Therefore, the delicate and precise adjustments of the intrinsic tissues of the vocal folds are probably dependent on equally precise abduction-adduction postures that change quite rapidly. In addition, the entire laryngeal complex is known to move inferiorly during speech production, probably in association with voiced consonant productions, and then return. Such action of the extrinsic laryngeal muscle complex undoubtedly contributes to, or must be accommodated by, intrinsic adjustments.

It would be easy to assume that the intrinsic laryngeal muscles are the prime contributors to intonation patterns, but, as just reviewed, the speech airstream must possess certain characteristics for variations in fundamental frequency. Moreover, intonation patterns are confounded with stress contrasts. As explained in the early comments on assessment and management in Chapter Five, stress changes also involve differences in vocal intensity and timing characteristics of the phonatory and articulatory mechanisms. The term prosody is frequently used to denote those complex attributes of the speech signal that include intonation and stress changes. It would appear, then, that normal speech prosody is dependent on the interaction of the muscle groups throughout the speech-producing mechanism, even though the perceptual characteristics of prosody may lead to the impression that it is due to laryngeal function.

Problems of Laryngeal Function. Attempts to phonate by a few severely involved cerebral palsied speakers result in simply a rush of air through the vocal tract with no phonation taking place. The behavior suggests strongly that the vocal folds are not being adducted into the midline of the glottis. Milder laryngeal dysfunction of this type may be manifested by phonation of weak intensity and breathy quality. In these cases, the vocal folds are not being adducted appropriately, and/or there is insufficient tension of the folds.

In other dysarthric cerebral palsied speakers attempts to phonate may result in what appears to be an effort to drive the speech airstream through a hyperadducted glottis, with the result that no phonation takes place. In such extreme cases there is always the possibility that this effortful type of behavior is, rather, the result of generalized muscular contractions throughout the entire speech-producing mechanism. To the extent that such is the case, the resulting generalized immobility and lack of airflow through the glottis may not be the result of attempts to force the airstream through severely hyperfunctioning vocal folds but rather a generalized immobility of the speech-producing system.

Specification of a laryngeal function problem seems defensible in some of these latter cases since there will be instances in which they are able to phonate. These instances may be characterized by what I tend to refer to as a "strained" vocal quality. Moreover, the phonatory segment frequently is initiated with what sounds like a glottal attack, as if hyperfunctioning vocal folds were suddenly blown into vibration. To the extent that such hyperfunction exists, the greater magnitude of subglottal air pressure needed for phonation would place a significant demand on the respiratory system of a speaker with cerebral palsy, and those speakers who manifest this vocal characteristic will routinely have difficulty prolonging phonation and utterances.

The earlier discussion that dealt with spastic diplegia pointed out that it is unlikely that involvement of the intrinsic laryngeal muscles exist even though spastic diplegic speakers may be dysprosodic. It was suggested that the contribution to the dysprosody that can be attributed to laryngeal dysfunction may be due to involvement of the neck musculatures. Laryngeal dysfunction due to extrinsic laryngeal muscle dysfunction would be expected during activities such as connected discourse but not during acts like phonating vowels.

The characteristics of the vocal tone may suggest reasonably normal laryngeal function during usual speech efforts. However, vocal characteristics strongly suggestive of laryngeal dysfunction may become apparent during speech acts for which the laryngeal activity deviates from that usage. For example, the vocal tone of a dysarthric cerebral palsied individual may be perceptually quite normal at a conversational level of vocal intensity; however, that same speaker may be unable to produce normal-sounding phonation at low or high levels of intensity. These deviations may be due to in part to respiratory dysfunction, but the speaker's behavior frequently suggests their basis to be at the level of the larynx.

Perceptible phonatory characteristics among cerebral palsied speakers can lead the examiner to conclude that there may be present a continuum of laryngeal dysfunctions from the severe hypofunction problems, to normal laryngeal function, to the severe hyperfunction problems in the population. Careful attention to the characteristics of the vocal tone during a variety of phonatory activities may result in confirmation that such a problem is present. However, in a large number of cases it may be impossible to draw firm conclusions in this regard.

Assessment of Laryngeal Dysfunction. Activities that are elicited specifically for assessment of laryngeal dysfunctions should be designed to eliminate, to the extent possible, the confounding effects of dysfunction of the other speech-producing musculatures on the laryngeal mechanism. The complexity of supraglottal activity associated with conversational speech efforts and the demands that those efforts place on the person's respiratory system frequently serve to affect laryngeal function adversely in the presence of neuromotor involvement throughout the respiratory, neck, and articulatory musculatures. Because of these effects, the presence of an abnormal vocal quality during connected speech may be misleading regarding dysfunction of the larynx.

The perceptual quality of the vocal tone during prolongations of a neutral vowel may well be the best indicator of intrinsic laryngeal musculature dysfunction. A neutral vowel is specified to offset the possibility that attempts by the speaker to adjust the position of the tongue will, through hypertonicity of the tongue-neck musculatures, alter the posture and function of the laryngeal mechanism.

As discussed in some detail in Chapter Five and mentioned in the above discussion of respiratory dysfunction, the frequent tendency of speakers with developmental dysarthria to substitute voiced for voiceless consonants may be indicative of an adduction-abduction problem of the larynx. Asking the speaker to produce short, discrete neutral vowels may assist in determining if this is the prime reason for consistent voicing. However, such productions are particularly difficult even for some physiologically normal speakers.

The speech testing may clearly indicate that this substitution pattern has been adopted primarily to maintain aerodynamic efficiency of the vocal tract. Even so, for speakers who demonstrate this pattern, the examiner may wish to select a voiceless consonant for which the voiced cognate is frequently substituted, elicit productions of that consonant in a VCV context, and coax the speaker to change the pattern to a voiceless production with changes in the speaker's rate, use of the respiratory system, and so on. The most usual result will convince the examiner that the voiced-voiceless substitution pattern has been adopted for the reasons given in Chapter 5 and that intrinsic laryngeal musculature dysfunction contributes very little, or not at all, to the problem.

Other potential indications of laryngeal dysfunction have already been mentioned. Routine glottal, or strained, initiation of phonation may be indicative of a hyperadduction or hypertension problem of the vocal folds. A relatively consistent breathy initiation of phonation, on the other hand, may result from a hypofunction problem.

Reduced pitch and loudness ranges, as well as differences in vocal quality as a function of pitch and loudness usage, also may be indicative of laryngeal dysfunction. However, the potential contribution of respiratory function to generation of pitch and loudness differences must be remembered.

The impressions of laryngeal behavior obtained through these observations should provide an indication of the limitations that the function of the speaker's larynx presents to his or her speech-production capability. Indications of the conditions under which the speaker seems able to modify his or her laryngeal behavior in a desirable way should be noted very carefully, as should conditions that seem to result in a deterioration of that behavior.

velopharyngeal port mechanism

Compared to the function of the respiratory and laryngeal systems, the function of the velopharyngeal port mechanism for speech production is relatively simple to conceptualize. The muscles of the soft palate and pharyngeal walls serve to elevate and stretch the soft palate posteriorly and to constrict the pharyngeal walls around the elevated palate to occlude the nasal cavity from the oral cavity. For most speakers of General American English, the velopharyngeal port in general is closed in association with all phonological units of speech except nasal consonants. For nasal consonants, the port opens enough to couple the nasal and oral cavities acoustically so that the air in the former will be set into vibration.

The port usually is closed prior to and throughout production of the nonnasal components of the speech signal. The frequency of nasal consonants, however, is sufficient to result in intermittent opening and closing of the port during most utterances.

Such patterns of velopharyngeal closure, however, vary considerably among normal speakers. Some show anticipatory opening to nasal consonants for which the velopharyngeal port begins the opening gesture in advance of production of nasal consonants, and the opening may be retained to some extent after production of those consonants. Also, the degree to which the soft palate elevates, and, hence, the degree to which there may be port closure may vary as a function of the height of the posterior tongue mass; it is usually assumed that the interconnection between the lateral posterior borders of the tongue and tissues of the soft palate by the palatal glossus muscles creates this relationship between movements of the palate and the tongue. As a result, there tends to be firmer port closure associated with high back vowels than, for example, high front vowels, for which the posterior portion of the tongue tends to be positioned low in the oral cavity.

As reviewed in Chapter Five, the acoustic coupling of the oral and nasal cavities leads to the perception of nasality, and hypernasality is often thought of as the clinically significant manifestation of velopharyngeal incompetence. For the present purposes, however, the prime consideration is that closure of the port is required for aerodynamic efficiency of the oral structures to produce many components of the speech signal.

Velopharyngeal Port Dysfunction. It is possible to use concomitant measures of intraoral air pressures and nasal airflow rates to calculate the area of velopharyngeal port opening at moments in time throughout a speech sample (Netsell, 1969 a). Use of this procedure for a number of years with dysarthric cerebral palsied speakers has indicated that there can be no generalization as to patterns of their velopharyngeal incompetency. For some there is substantial, consistent opening throughout all utterances. For others there are moments of closure, usually associated with nonnasal consonant productions; however, these moments of closure may lag in time the other associated articulatory gestures, so there is significant port opening at those times when relatively large magnitudes of intraoral air pressure should be generated. There may be closure in association with high back vowels and proximal consonants; but not for high front and neutral vowels and consonants adjacent to such vowels. In other cases, there may be more competence at rapid than at slow speaking rates or vice versa. In still others, the effect of rate is the reverse. Some dysarthric speakers show competence, or minimal incompetence, during the first few syllables of an utterance, after which the function of the port mechanism deteriorates.[5]

[5]A relatively frequent pattern of velopharyngeal function of speakers with developmental dysarthria is that the port closes in association with voiceless consonants, but there is a relatively small opening over the remainder of an utterance. This pattern of closure apparently is a result of the speaker's mechanism developing velopharyngeal port closure in conjunction with those articulations for which generation and maintenance of intraoral air pressures are most needed. Of course, it tends to result in perceived hypernasality. However, in those cases where development of intelligible speech is the prime consideration and hypernasality may be viewed as clinically insignificant, this pattern of velopharyngeal closure may also be viewed as insignificant.

In still other cases, patterns of velopharyngeal closure are compounded by head position. Velopharyngeal port function may be reasonably good when the cerebral palsied speaker's head is held in what might be thought of as a normal, forward-looking position. However, when the head is tilted backward, the anatomical relationship of the palatal plane and posterior pharyngeal wall may be such that consistent port opening exists. This may be a critical problem, for example, for the dyskinetic child whose pattern of neuromotor involvement causes him or her to routinely hold the head back and to the side in what might be considered a manifestation of the asymmetrical tonic neck reflex.

   Assessment of Velopharyngeal Incompetence. As is the case for evaluation of respiratory dysfunction, speech-language pathologists do not routinely have available the instrumentation needed for precise determination of velopharyngeal incompetence. Again, however, a number of observations that may be made without the use of such instrumentation will provide, in the usual case, enough information to determine the presence of significant incompetence.

   Some strong cautions, however, are in order. Firm, accurate conclusions regarding the presence or absence of incompetence cannot be made on the basis of (1) perceived hypernasality or (2) audible emission of air through the nostrils. With respect to the former, factors operating within the vocal tract of dysarthric speakers frequently obscure the perception of obvious hypernasality, even though gross, consistent incompetence is present. I can only speculate as to what these factors may be, and such speculations are not particularly helpful. The fact remains that some cerebral palsied speakers, who have highly significant incompetence may be perceived as minimally hypernasal. With respect to the latter caution, relatively large velopharyngeal port opening may be consistently present; the speaker may be unable to generate needed intraoral air pressure for production of some consonants, relatively large volumes of air may flow through the nasal cavity during utterances, and yet that airflow may not be audible.

   Also, it is impossible to determine the extent to which the soft palate is making contact with the pharyngeal walls by viewing perorally the velopharyngeal mechanism as the speaker phonates vowels. The anatomy of the area precludes making such an observation. Extensive palatal and pharyngeal wall movement may be observable. Nevertheless, in numerous cerebral palsied speakers in which that is the case, other observations will show that significant incompetence during speech production is present.

   The one noninstrumental procedure on which I rely most heavily involves, simply, holding a mirror under the individual's nostrils as he or she produces a variety of speech acts. The edge of the mirror that is held next to the speaker's face should be curved so that it follows to some extent the contour of the upper lip; otherwise, fairly substantial amounts of air may flow laterally through the opening between the straight edge of the mirror and the lateral surfaces of the upper lip. The observation to be made, of course, is the extent to which the nasal emission of air fogs the mirror during speech production. Since expiratory air is at body temperature and moisture-laden, having the mirror at room temperature is usually sufficient to bring about observable fogging, and the area of fogging will become larger and smaller throughout an utterance as nasal airflow rates vary. The mirror may be waved away from the client's face between speech acts to evaporate completely the collected moisture prior to the next activity.

Nasal airflow during vowel productions is so minimal that fogging of the mirror usually will not be associated with vowel productions even if the velopharyngeal port is open. In contrast, of course, nasal airflow should be detectable with each production of a nasal consonant. Even with many normal speakers, fogging of the mirror can be observed during production of nonnasal consonants just prior to or after nasal consonants.

I have come to ask dysarthric speakers routinely to count from one to ten for an indication of the general velopharyngeal function during speech production. Of course, fogging of the mirror should be detectable in association with the /n/ in the word *one;* the fogging may continue to expand as a result of the retentive opening of the port as the individual produces the /t/ in *two.* However, no detectable nasal emission of air should be associated with the consonant productions thereafter until the word *seven* is produced. Even for some normal speakers, anticipatory port opening may be observable for the /s/ in *seven*, and with retentive opening after that nasal and the anticipatory port opening associated with the following /n/s in the words *nine* and *ten*, there may be consistent fogging of the mirror throughout the remainder of the act.

Indicators of the variables that affect the velopharyngeal function of a dysarthric speaker may be obtained by using CV syllable trains in which consonants are varied according to manner and place of articulation in combination with vowels of different tongue heights. Again, the specific consonants to be used depend on the facility with which a given dysarthric speaker can produce those consonants. If possible, a continuant voiceless consonant and voiceless-voiced pairs of stop consonants also should be used in repeated CV syllables. At least one pair of CV syllables should be repeated at different rates of utterance, and one pair also should be elicited with vowels for which there are extreme tongue positions (e.g., /i/, /ɑ/, and /u/). Determination of the effect of head positioning on velopharyngeal port function is crucial if the cerebral palsied speaker tends to hold his or her head in some unusual position.

Reservations have already been offered regarding the extent to which peroral observation of palatal elevation is helpful. However, as will be reviewed in Chapter Seven, if some type of prosthetic or surgical management of the velopharyngeal incompetence is anticipated, such observations may be helpful. It will be even more helpful to observe velopharyngeal wall movement during phonations.

There are a number of methods for determining velopharyngeal closure with relatively elaborate instrumentation that may be available to some speech-language pathologists, and these methods may be used to improve the precision and understanding of the incompetence that may be detected. Many of these procedures have evolved through work with the cleft palate population. Some of these procedures, however, must be used with caution with dysarthric speakers.

Lateral head X-rays may be taken during prolongations of continuant consonants and vowels. The resulting views may confirm the presence of incompetence during those acts, and they are especially helpful in determining the presence of an anatomically short palate. However, there are numerous cases in which the soft palates of cerebral palsied speakers make contact with the posterior pharyngeal wall as seen on such X-rays; yet, there may be substantial opening through the lateral ports of the velopharyngeal aperture.

Of course, if it is possible to make arrangements to use motion picture X-ray that provides a lateral view of the oral structures, such cinefluorography will be helpful in selected cases where it seems important to identify the patterns of palatal movement during speech production. Again, however, even this procedure probably will only confirm, or make more precise, information regarding velopharyngeal port dysfunction that can be obtained in the usual clinical situation.

Because of the historical emphasis on doing so, most speech-language pathologists will be inclined to determine the extent to which a gag reflex can be elicited. As was also discussed earlier, presence or absence of this reflex may have absolutely no predictive value as to palatal function during speech production. Determination of the presence of the gag reflex will be helpful, however, for assistance in determining possible difficulties in prosthetic management of velopharyngeal dysfunction.

The significance of any velopharyngeal incompetence that is present during speech production will depend in many cases on the degree to which there are other aberrations of speech physiology. If the velopharyngeal port remains open during all utterances, that incompetency will be highly significant, just as it is in the cleft population. However, if there is substantial dysfunction of the speaker's respiratory system and restricted mobility of the other articulators, what might otherwise be considered minimal incompetence may also be highly significant.

lips, jaw, and tongue

Although it is somewhat trite to state it, the synchronous activity of the lips, jaw, and tongue during speech production is exceedingly complex. The muscular activity and the movements of these structures that result have been intensively studied. Such study will undoubtedly continue since a number of issues regarding the movement patterns of these articulators are yet to be resolved.

The knowledge that has been gained, however, speaks strongly against conceptualization of the articulatory process as a series of discrete gestures, one for each phone-type (or speech sound). Rather, it appears that speech articulation consists of a process of ongoing movements for which target positions are accomplished with considerable efficiency. The lips, for example, may begin moving toward a target position well in advance of when that position is associated with production of a given phone if there are no lip gestures associated with intervening phones. This phenomenon of "forward coarticulation" may cross syllable and word boundaries. To the extent that this phenomenon is representative of the organization of neuromotor processes of speech articulation, an orientation of that process as a series of discrete movements is inappropriate.

It seems reasonable to postulate that there is disruption of the forward coarticulatory movements and other dynamics of articulatory movements in the speech-producing process of many dysarthric speakers. It is difficult to state with equal confidence that such disruption should be given attention in the clinical process. I know of no way in which that attention will pay dividends. However, the phenomenon of forward coarticulation ·exemplifies that assessment of the function of the lips, jaw, and tongue of a cerebral palsied speaker must extend beyond the traditional view of assessing the ability to perform discrete movements.

In addition, as might be anticipated from the bias expressed in Chapter Five, the assessment should concentrate on the movements of these structures during speechlike activities. The assessment process must consider the extent to which tongue, lips, and jaw movements can adequately (1) valve the speech-producing airstream in certain specified ways to generate the noise components of the speech signal and (2) form resonance chambers within the vocal tract for production of vowel formants and transitions. In that regard, the clinician should not overlook the fact that the transitions of the vowel formants contribute more to intelligibility than do the acoustic characteristics of the noise components of the speech signal.

The most useful and practical clinical information regarding the adequacy of articulatory movements can be obtained from an analysis of a speaker's ability to produce specific phone-types (or speech sounds). The results of articulatory inventories (tests) that assess a speaker's ability to produce specific consonants, consonant clusters, vowels, and diphthongs in specified phonetic contexts must be viewed, however, within a frame of reference that recognizes the dynamic nature of the articulatory process.

Problems of Lips, Jaws, and Tongue Function. Patterns of disordered movements of the lips, jaws, and tongues of dysarthric cerebral palsied speakers are extremely heterogeneous. Some general patterns, however, are seen.

General immobility of the lips is the most frequently observed problem of lip function for speech production. Lip gestures associated with vowel productions are reduced, and lip protrusions associated with consonants such as /w/ and /ʃ/ may be minimal. These particular manifestations of immobility may not adversely affect the intelligibility of speech. Lip involvement may interfere with bilabial and labial-dental contacts, but the speaker may be able to compensate with jaw movements.

That is not to say that mobility of the jaw is normal in most of these speakers. It is not. Jaw movements are typically slowed. Nevertheless, mandibular function frequently is good enough so that compensatory movements can be accomplished to assist with lip and tongue gestures.

Occasional cases, however, may show extensive mandibular dysfunction. The most frequent of these problems is what has been referred to as the "extensor thrust" of the jaw that is sometimes associated with dyskinesia. An extreme opening of the mouth may precede most acts associated with mouth opening. Milder forms of this problem may, of course, interfere with jaw movements, but in its extreme form the condyle of the mandible may actually be dislocated from the mandibular fossa. A relatively few cerebral palsied speakers with this problem may find it difficult to close the jaw once this dislocation occurs. In relatively rare cases, the oral behavior of the cerebral palsied speaker suggests that the jaw routinely tends to close with too much force.

The more usual case is that mandibular movements appear to assist the speaker in accomplishing articulatory gestures of the tongue. In fact, tongue gestures seem directly linked to jaw movement in many cerebral palsied speakers, and achieving articulatory target positions may be dependent on mandibular positioning.

The tongue frequently seems to move, as mentioned earlier, in a relatively inflexible mass. The tongue may hump somewhat anteriorly with lingua-alveolar contacts actually being made with the blade of the tongue against the alveolar ridge, with no discernible elevation of its tip. Similarly, the tongue may hump somewhat posteriorly for lingual-palatal contacts, but in both cases a major contribution to the tongue's elevation may be jaw movements.

A "tongue thrusting" type of activity may be seen in some dyskinetic speakers. The movement pattern appears to resemble the thrusting type of lingual behavior seen in infants during swallowing.

The severity of restriction of tongue movement may range from the extreme in which movements of a relatively inflexible tongue are barely perceptible to mildly impaired gestures that appear only slightly slowed and imprecise. Of course, the degree to which gestures associated with stop consonants and formation of various tongue configurations for valving the speech-producing airstream will vary accordingly. Retroflection of the tongue for /l/ may, or may not, be possible, and appropriate tongue positioning for the consonant /r/, the vocalic /ɝ/, and various vowels may appear impossible for the speaker.

Assessment of Lips, Jaw, and Tongue Function. Counting rates of reciprocal nonspeech movements of the tongue, lips, and jaw has been emphasized historically in assessment of dysarthria, and rates at which normal speakers can perform such movements have been assessed. Normal speakers show wide variation in such rates, and that variability works against establishing cut-off rates that are clearly indicative of abnormal function among different speakers. It may be impossible to specify those rates of movements that differentiate normal from abnormal behavior in other than the already obviously abnormal cases. There is a relationship between these rates of reciprocal nonspeech movements of the articulators and the severity of the speech problems in the cerebral palsied population. However, that relationship is only moderately strong for group data, and it is quite weak in numerous individual cases.

Deviations from normal lip, jaw, and tongue mobility frequently can be seen in speakers with cerebral palsy when they attempt to protrude and/ or spread the lips, lateralize the tongue when it is protruded, open and close the jaw, open and close the lips while the teeth are held together, and elevate the tongue tip to touch the alveolar ridge while the jaw is being held open. Observation of those deviations, as well as determining that a given cerebral palsied speaker can repetitively elevate only very slowly the tip of the tongue to the alveolar ridge or is unable to protrude it beyond the plane of the anterior teeth are strongly suggestive of neuromotor involvement of the musculatures used for those movements. The presence of such irregularities may serve to support the conclusion that deviations from expected lip, jaw, and tongue movements during speech production are due to that involvement. However, noting the existence of these movement irregularities during nonspeech acts as indicators of the presence of neuromotor involvement is quite different than making the assumption that the extent of the irregularities of these movements reflects the severity of the restriction of articulator movements during speech production.

This is not to say that the examiner should not determine the abilities of the speaker to perform these nonspeech movements of the lips, tongue, and jaw. A rather systematic appraisal of such abilities should be made. The discussion in Chapter Eight reviews the concept of developmental speech apraxia, and a determination of what the speaker does in response to requests to perform nonspeech movements with the lips, jaws, and tongue may be important to differentiating between that problem and a dysarthria. The important points here are that a speaker's ability to perform nonspeech movements of those structures may serve primarily only to (1) confirm the existence of neuromotor involvement of the musculatures associated with those movements and (2) provide the examiner with an idea of difficulty that may come later if the management program is to involve asking the speaker to place these articulatory structures in specified positions in the process of improving his or her speech skills.

Just as I believe that assessing a speaker's ability to perform nonspeech movements or so-called movements on the voluntary level, has limited usefulness, I also believe that assessing function of the oral structures at the so-called vegetative level may have even more limited utilization. As a consequence, I am disinclined to use observation of chewing and deglutition behaviors as a routine part of the assessment process. The fact that a child with cerebral palsy has difficulty chewing, managing the bolus of food in the mouth, and swallowing usually will be confirmatory of a neuromotor problem involving the oral structures, and such observations may be helpful in selected instances in the clinical process. However, the idea that the severity of chewing and swallowing difficulties reflect the severity of the speech physiology problems in the individual case may be very misleading.

Even though a strong relationship has been demonstrated between rates of repetition of consonant-vowel syllables and general levels of severity of dysarthria in cerebral palsy, caution should be used in attributing slow rates of consonant-vowel syllables to involvement of the musculatures that control the prime articulator(s) associated with production of the specific consonant. It might be assumed, for example, that slow repetition of /t / and /dʌ/ is due to a problem of tongue mobility. Such an assumption overlooks other explanations. Some of these speakers may start the syllable train relatively rapidly, but as they quickly exhaust the volume of air available for speech production, they slow their rate in what appears to be an extreme effort to drive the vocal tract; an entire syllable train may be produced very slowly for the same reason. Reduced jaw function may result in slow rates of repetition of any CV syllable.

Many tongue gestures are unobservable as a speaker talks, and there is not a direct correspondence between configurations of the vocal tract and the acoustic product. Nevertheless, observation of movements of the lips, jaw, and tongue where possible, along with careful synthesis of the perceived characteristics of the speech signal during a variety of speech acts should lead to a reasonably good idea of limitations of lip, jaw, and even tongue movement for speech production. The speech testing that will provide the prime information for that synthesis will be described shortly.

Before discussing that testing, however, some comments must be made regarding the anatomical relationships of the structures of the oral cavity. Even relatively gross anatomical deviations of those structures may be present in physiologically normal individuals with no discernible effect upon their development of speech production. For example, although severe malocclusions may appear to interfere to some extent with a normal child's learning articulatory skills, the speech learning of many such children is unaffected. In the presence of even mild neuromotor involvement of the oral musculatures, however, otherwise insignificant deviations may preclude needed articulatory contacts and configurations. A higher than normal palate with a narrow maxillary arch, for example, may present no problem whatsoever to a physiologically normal child's producing /k/, /g/, and /ŋ/. That configuration is often seen in dyskinetic cerebral palsied individuals, and in combination with the restricted mobility of their tongues, the articulatory contacts for those consonants may be impossible. Therefore, it is important to note deviations of structural relationships of the oral structures as a part of the assessment of lip, jaw, and tongue function. The presence of any such deviation should be considered in the determination of what may, or may not, be a physiological limitation on the speaker's ability to articulate.

beginning the assessment: speech testing

As with any type of communication handicap, the initial conversation with the client can provide considerable information regarding the nature and needs for assessment of specific aspects of the problem. An initial conversation with a cerebral palsied speaker also should provide indications of how he or she routinely uses the speech-producing mechanism, and that use can be contrasted with later determination of the optimum manner in which the mechanism may be used to produce the speech signal.

In view of the earlier discussions relative to (1) function of the entire speech-producing mechanism in the intonation, stress, and timing changes that comprise prosody and (2) the usual distribution of neuromotor involvement in cerebral palsy, it is not surprising that dysprosody is a distinctive characteristic of developmental dysarthria. There are a few cases in which speakers (1) are diagnosed as having cerebral palsy, (2) have a speech-production problem, (3) show unmistakable signs of dysfunction of selected speech musculatures, but (4) speak with good prosody. However, such cases are infrequent enough that the presence of acceptable prosody usually indicates that the speech problem is not due to a neuromotor disorder.

The dysprosody usually will be readily apparent even in cases of mild involvement. The source of the dysprosody may be perceived as primarily reduced fluctuations in intensity, fundamental frequency, or timing characteristics of the speech signal; however, there usually is reduction in the variation of all these parameters. There frequently will be deviations of other aspects of the speech signal in mildly involved cases, such as generally imprecise articulation and articulation errors that will vary according to the pattern of neuromotor involvement and the manner in which the speaker has learned to use the speech mechanism.

For most cases of moderate, or somewhat more severe, involvement of the speech-producing musculatures, whether or not a dysarthria is present will be unequivocal, and the dysprosody will be only one of the characteristics of the problem. A prime contributor to the perception of the dysprosody may be a tendency for voicing to be present throughout utterances. Some speech-producing behaviors that are general deterrents to good speech may be easily identified. The speech rate may be too rapid to permit completion of articulatory gestures of the involved lips, jaw, and tongue; the tendency to speak rapidly may, or may not, be confounded with what appears to be the use of extreme physiological effort with each expiratory-speech segment.

For the more severely involved speakers, conversation may be impossible, and it may be obvious that numerous aspects of the assessment procedures are not warranted. In these cases the examiner should choose among the selected activities that have been, or will be, described and that appear appropriate for the speaker's capabilities.

Regardless of the degree of severity of involvement of the speech-producing musculatures, the presence of other general contributory factors may be apparent. If the speaker's head is routinely held in an abnormal position, for example, simply holding it in a normal position may demonstrate that either a program for training the speaker to hold such a head position is called for or, in more severe cases, a general positioning program may be needed.

Other general factors may be more difficult to ascertain readily. Changes in the manifestation of the neuromotor disorder as a function of affective state may be obscured; the speaker may be reacting to the assessment session in a manner that brings about the increased problem. On the other hand, a generalized increase in the neuromotor dysfunction and associated deterioration in speech may be apparent as a child enthusiastically attempts to talk about something of keen interest, such as a pet.

Once a reasonable clinical relationship seems to have been established and a global impression of the individual's speaking abilities and use of the speech mechanism has been obtained, the assessment of speech skills should proceed in a relatively systematic way. The following procedures provide suggestions for a set of activities that may be used to begin delineating the manner in which the speaker uses, and is capable of using, his or her articulatory mechanism for the numerous cases that present articulatory problems.

Assessment of Articulatory Function. These suggestions for assessing the function of the articulatory structures may be useful for even those cases that demonstrate only generally imprecise articulatory patterns. The rationale for the procedures is to elicit the speaker's ability to produce each phone-type in contexts that impose reduced levels of demand on the speech-producing mechanism while providing a systematic review of physiological restrictions to articulatory gestures. The procedures call for eliciting the manner in which the speaker produces (1) all consonants and consonant clusters (blends) in words, (2) those consonants and clusters in combination with a neutral vowel, and (3) all vowels and diphthongs in combination with all consonant gestures that can be produced reasonably well.

A relatively fine phonetic transcription system should be used in order to reflect as precisely as possible the misarticulations that are heard. The results should be displayed in a manner that provides easy comparison of the effects of place and manner of articulation.

Testing Articulation of Consonants. There are numerous commercially available tests of articulation skills that might be used for the assessment of consonant productions in words, or the examiner may construct a test to suit his or her particular approach to the task. I have not found testing the production of consonants in the historical medial position to be informative, and I use single-syllable test words wherever possible. A more representative articulatory pattern to that which is usually used may be obtained if the test words can be elicited without the speaker's reading or hearing them, but I do not hesitate to present them orally or for reading if doing so is necessary and efficient for their elicitation.

The results may be dramatically different from that which would be anticipated from the conversational abilities of the speaker. There are selected cases in which the dysarthric cerebral palsied speaker may have poor intelligibility during conversation and yet manifest what must be transcribed as normal articulation of most consonants throughout the articulation survey. Numerous possible reasons for such a difference have been given. The demand placed upon the respiratory system for continuous speech and the use of a number of deleterious speaking behaviors to compensate for that physiological demand for prolonged utterances are examples.

Patterns of physiological problems of articulation may be observed in the test results. Lingua-palatal consonants (/k/, /g/, and /ŋ/) may be omitted or misarticulated, which suggests inability to elevate the dorsum of the tongue sufficiently for the needed contact. Consistent omission or misarticulation of voiceless consonants suggests velopharyngeal incompetence in this and the cleft palate population, and the frequent pattern of voiced for voiceless consonants may be a compensatory behavior for that and other sources of aerodynamic inefficiency of the vocal tract in developmental dysarthria.

There are some general patterns of misarticulation associated with developmental dysarthria that can be anticipated in addition to the tendency to voice all consonants. It has long been known (e.g., Byrne, 1959) that consonants developed later by normally speaking children are more likely to be misarticulated by children with developmental dysarthria. While there have been various explanations for the normal developmental sequence of consonants, the extent to which various consonants tax the aerodynamic-mechanical ability of the involved speech-producing musculatures probably is a prime contributor to this pattern in cerebral palsied speakers. There also will be a tendency for consonants to be misarticulated more in the postvocalic than the prevocalic position. Speech production undoubtedly requires more physical effort for the dysarthric cerebral palsied speaker than for the normal speaker. Therefore, such a speaker may have adopted a speech pattern of not maintaining the physiological effort required to completely articulate a syllable that has a postvocalic consonant.

Some reasons for the disparity between conversational speech and production of single words may be evident from the articulation inventory. Although the perception may have been formed that the speaker routinely used voiced for voiceless consonants during conversational speech attempts, he or she may have produced most voiceless consonants correctly during the single-word articulation inventory. In those cases it might be assumed that the voiced for voiceless substitution pattern is, indeed, learned behavior as described in Chapter Five.

It would be premature, however, to assume that the articulations in single words compared to those in running speech represent all of the patterns of functional overlay of articulation that might be present. The speaker may show even greater ability to articulate correctly when the production of phone-types is elicited in an even simpler context. Consequently, attempts should be made to elicit each consonant in a single CV syllable context in which the vowel is a neutral. The speaker's ability to produce consonant clusters in CCV, CCCV, and VCC syllables also may be determined. The speaker may correctly articulate some of the consonants and clusters in these syllables that he or she produced incorrectly in the single-word articulation test.

Testing Production of Vowels and Diphthongs. Under the assumption that problems in producing vowels during conversation and production of words may result from difficulty with tongue gestures of proximal consonants, the speaker's ability to produce vowels should be assessed in phonetic contexts that, to the extent possible, are not associated with such gestures. However, isolated steady-state vowels are relatively difficult to perceive accurately; moreover, as mentioned earlier, the transitions from consonant articulations to the target positions for vowels may be as important to speech intelligibility as other components of the speech signal.

Using those consonants that are produced well in the above-described production of CV syllables, the examiner may consider eliciting them again in CV syllables with vowels that represent the extremes of the vowel triangle (i.e.,/i/, /ɑ/, and /u/). The production of all diphthongs also might be elicited in CV syllables with those consonants.

This type of testing could be carried on to the extreme by use of each vowel in combination with each consonant. However, using the three vowels that call for extremes of tongue positioning should give an indication of the speaker's ability to move the tongue to form the appropriate resonance chambers for production of vowel transitions and vowels.

Patterns of Physiological Dysfunction and Functional Overlay. From the display of misarticulations by manner and place of consonants and place of vowels, patterns of dysfunction of the articulators may be even more apparent than from the results of only the single-word articulation test. A somewhat selective problem of elevation of the tongue tip might be suggested by omission of misarticulation of /t/, /d/, /n/, /s/, /z/, /tʃ/, /dʒ/, and /l/. That problem might be confirmed by misarticulation of /i/ (e.g., consistent substitution of /I/ in conjunction with all consonants, including bilabials, which place minimal physiological constraints on the tongue for vowels that are proximal to the consonant.

In addition to revealing such patterns of physiological dysfunction, the results of the assessment of consonant articulations and vowel productions may also give a hierarchy of functional overlay to the physiological restrictions to such articulations and productions. All of the above listed consonants may have been misarticulated in the single-word articulation test, but /t/, /d/, and /n/ may have been articulated well in the CV syllables; moreover, the vowel /i/ may have been produced well in conjunction with those correct articulations. The implication of this type of finding is, of course, that the speaker has shown physiological capability of making lingua-alveolar stop contacts for articulations under certain circumstances and, theoretically, he or she should be able to learn to use those contacts consistently. That may or may not prove to be the case.

The procedures described earlier in this chapter for determining the contributions of respiratory system and velopharyngeal port function to the speech problem call for production of CV syllables that are produced reasonably well. Those CV syllables may be chosen from the results of the procedure described immediately above. As is the case for the above suggestions for assessing the speaker's ability to produce vowels, selected speakers with developmental dysarthria for whom all of these procedures are appropriate may not produce consonants well enough to form the called-for sets of CV syllables. When that circumstance arises, the examiner should use CV syllables that will best meet the criteria of approximating normal articulatory gestures where it seems reasonable to do so.

There are additional steps to determining the extent of functional overlay of articulatory function and other general aspects of speech generation that involve instructing the speaker to change his or her method of using the speech mechanism. Therefore, it may be best to defer those steps until at least the manner in which the speaker usually uses the respiratory and laryngeal systems, as well as the function of the velopharyngeal port mechanism, has been determined as described earlier.

Further Assessment of Functional Articulatory Overlay. When the point is reached in the assessment where the speech-language pathologist begins to determine the extent to which the speaker can make changes in his or her speech, it may be desirable to return to elicitation of CV syllables. The speaker may be coached to articulate more accurately those syllables that were not well articulated. With such coaching, which may include demonstrations by the examiner, the speaker may improve some of the consonant articulations and vowel productions over the earlier attempts. Again, an indication of the physiological capability of the speaker will have been determined.

Effects of Speaking Rate and Effort. Coaching and demonstration of changes in speaking behavior should include attempts to have the speaker vary his or her speaking rate and effort. The speech samples may be any words, phrases, or longer utterances that the examiner can elicit in a manner that the speaker may produce repetitively and for which the examiner has a good impression of the general quality with which they are produced without special instruction.

The speech of many speakers with developmental dysarthria will improve spontaneously when they slow their speech rate. Such improvement is unlikely when they attempt faster speech rates.

Some cerebral palsied speakers who routinely seem to be attempting to drive the speech airstream through a hyperfunctioning laryngeal mechanism and/or moving the oral structures laboriously within what appears to be a background of generalized muscle contraction may improve the quality of their speech substantially when they are instructed or coached to speak at a reduced intensity level and with instructions such as, "Don't try so hard." For those who seem to be speaking with insufficient effort, improvement may result from their attempting to increase their overall vocal intensity, such as when they are asked to talk loudly to the examiner from across the examining room.

A distinction should be made between the variable of the physiological effort with which the speech signal is generated, as described above, and maintaining an appropriate effort throughout an utterance. As mentioned previously, the tendency for speakers with developmental dysarthria to omit or slight postvocalic consonants frequently seems to be a result of the latter. It may be possible for these speakers to articulate such consonants reasonably well when their attention is called to the desirability of maintaining the effort that is needed to produce all components of an utterance.

The greatest degree of spontaneous speech improvement may be realized through varying simultaneously both rate and effort (e.g., slowing the rate and speaking with greater and sustained effort). Also, the examiner may notice that the speaker is changing the manner in which he or she is using the speech physiology mechanism to bring about these rate and effort differences. For example, if a child is successful in speaking at a slower rate with more desirable, greater effort, the examiner may observe that he or she also is increasing the depth of inhalations prior to each phrase or utterance. Regardless of how the speaker has accomplished such changes, an indication of a potentially realistic management goal will have been obtained when the speaker can readily modify rate and effort, with the result of improved speech.

planning the management program

Careful integration of the perceived characteristics of the speech signal and observations of speech-producing behaviors that have been obtained should make it possible to outline reasonably specific goals for management. Moreover, some of these goals may be established as achievable in a shorter period of time than others.

The relatively short-term goals usually will be in reference to changes in the deleterious speech-producing behaviors discussed in Chapter Five as functional overlay to the developmental dysarthria. Among those goals, highest priority should be given to changing those general aspects of speech behavior that should lead to overall improvement in the quality of speech production and those that may lead to elimination of other deleterious speech-producing behaviors. These may include production of relatively short phrases or utterances at appropriate levels of the lung volume, reduction in speech rate, and use and maintenance of appropriate physiological effort for speech production. As will be emphasized in the following chapter on management programs, attaining habitual changes in even those behaviors will usually require management of reasonably long duration due to the presence of the neuromotor disorder and the difficulty the speaker may have in establishing any such changes as a routine part of his of her speaking behavior.

Goals for changing the speech-producing motor patterns that seem to require expanding the physiological limit of the mechanism probably will require an even longer duration of management. Frequently, these long-term goals may prove unrealistic, as may some of the short-term goals.

The tenability of some of the goals can be judged by careful review of all of the assessment findings. For example, even though a speaker may have shown better ability to articulate some consonants in CV syllables as compared to words, a review of those consonants may reveal that some are those with which maintenance of intraoral air pressures is associated; in addition, there may be firm indications of some velopharyngeal incompetence. It would seem unlikely that improvement can be expected in the routine articulation of those consonants in longer speech segments that also have components requiring generation of intraoral air pressures. The speaker may be unable to compensate for the incompetence for more than one syllable on an expiration, particularly if he or she has significant respiratory dysfunction.

statement of prognosis

The speech-language pathologist should discipline herself or himself to make a prognostic statement whenever the assessment has proceeded to the point where potentially realistic short-term and long-term goals can be established. Of course, specification of such goals is, in and of itself, a declaration of prediction of improvement.

It should be assumed that any set of management goals, and the implied prognosis, will be subject to change as the management proceeds. Impressions that were formed early will be revised, and specific aspects of motor behavior that seemed rather easily subject to change will prove not to be so; some motor behaviors that appeared highly resistant to change will prove to be changeable. As a result, any prognostic impressions also will be subject to change, but there should be a rigorous attempt made to keep a realistic total outcome of the management program in mind.

associated disabilities and problems

Of course, the assessment process will not be complete until it has been determined whether those associated disabilities and problems discussed in Chapter Eight are confounding the dysarthric problem. As emphasized earlier, the presence of any such associated disability or problem is likely to affect adversely the prognosis that would otherwise be predicted for a general case of developmental dysarthria.

The most crucial aspect of the clinical process regarding developmental dysarthria is assessing the problem. That assessment should lead to determination of therapeutic goals and suggest the management program that will achieve those goals.

There are patterns of distribution of the neuromotor involvement in cerebral palsy that are predictable for large numbers of cases in which the predominant neuromotor disorder is spasticity or dyskinesia. There are also deviations from these general patterns that are seen frequently. As a consequence, it is possible to predict many of the characteristics of the general case of developmental dysarthria based upon these commonly seen patterns of distribution and characteristics of the neuromotor disorder throughout the speech-producing musculatures. The general nature of the problem also can be described for other types of neuromotor disorders within the cerebral palsied population.

The assessment process entails eliciting a variety of speech activities that are designed to ascertain (1) the specific characteristics of the speech-production problem, (2) the manner with which the speaker usually uses his or her speech-producing system, and (3) ways in which that use can be modified to improve the speech signal. Although the results must be integrated in a way that reflects the activity of the speech-producing system, it is helpful to analyze the problem from a base of knowledge regarding the operation of the respiratory, phonatory, and articulatory mechanisms of the normal speaker and the expected deviations that may be found in speakers with developmental dysarthria. The assessment process also should include procedures to ascertain the physiological limitations of those mechanisms for speech production.

The assessment procedures also should reveal the presence of deleterious behaviors that the speaker has developed in the attempt to produce speech in the presence of his or her speech-physiology problems. The extent to which the speaker can modify those behaviors and the indications of the physiological limits of that speaker's speech producing mechanisms may be used to outline a set of short-term and long-term management goals. This initial plan of the management program should also lead to a statement of the prognosis of the extent to which the speaker with developmental dysarthria can be expected to improve his or her speech-producing capability.

These guidelines require modification to the extent that the individual case also has any of the numerous other disabilities and disorders that are frequently associated with cerebral palsy and that also affect the individual's ability to respond to a speech habilitation program. Of course, the design of the management program and the anticipated outcome also will frequently require modification as the clinical program is carried out.

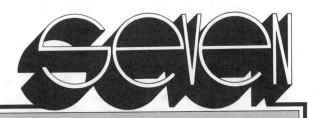

Management of developmental dysarthria: The general case

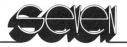

The bulk of the material in this chapter should be generally applicable to school-age and adult persons with cerebral palsy who have speech production problems due to obvious neuromotor involvement of the speech-producing musculatures and a reasonably good prognosis for improving their oral communication. A later section will deal with additional considerations for individuals who have relatively mild involvement of the speech-producing musculatures and for whom the overall management goal will be to improve the quality of the speech signal in the presence of usual intelligibility. Suggestions for work with infants and younger children and the individual with extremely severe neuromotor involvement of the speech-producing musculatures will be discussed in later chapters.

The management program and therapeutic activities described are those that are most appropriately carried out by, or under the direction of, the clinical speech-language pathologist. Under the assumption that the clientele of most readers of this book will be children of elementary school age, a number of the specific therapeutic activities will be described in the context of that age group. The goals of a management program for most older individuals and the changes to be made in their speech-producing behaviors are comparable.

The discussion of management in this chapter deals with the general case for improvement specifically of developmental dysarthria. Selection of the activities to be used and the expectations of the outcome will be different for cerebral-palsied children who have additional disorders and disabilities, such as mental retardation. The statements that are made also may need qualification as a result of a concomitant program of management of the overall neuromotor problem (e.g., a positioning program). Such considerations must be integrated into the management programs of the speech-production problem that are given here.

○ PLANNING MANAGEMENT

The concluding statements in Chapter Six referred to the possibility of establishing what were called short-term and long-term goals. The former term was used in reference to modification of those deleterious speech-producing behaviors that seem to be currently within the physiological capability of the speaker. The latter referred to objectives that call for establishing speech-production behaviors that are not within the current capability of the speaker. These concepts should be quite useful in designing a management plan.

priorities for management goals

From among those deleterious speech-producing behaviors that appear to be within the capability of the speaker to change, it frequently will be possible to determine those that (1) seem most subject to modification, (2) will contribute most substantially to overall improvement in the speech signal, and (3) will permit the speaker to make other desirable changes. Slowing the speech rate, for example, may make it physiologically possible for the speaker to accomplish a number of other desirable changes. As a consequence of such relations among potential goals of management, priorities for emphasis within the management goals can be established. Although, as will be discussed later, a number of aspects of the speech-production problem probably should receive attention concomitantly, those that meet the above criteria should be given primary emphasis in the clinical regimen.

If the results of the assessment indicate that a cerebral palsied speaker can routinely use lung volume levels for speech generation over which the respiratory system has better capability to drive the inefficient vocal tract, a number of additional realistic short-term goals may be established. Generalized overflow of undesirable muscle contractions may diminish; as a result, the individual may be able to control the magnitude of the general physiological effort with which he or she produces speech. That more appropriate physiological effort may result in improved prosody and vocal quality, the individual may be better able to control vocal pitch and intensity, and most important, it may be possible for the individual to maintain much better the air pressures within the vocal tract that are requisite to speech-sound articulation. Thus, by establishing a prime goal for modification of speech breathing, a number of other management goals may be feasible.

As given in the example above, there may be strong indications that the individual can improve his or her speech by using a slower speaking rate. Slower speech rates will frequently result in a general improvement in the precision of consonant articulations and vowel productions. The individual may be able to eliminate omissions of some phone-types, and a pattern of routinely omitting production of postvocalic consonants may not be subject to change until the speech rate is slower than that which the speaker routinely uses. Although the speaker may have adopted a pattern of using voiced for voiceless consonants primarily to conserve the aerodynamic energy that his or her respiratory system must generate to drive the vocal tract, a reduction in the speed with which the vocal cords can abduct may have been a contributor to the speaker's having learned that pattern. At slower speech rates, use of voiceless consonants may be possible, and production of those consonants may be facilitated even more by improved use of the respiratory system for speech production.

A number of the examples of potential assessment results given in Chapter Six suggests another frequently desirable general goal, namely the duration of utterances produced between inspirations should be relatively short. As will be emphasized, production of relatively short segments of speech on one expiration may lead to overall improvement of some aspects of speech production even though a speaker seems unable to modify use of the respiratory system.

Remediation of specific sets of articulatory errors will seldom result in a generalized improvement of the individual's speech. Nevertheless, to the extent that the assessment procedures have identified specific misarticulation patterns that the speaker appears to be capable of modifying quite easily, such modification may be incorporated into the early stages of the management process. Later discussions of therapeutic activities will review how work on specific articulatory errors can be accomplished in conjunction with activities designed to modify the more general deleterious speech-producing behaviors. There is no implication intended that attention to specific articulatory problems should be deferred until some degree of change has been accomplished in other aspects of speech production. To the contrary, as the potential for modification of misarticulation behaviors becomes apparent, and as the capability of the speaker to respond to therapeutic activities is learned, it will be natural to begin directing more and more attention to those misarticulations. The point is that modification of misarticulation patterns infrequently should be established as an initial, sole short-term management goal that receives primary emphasis for cases of developmental dysarthria.

It should be obvious that those changes in speech-producing behaviors that might be classified as long-term goals may be very difficult to accomplish. Months of carefully planned therapeutic activities may demonstrate that it is extremely difficult for a speaker with developmental dysarthria to extend the physiological limits of selected aspects of his or her speech-producing mechanism.

This discussion may imply that those changes in speech-producing behaviors that are referred to in the context of short-term goals will be easy to accomplish. No such implication is intended, and it would be unrealistic to anticipate such an outcome of therapeutic activities.

Even those changes that can be brought about relatively easily in clinical sessions may prove very difficult for the speaker to incorporate into his or her habitual speech. The problem of "carry-over" from the clinical situation is usual with any type of speech-production problem, and the special problems of carry-over with this population will be treated later. The point here is that as long as the speaker domonstrates an ability to use a new and desirable speech-producing skill in the clinical situation, routine use of that skill should be maintained as a management goal.

revisions of goals

Continual reappraisal of initially established goals is requisite to efficacious management. The concluding discussions of Chapter Six gave an example of how the presence of highly significant velopharyngeal incompetence might eventually require modification of what initially were thought to be realistic short-term goals. Revisions of management goals, however, are not always in a negative direction. A child who has habitually come to attempt speech by what might be called surges of generalized physiological effort may have been unable to modify significantly his dysprosody and strained vocal quality throughout the assessment and early management program. However, if improvement in articulation was noted when he attempted to produce speech at relatively high levels of the lung volume, that use of the respiratory system might have been established as a management goal. As progress is made toward achieving that goal, that use of a more appropriate physiological effort for speech production may become possible, with a resulting diminution of severity of the dysprosody and deviant voice quality. The management goals should be revised accordingly.

Continuing reappraisal of the results of work toward a short-term goal may show, at any stage, that progress is slowing. The speaker's current physiological capability to improve that aspect of his or her speech production may have been reached. Whether that limit is recognized initially, or whether it becomes apparent from work in progress, the clinical process will then require motivating the speaker to engage in repetitions of motor behaviors over a long period of time with minimal immediate rewards.

Continued objective analysis of the results of the management program may strongly suggest that work on a particular aspect of the problem should be given lower priority or be terminated. Lowering the priority of or even terminating work on one aspect of the problem is not necessarily an indication that further progress cannot be achieved with other aspects.

○ GENERAL CONSIDERATIONS FOR MANAGEMENT

General considerations that are applicable to both assessment and management of developmental dysarthria were reviewed in Chapter Five.

There are other general considerations that relate primarily to the management process.

maintaining records

Realistic reappraisal of management goals and the prediction of the outcome of management will usually be dependent on maintaining clinical records of all types that will promote objective analysis of progress or lack thereof. The inherent long durations of these programs require extra efforts to maintain objectivity.

It is very easy to become persuaded erroneously that significant progress is being made. An engaging personality of a child, consistent efforts on his or her part to perform therapeutic activities, and the clinician's familiarity with the child's speech pattern can contribute to such deception. Tape recordings of structured speech samples that have been made over a period of months may indicate that progress has been made in performance of therapeutic activities, yet recordings over that period of attempts at spontaneous conversation for which the context is not known may demonstrate that minimal progress is being made toward intelligible functional oral communication.

On the other hand, notes and tape recordings can demonstrate that significant progress is, in fact, being made. Parents, because of their consistent contact with their child, may fail to appreciate their child's slow steady improvement. Their listening to tape recordings made some months in the past may be very encouraging to them. Such notes and recordings may also demonstrate significant long-term progress to professional persons who may be working with the speaker.

working toward goals simultaneously

I have come to believe firmly that the management plan for improvement of developmental dysarthria should involve concomitant work on as many aspects of the problem as is possible. This belief may seem to violate a general principle of management to which many speech-language pathologists strongly subscribe. Programs of management for children with functional articulation problems routinely call for concentration on selected sets of phone-types at one time. That approach may be appropriate for the child who has no difficulty in modifying his or her motor patterns, and it is reasonable to expect that when such a child incorporates improved production of some phone-types into his or her spontaneous speech that the management program can then move to improvement of other phone-types. Moreover, it also is reasonable to assume that when the bases of a speech-learning problem include, for reasons that may not be known, confusion on the part of a child in learning the speech-articulatory process, the introduction of a variety of articulations into the management program may unduly delay progress. Such an approach should not be generalized to management of the speech-production problems associated with developmental dysarthria. As has been emphasized strongly, improvement in any aspect of producing the speech signal with this population is likely to be slow, and the most efficacious plan of management usually calls for achieving a number of goals simultaneously.

Specific therapeutic activities may be designed to achieve one specific goal (e.g., training a child to slow his or her speech rate). However, if it has been determined that a child can realistically be expected to improve specific articulations, the speech samples used in the activity for rate change can, and probably should, include those particular phone-types. It may be surprising to find that even relatively young children with developmental dysarthria can productively concentrate on simultaneously improving a variety of speech-producing behaviors.

The probability of confusing a child by working toward a variety of goals simultaneously is highest in the area of articulatory remediation. Nevertheless, where there are strong indications that a child is physiologically capable of improving his or her articulations of a number of phone-types, serious consideration should be given to simultaneous work for remediation of a number of those misarticulations. The approach should be that the speaker's ability to tolerate work toward a number of goals at the same time should be tested.

avoiding maximum physiological efforts

From my point of view, engaging speakers with developmental dysarthria in therapeutic activities that promote maximum physiological effort is to be avoided. The potential deleterious effects on motor behavior that has been referred to as overflow has been discussed. The possibility that this type of reaction may result from maximum efforts should be sufficient to cause the speech-language pathologist to consider with great caution the use of activities that call for such effort.

In addition, the muscular activity associated with speech production represents an exceedingly precise type of motor activity involving delicate, rapid adjustments of muscle tension. The most efficacious type of training for such motor skills seldom involves activities that call for maximum effort in either rate of movement or force of muscular contractions. Rather, such training probably should concentrate on accuracy of appropriate gestures and achieving target positions at a rate that is within the capability of the system. After the motor patterns are reasonably well established, the training may be directed toward increasing the rate of performance and use of varying degrees of force to refine that performance. The design of therapeutic activities for motor speech training should include these considerations.

monitoring speech production

There may be a strong inclination to assume that speakers with developmental dysarthria monitor their own oral output well enough for them to appreciate the need for many desirable changes in specific aspects of their own speech signal. The assumption is quite natural in view of the nature of the problem.

These speakers, however, are frequently unaware of even relatively gross deviations in their own speech. They may have strongly negative reactions to hearing their own speech from a tape recorder. They may work with considerable concentration toward achieving desirable changes in a specific thereapeutic activity. Yet, when they are participating in some other activity, they may be unable to indicate whether or not they have used those changes when they were talking during the second activity.

Therapeutic activities may include negative practice in which the speaker with developmental dysarthria is purposefully directed to produce some aspect of his or her speech in the premanagement manner and contrast that with the production of the improved manner. Frequent checking, by any means that may be devised to determine that the speaker is monitoring well his or her own speech, should be a component of the management program. Moreover, it cannot be assumed that appropriate monitoring will continue without continuing supportive assistance with that skill. Carry-over of newly learned skills and maintenance of gains that have been made in a management program may depend on such assistance.

programs for carry-over

A number of factors have been mentioned that may contribute to problems of carry-over to other speaking situations of desirable speech-producing behaviors that have been established in clinical sessions. The inherent difficulty in changing motor patterns in the presence of a neuromotor disorder in and of itself requires that carefully designed programs for carry-over should be considered as a part of the management program.

To the extent possible, all of those professional persons who are involved with the cerebral palsied individual's management should be made aware of the goals of the program and the progress that is being made. Those who are in a position to assist directly should be provided with the needed specifics of the plan. For children, of course, parents should be involved to the extent that seems reasonable and practical within each family's circumstance.

Because of the complexities of the speech-producing behaviors that are involved, it probably is unreasonable to expect that other professional people, parents, or care personnel can adequately participate in the management program simply on the basis of plans that are provided through discussion or written communication. To the extent that it is possible to do so, the speech-language pathologist should work with the speaker in those persons' presence, demonstrating the specific behaviors that can be expected outside of the clinical situation. Not only will all concerned have a better understanding of what is to be expected on the part of the speaker, but the speaker also will be aware of the expectations for his or her speaking behaviors outside of the clinical situation. There may be limits to which that awareness can be maintained in younger children. However, if the expectations for the desired changes and any associated reward program are used with a great deal of consistency, even young children will come to anticipate those expectations, and the probability that they will respond favorably will be increased.

Care should be taken in determining the number and variety of changes to be routinely expected outside the clinical situation. A cerebral palsied child should not be expected to concentrate on his speech-producing behaviors to the detriment of performance in classroom activities. Recommendations for direct participation with care workers or parents also should take into account that a child needs some relief from consistent attempts to improve a behavior. The classroom teacher, physical therapist, and other professional persons must also concentrate on helping the child develop other skills. It is easy to assume that parents should be able to devote considerable time to working on their cerebral palsied child's speech; however, parents may in fact find it very difficult to devote time to a home speech program to the extent that may be desirable. As will be emphasized later, the speech-language pathologist must *never* forget that professionally recommended programs should not be imposed on interactions in the home that may jeopardize desirable parent-child relationships.

○ THERAPEUTIC PROCEDURES

As in the discussion of assessment procedures in Chapter Six, some of the following discussion of therapeutic procedures is organized within topic headings that call attention to selected mechanisms of the speech-producing system. Again, this editorial organization is not meant to imply that work toward improving the function of one portion of the system (e.g., the respiratory mechanism) should proceed independently from consideration of other mechanisms (e.g., the lips, jaw, and tongue). Even though specific management goals and therapeutic activities relate to one specific aspect of speech production, constant attention must be given to the effect of the changes in that one aspect on the total speech-producing system.

Improving use of the respiratory system

I have become quite pessimistic regarding the possibility that the capability of the respiratory systems of persons with developmental dysarthria to drive the vocal tract can be extended to any significant degree. I have not achieved success through use of blowing exercises or any type of non-speech-producing maneuvers of the respiratory system, and I have not been satisfied that others whom I have observed using such procedures were obtaining sufficient results to merit the activity.

Use of abdominal corsets has been suggested (Westlake and Rutherford, 1961). I have never witnessed the use of such devices, nor am I aware that their use has received general acceptance. If such corsets were elastic and fastened tightly around the abdomen, they might assist with expiration through contraction of the abdomen, which would force the diaphragm into the thoracic cavity. Such a device would also serve to reduce the ability of the individual to inspire, and as a consequence, the volume of air that could be inhaled would be restricted. Since there is the potential that the individual's ability to inspire may be reduced, such a procedure should be used with great caution and probably under the supervision of a physician. Frankly, I do not recommend it.

Another procedure that I have frequently seen used is to work with the speaker in a supine position. When the body is upright, gravity pulls the abdominal contents down and thus flattens the diaphragm. In a supine position, those contents will tend to push the diaphragm into the thoracic cavity and thus assist in expiration. There is, again, a trade-off, in that inspiratory ability will not be as good since the diaphragm must push against the abdominal contents for inflation of the lungs. Therefore, as with the use of elastic abdominal corsets, even if an improved capability for generating expiratory air pressures is realized, a reduced ability to inspire would shorten the duration of utterances over which the respiratory system could be expected to drive the vocal tract. However, there is little difference in the respiratory function of cerebral palsied speakers who have extensive involvement of the respiratory system as a result of static differences in posture (Hardy, 1964). Evidently, because of the restricted flexibility of their torso wall muscles, there is little change in the respiratory function capability of such speakers whether they are lying prone, sitting, or lying supine.

During the era of accelerated interest in cerebral palsy, mentioned in Chapter Two, respirators and an instrument called the electrolung were used in attempts to modify the speech-breathing function of this population. That procedure actually reduced cerebral palsied children's ability to generate expiratory air pressures.

It is more practical to assume that these speakers may be better able to drive their vocal tracts by speaking at the upper levels of the lung volume, where greater expiratory air pressures are possible, than it is to assume that any procedure will increase their ability to generate the needed air pressures. The desirability of training cerebral palsied speakers to inflate their lungs to relatively high lung volume levels prior to initiating speech is not a newly expressed idea (e.g., McDonald and Chance, 1964). Moreover, such training frequently includes prolonging the ensuing speech production for as long as possible on one expiration, and the usual activity for working toward prolongation of speech production on one expiration is to have the speaker sustain a vowel. As pointed out in Chapter Six, a sustained vowel probably represents the optimum condition of valving the speech-generating airstream; therefore, prolonging vowels is not comparable to the physiological activity of the vocal tract during conversational speech.

For reasons already cited, asking the speaker to prolong any type of speech on one expiration in a way that requires maximum expiratory efforts is probably contraindicated. The most effective procedures for reducing the effect of respiratory dysfunction, therefore, may be to train the speaker to produce speech within the limits of the respiratory system.

Speaking within Limits of the Respiratory System. The assessment procedures to determine the contribution of respiratory dysfunction to the developmental dysarthria described in Chapter Six will demonstrate if there will be general improvements in speech when relatively high lung volume levels are used. They will also indicate the length of utterances that can be produced before the lower level of the lung volume is reached, causing those general improvements to begin to deteriorate. In the numerous cases where this will be the finding, a reasonable management goal may be to establish the following use of the respiratory system for speech production: (1) Prior to each phrase or utterance that is to be produced over one expiration, there should be an inspiration to a relatively high lung-volume level where the relaxation recoil of the respiratory system will assist in generating the needed air pressures within the vocal tract in the presence of a relatively continuous reduction in volume; (2) since the lung volume levels over which such pressures can be generated can be expected to be relatively restricted, and since the volume of air expired in producing even such short utterances may be excessive due to inefficient valving of the speech-producing airstream, the length of the phrase or utterance to be produced on one expiration must be kept relatively short; (3) there should be an inhalation back to the higher level of lung volume prior to production of the ensuing phrase or utterance.

By "an inhalation back to the higher level of lung volume," I do not necessarily mean to imply a maximal inspiratory effort in all cases. Even some older cerebral palsied children, who can respond to direct instructions and demonstrations of how to use their respiratory systems, seem to have significant problems in maximally inflating their lungs and then controlling the generation of the speech airstream against the elastic recoil of the respiratory system. They routinely expire some air prior to beginning such a phrase for utterance. Thus, the additional potential of aerodynamic energy that might be gained by maximum inspiratory effort is, in fact, lost before they begin the utterance. Also, the principal of avoiding maximum efforts that result in increased dysfunction applies. On the other hand, many speakers with cerebral palsy seem to be continually able to inspire maximally between each phrase or utterance and to begin speech production with the initiation of expiration.

Whether the inspirations used are maximal or not, the utterance that is produced should not be so extensive as to deflate the lungs to levels where the needed air pressures within the vocal tract can be produced only with extreme physiological effort. It should also be recognized that the duration of such utterances will vary as a function of the phonology of the utterance. Recall the statements made earlier that greater magnitudes of airflow are associated with some phone-types (e.g., voiceless sibilants and fricatives) than others (e.g., voiced stops).

There usually is little difficulty in motivating older children to respond to direct instructions and demonstrations of how they should modify their speech-breathing patterns. However, younger children in the elementary-school age range may experience considerable difficulty in responding to direct instructions to inhale more deeply prior to each phrase or utterance of limited length. Of course, this is also the age where gamelike motivating activities may be most successful.

Under no circumstance, and for the reasons explained in Chapter Five, would I use procedures to bring about deep inspirations through inducing yawns. Neither would I use a procedure that has been recommended of holding a child's mouth and nostrils closed momentarily to prohibit them from inspiring so that when they are permitted to do so their inspirations will be relatively deep. I have seen that procedure used, and I have been convinced that it is routinely frightening to children, no matter how good the clinical relationship.

I also have observed activities in which the child inspired and produced speech in an enclosed respirometric system such as a spirometer, with a face mask covering the child's mouth and nose to trap all air. The object of the activity was to lower the spirometer bell as much as possible through a deep inspiration prior to the speech-producing effort. Such an activity cannot be maintained for many repetitions of inspiration and production of utterances unless there is some type of carbon-dioxide-absorbing material in the spirometer bell; otherwise the child's oxygen uptake will exhaust the oxygen in the device. Also, some physiologically normal individuals, including adults, have adverse reactions to breathing into a closed respirometric system that adds mechanical dead space to respiratory function. Other than those two potential difficulties, such an activity may be staged in a manner that does motivate the child to use the respiratory system in the desired manner, but because of the covering face mask, there is no opportunity to observe and monitor the accuracy and precision of the speech being produced.

It may be possible to construct a number of gamelike activities that will motivate young children to participate enthusiastically in work that is designed to modify the use of their respiratory system. Monitoring of their inspiratory and expiratory efforts during such activities may be accomplished by placing a hand over the epigastrium, with the fingers spread so that movements of both the thorax and abdomen may be felt. While carefully observing these movements, the clinician may engage the child in a number of inspiratory and expiratory activities. A tissue may be held suspended a few inches from the child's mouth, and a game may be made of sucking it toward and blowing it away from the mouth. Any light object that will move with a respiratory airstream of minimal force can be used, such as a ball of cotton suspended on a string.

The objective of such activities is not to improve the child's force of inspiration or expiration. Rather, these activities have two objectives: (1) the clinician should come to have confidence in determining the correspondence between contraction-expansion characteristics of the torso and the direction of the respiratory airstream, and (2) depending on the age and the ability of the child to comprehend the activity, the child's attention may be directed to consciously attending to his or her respiratory efforts. With regard to the latter, a child's perception of his or her respiratory maneuvers may be enhanced by feeling the pressure of the clinician's hand. With respect to the former objective, the clinician should not be surprised if the torso wall movements feel bizarre relative to what is expected. The torso wall of a child with dyskinesia, for example, may be felt to be writhing subtly under the hand on the epigastrium, but the respiratory airstream may be well controlled and of steady force.[1]

Once the clinician has confidence in monitoring when inspiration and expiration is taking place, activities designed to enhance further the speaker's awareness of respiratory maneuvers and modify the use of the respiratory system for speech production may begin. For example, by using a crayon to draw on paper, or chalk on a chalkboard, a wavy line may

[1]Much of the early study of speech breathing of cerebral speakers was done through observations of the expansion-contraction patterns of the torso walls with an instrument called a pneumograph. The limitations of that instrument notwithstanding, and there are many, a direct correspondence cannot be expected between the patterns of the torso wall and direction and speed of the respiratory airflow as measured by some instrument that directly senses that airflow. Even though their torso walls may show various patterns of contraction and expansion, the speech airstream usually will be steady and well controlled. Exceptions and their implications have been mentioned in Chapter Six.

be drawn across the paper by moving the crayon upward during inspiration and downward during expiration. Later, an object of such a game may be for the child to inspire and expire as the clinician moves the crayon through a predrawn path over "mountain tops" with the crayon moving up to the peak during an inspiration, and down to the next valley during an expiration. A toy monkey can be made to go up and down poles; toy superheroes can fly to the top of objects and back down. Even for children of elementary-school age, who can readily respond to direct instructions regarding respiratory maneuvers, it may be helpful to devise such games for respiratory speech-production activities.

At some early stage, phonation should be introduced on the expirations. The phonatory act that is to be a part of these activities may initially be a sustained vowel. However, other speech acts, such as CV syllables, should be introduced as soon as possible. The consonants and vowels that make up those syllables should be easily within the capability of the child. Later, when the child is engaging in activities designed to make such use of the respiratory system a habitual part of the child's speech-producing behaviors, the consonants and vowels whose production the child is attempting to improve can be used. Their production in single-syllable words that are repeated throughout the expiratory phase of the activity should be incorporated into the activity as soon as possible. Phrases used may include short sentences, and this respiratory training may be used to assist the child to produce various pitches and loudness levels if that type of voice training is a management goal. Even exercises related to speech rate may be incorporated; a toy clown may be made to go smoothly up an incline during inspiration, but in progressing downward, it must go slowly over a series of steps, with each step associated with a syllable.

To keep any child motivated to participate in these types of respiratory–speech-producing activities, the variety of activities must be extensive. Moreover, they must be presented in such a way that the child realizes that the prime task is to use his or her respiratory system in the desired manner. The quality of the speech act that is involved may not be a prime consideration initially; however, as soon as it is possible to do so without detracting from the respiratory maneuvers, the best quality of articulation and/or phonation should be required.

As a speaker begins to use the desired speech-breathing pattern habitually, consideration may be given to attempting to extend the physiological limit of the respiratory system for speech production. Work may be initiated to have the speaker fully inflate the lungs and begin speaking immediately upon beginning the expiration, or efforts may be made to have the speaker continue utterances over the lower levels of the vital capacity. As indicated earlier, more success is likely with the former. Nevertheless, I recommend that work toward even gradually extending that portion of the lung volume over which speech can be produced with ease be deferred until it is certain that the speaker is producing most other speech behaviors optimally within the limits of his or her neuromotor capability. It probably is counterproductive to ask that speech be produced at those levels of the lung volume at which improved characteristics of the speech signal deteriorate. Unfortunately, work over a long duration may show that with a large number of cases it is unrealistic to expect to be able to extend the levels of the lung volume over which optimally intelligible speech can be generated.

The probability should not be overlooked that by improving other aspects of speech production a speaker may reduce the contribution of the respiratory function problem to the dysarthria. As the precision of articulation improves, for example, the respiratory system may be better able to drive the vocal tract, and the number of syllables that can be produced relatively easily on one expiration may increase. For those speakers with developmental dysarthria whose respiratory musculatures are severely involved and their respiratory systems are incapable of producing more than one or two syllables on an expiration, the most realistic approach to improving their ability to produce longer phrases may be through improving the efficiency with which the structures of their vocal tracts valve the speech airstream.

Phrasing of Utterances. The potential need for a speaker with developmental dysarthria to produce relatively short utterances between inspirations has been mentioned in a number of contexts. This need should be considered initially in management programs of most speakers with developmental dysarthria.

No matter what the prime purpose of a given clinical activity, whenever a speech activity is elicited, the duration of the speech produced on one expiration should be within the limits of the speaker's respiratory system. The number of words to be repeated as parts of an articulation drill should be so phrased. When the sample is composed of grammatically intact words (e.g., subject-verb phrases, prepositional phrases), the speaker should be trained to recognize these logical phrase divisions and to use them in any attempt at oral communication. For some speakers, of course, linking such phrases to produce sentences on one expiration may be possible. For the more severely involved, for whom only one- or two-syllable phrases may be reasonable, not only may the grammatically organized phrases need to be divided, but even multisyllable words may have to be produced on more than one expiration.

My experience suggests that even relatively young children rather easily come to understand logical phrase divisions. However, probably because such phrased speech is unnatural compared to that which they routinely hear, it may be difficult to motivate them to attend routinely to this aspect of their oral communication attempts. That may be so even though with appropriate phrasing they are more intelligible.

management of laryngeal dysfunction

Some cases will be encountered in which laryngeal dysfunction appears to be the prime limiting factor to intelligible speech. The relatively rare cases in which there is apparently inability to adduct the vocal folds or the somewhat more frequent cases of inability to drive hyperfunctioning vocal folds into phonation are examples. However, the more frequent type of limiting laryngeal dysfunction is that of severe hyperfunction, in which the phonation that is possible seems to require extreme degrees of physiological effort. Phonatory efforts may be described as sounding "strained," and the individual may be able to do little more than produce a relatively undifferentiated vowel.

All of these extreme cases of laryngeal dysfunction usually coexist with relatively severe degrees of involvement of other speech-producing musculatures. The impression is frequently gained, however, that if the laryngeal behavior could be modified, some functional intelligible speech would be possible. It has been my experience, unfortunately, that such modification is extremely difficult. Even though a trial period of management probably should be attempted, the presence of these laryngeal behaviors is an indicator of a negative prognosis for development of functional oral communication.

For somewhat less severe cases of laryngeal dysfunction, the assessment results may indicate that some improved vocal quality can be expected within a relatively restricted range of pitch and loudness levels. Moreover, it will frequently be found that such phonatory improvement occurs only in conjunction with appropriate use of the respiratory system, as described above. There will appear to be a very delicate balance between the force with which the speech airstream must act with the vocal folds within the limited pitch and loudness levels. It may be extremely difficult for the speaker to maintain that balance when sustaining vowels, much less use the resulting improved phonatory behavior for speech production. Since there routinely are other aspects of speech production that must be modified before intelligible speech is obtained, it may be better to defer emphasis for improvement of phonation in these cases, and the prognosis may be for intelligible speech accompanied by some type of abnormal vocal quality.

An exception will be cases in which voiced consonants tend to be substituted consistently for voiceless consonants. If there is any indication that the speaker can produce voiceless consonants, I frequently will establish such production as an early management goal, as will be discussed later.

When at least some laryngeal muscle involvement is present, progress may be obtained in voice quality, initiation of phonation, and general voice usage as long as the therapy activities are restricted to vowel productions. For a number of speakers, incorporating these changes into speech production may be difficult. That is particularly so for the contributions that the laryngeal mechanism seems to make to prosody. It is with some reluctance that I offer these discouraging comments about modification of problems of voice usage in developmental dysarthria. Nevertheless, my experience dictates that I do so.

In those cases in which phonatory problems seem to be primarily the result of functional overlay, improvement of voice usage may realistically be established as an early management goal. Therapeutic activities designed to establish easy initiation of phonation, better pitch usage, and improved loudness usage may be comparable to those used with functional voice cases. Response to the voice therapy, however, seldom will be as good as with those cases. I tend to attribute this slow or limited progress to the inflexibility with which the speech airstream can be used, restricted mobility of neck musculatures, and/or problems of supralaryngeal muscle function that are imposed on the laryngeal complex. Again, substantial progress may be dependent on obtaining success in optimum use of the respiratory system and magnitudes of speech production effort.

There are notable exceptions. In some cases when other improved speech-producing behaviors begin to be used, relatively severe problems of voice quality and other undesirable aspects of voice usage may spontaneously improve to a remarkable degree. A voice that sounds "strained" and invariant in pitch may become more normal-sounding, and the speaker may be able to use some intonation changes after finding that it is unnecessary to attempt speech with extreme effort. That effort may have resulted in generalized muscle overflow throughout the speaker's musculatures, and generation of the maximum amount of force of the speech airstream may have seemed necessary to drive the hyperfunctioning vocal folds. Such changes may also result from improvement in supralaryngeal activity. A breathy voice and an articulation pattern that sounds as if voiced consonants are also produced with incompletely adducted vocal folds may become much less breathy as the aerodynamic inefficiency of the articulatory structures is reduced. This type of change is particularly evident in some cases where velopharyngeal incompetence is managed in some manner; the change in vocal quality may lead to the conclusion that, in the presence of the open velopharyngeal port, these speakers have attempted to compensate by forcing air through the vocal tract with great force and the vocal folds were remaining less than optimally adducted in order to permit the excessive airflow. In any cases of these types, incorporating specific voice therapy procedures to reinforce the improvement may bring about even better voice usage.

management of velopharyngeal dysfunction

For the reasons given in Chapter Five, management of velopharyngeal dysfunction is requisite to significant speech improvement in a number of individuals with developmental dysarthria. Recognition of that requirement led me to participate in surgical management of the problem in the late 1950s (Hardy et al., 1961). After the results of that program proved disappointing, palatal lift prostheses proved to be a viable alternative (Hardy et al., 1969), and I have continued to use prosthetic management of these cases of velopharyngeal incompetence since that time (LaVelle and Hardy, 1979).

Many of the potential benefits of resolution of velopharyngeal incompetence that are associated with developmental dysarthria are now recognized. Providing the speaker with the ability to generate and maintain the needed intraoral air pressures for consonant productions and generally increasing the aerodynamic efficiency of the vocal tract were assumed initially. As a result of the latter, an increase in the duration of utterances on one expiration and an increase in oral output also are frequent results. Undesirable phonatory behaviors also may diminish spontaneously in selected cases, as was mentioned in the discussion of laryngeal dysfunction. The discussion that follows regarding management of articulatory errors points out that there are occasions when the general ability of a speaker with developmental dysarthria improves, and some movement patterns begin to develop that previously seemed not to be within that speaker's capability. That phenomena may be observed in the behavior of the remainder of the articulatory structures of some of these speakers subsequent to management of their incompetence.

The tongues of cerebral palsied children tend to adopt a more normal position for vowel productions rather quickly after prosthetic management of their incompetence (Netsell, 1969b). That is so even in the presence of the restricted mobility of their tongues. The accoustic decoupling of the oral and nasal cavities evidently results in the mechanisms being used very quickly as a more normal acoustic generator.

That decoupling, of course, also eliminates hypernasality, the most frequently recognized symptom of the deficit. However, as has been strongly emphasized, the presence of hypernasality may be a relatively insignificant clinical problem of speakers with developmental dysarthria compared to the profound effect that incompetence has on the aerodynamic-mechanical integrity of the speech-producing system.

The significance of velopharyngeal incompetence that is associated with dysarthria is becoming generally recognized. Johns and Salyer (1978) have provided a comprehensive review of the literature and their experiences relative to its surgical and prosthetic management. Their discussion covers work both with adults who have acquired dysarthria and speakers with developmental dysarthria. Those authors' concluding remarks suggest that they believe pharyngeal flap surgery to be the procedure of choice.

Johns and Salyer mention an idea that has been expressed by others, namely, that palatal lifts facilitate the development of competence. After following over one hundred dysarthric speakers who have worn palatal lifts for a few years or more, I am convinced that the probability is quite low that permanent, improved velopharyngeal function will be realized. There is no doubt that after wearing one of these prostheses for a period of months, the velopharyngeal mechanisms of some dysarthric speakers may show substantial improvement in function for speech production, and I refuse to speculate as to the reasons for that improvement. Nevertheless, after those speakers have discontinued wearing their appliances for a number of months, the incompetence usually returns.

It is not the purpose here to debate the efficacy of either surgical or prosthetic management. I have observed persons with cerebral palsy and persons with an acquired dysarthria for whom palatal lifts have been constructed with minimal success. In addition, I have been involved with the design and construction of palatal lift prostheses for individuals from both groups of dysarthric speakers for whom the construction of the appliances was complicated by the presence of an ineffective pharyngeal flap. The success of either procedure is very likely to be dependent on a variety of characteristics of each speaker and the experience and skills of the professional people involved.[2]

There is no question that pharyngeal flap surgery is the procedure of choice where predictors of success are reasonably good. The wearing of an intraoral prosthesis is inconvenient, to say the least. Good intraoral hygiene is necessary; persons with restricted mobility of arm, hand, or fingers, will need assistance in extracting and inserting the appliance. Even so, I have come to recommend the use of palatal lift prostheses almost exclusively for cases of developmental dysarthria.

Johns and Sayler review the earlier problems that my colleagues and I experienced from pharyngeal flap surgeries with this population of speakers. There are strong indications, for example, that in order to be successful, the pharyngeal flap must be superiorly based. I would now add other requirements. The openings that are left between the lateral borders of the flap and the lateral pharyngeal walls must be exceedingly small, and there must be enough mesial movement of those lateral walls

[2]My preference for use of palatal lift prostheses undoubtedly results in large part from successful collaboration with prosthodontists. James W. Schweiger, who is currently affiliated with the Veteran's Administration Hospital in Wilmington, Delaware, was initially involved in developing this program. I have been working with William E. LaVelle, Department of Otolaryngology, at the University of Iowa, since 1972. Dr. LaVelle and I both evaluate and work together in design and construction of palatal lift prostheses. When a speech-language pathologist can be present during the actual molding of the velar portion of these appliances, the immediate effects of modifications of the appliance on the speech physiology status of the speaker can be judged. Moreover, the appliance can be recontoured until it appears that a maximally efficacious result has been obtained. It is unlikely that the positive results that I have observed would be possible without this collaboration. Also, I must acknowledge Ronald Netsell, Speech Pathologist, Boys Town Institute for Communicative Disorders, for his contributions to this program in its earlier stages.

during speech production to occlude even those openings. Otherwise, the remaining apertures may continue to (1) prohibit the ability to generate and maintain the intraoral air pressures needed for consonant productions and (2) permit sufficient loss of air through the nasal passages to seriously tax the respiratory systems of persons with cerebral palsy. In contrast, palatal lift prostheses usually can be constructed to lift the tissue of the soft palate into the lateral ports of the velopharyngeal port and, thus, provide complete occlusion of that port in cases where there is little or no lateral pharyngeal wall movement.

I personally have been involved with a few children with cerebral palsy whose velopharyngeal port mechanism seemed to respond to a clinical management program over a period of time. In each case, their ports closed, or approximated closure, intermittently during utterances. The procedures that appear to have resulted in improvement from that status have varied. In some cases, no special attention was devoted to this aspect of the problem; rather, as the speech remediation program proceeded, with concentration on general improvement of a number of characteristics of the speech production problem, the velopharyngeal port mechanism appeared to begin to function better as almost an artifact of concentration on and attending to improved speech-producing skills.

Some children respond favorably to working with a mirror held under their nostrils, as described in the discussion of assessment techniques for velopharyngeal incompetence in Chapter Six. After production of a syllable or two, the mirror can be raised to where they can view it easily so that they can determine if the mirror was clouded. Feathers or other light objects can be placed on a piece of thin cardboard or file card under the nostrils during a syllable or word production; the object, of course, is to produce the speech sample without the feather, or object, moving.

If therapeutic management of incompetence is to be undertaken, a number of cautions are in order: (1) it must be assumed that the dysfunctioning velopharyngeal port mechanism of some speakers with developmental dysarthria will not improve as a result of any type of speech remediation procedures; (2) if the incompetence is severe enough to negate the development of intelligible speech, it may be better to proceed immediately with a program of prosthetic and/or surgical management than to anticipate alleviating this prime speech physiology deficit over a long period of clinical work; (3) in cases where other speech physiology deficits are severe, and where there is question that management of the velopharyngeal dysfunction will enable the individual to develop intelligible speech, moving to a system of nonoral communication as described in Chapter Ten should be seriously considered; (4) where there seems to be a possibility that improvement can be achieved through clinical work, speech production should be used in the therapeutic activities; and (5) concentration on developing port closure for voiceless consonants is indicated since it is for those speech sounds that generation of intraoral air pressures is most needed.

For the reasons emphasized in Chapters Four and Five, I would never use a regimen of repeatedly eliciting a gag response under the assumption that such a regimen will lead to improved velopharyngeal function for speech production. Neither would I use blowing exercises under the assumption that directing the expiratory airstream orally will lead to the mechanism's occluding the oral from the nasal cavities. I have used such exercises with cerebral palsied children under the assumption that, with the presence of anatomically sufficient tissue to close the velopharyngeal port, directing the expiratory airstream orally during blowing would have a beneficial effect; I have become convinced that such a procedure is *not* effective in promoting palatal movement during speech with this population.

Throughout the discussion of the ramifications of velopharyngeal port dysfunction in Chapter Five, assessment of its presence in Chapter Six, and the discussion of its management here, the phrase "significant incompetence" has been used without precise definition. A critical area of velopharyngeal port opening that will create an insurmountable aerodynamic problem for speech production cannot be specified across speakers. For some cerebral palsied speakers who have reasonably good respiratory function, a consistent port opening of only a few square millimeters seems to be devastating; when the port is closed, as with a palatal lift prosthesis, the relatively immediate speech improvement may be remarkable.

changes in speech rate

Most speakers with developmental dysarthria produce speech at relatively slow rates. Nevertheless, it may be totally unrealistic to anticipate that such slow rates can be increased without further deterioration of speech intelligibility. The presence of the neuromotor disorder dictates an orientation toward not expecting normal rates of speech production. The discussion in Chapter Four of the underlying basis for spasticity points clearly to the high probability that increased rate of muscle stretch will be a stimulus for greater hypertonus in the presence of spasticity. Speakers with developmental dysarthria whose prime problem is spasticity, therefore, probably are working futilely against the limits of their neuromotor systems when they attempt increased speech rates. Most of the group with developmental dysarthria whose prime problem is dyskinesia must perform movements relatively slowly if they are to achieve desired articulatory target positions in the presence of their disordered neuromotor systems.

For these reasons the earlier-described assessment procedures and the discussions of formulations of management goals stressed and discussed the potential need for these speakers to slow their speech rates even further. Beneficial effects of that rate change will be observed with most of these speakers during the assessment. Those desirable effects may be so contributory to improvement in a number of aspects of speech production that establishing a slower speech rate should be seriously considered as an initial management goal. This is not to say that after a number of improvements have been incorporated into the individual's speaking behavior that the established slower rate cannot then be increased without a deleterious effect upon intelligibility.

Just as a clinician may be reluctant to work toward reducing the speech rate of a speaker who already has abnormally slow speech, many speakers with developmental dysarthria seem strongly disinclined to speak more slowly. As has already been mentioned, many of these speakers evidently adopt a speech rate that is too rapid for their physiological capability due to their inclination to produce as much speech as possible on one expiration in the face of limited respiratory capability. In addition, of course, it is likely that many of these speakers attempt to match the speech rate of normal speakers not only to duplicate that model but also to compete in their verbal society.

This strong recommendation to consider slowing the speech rate may seem contradictory to the previous emphases on the limits of the respiratory volume that may be available for speech production. It was said that the volume of air on one expiration is likely to be limited and that the duration of an utterance on one expiration should be short enough to accommodate that limitation. Now, it is being said that speech rate should be slowed. The result of the latter, then, would intuitively predict that fewer units of the speech signal can be produced on one expiration with the slower rate. That is not necessarily so. In fact, the relation between rate of a dysarthric speaker's speech production and the amount of air expired per unit of speech (e.g., per CV syllable) is not particularly strong. Since phonation is present throughout most of an utterance, decreasing speech rate prolongs proportionately more phonated elements of speech for which valving the respiratory airstream is most efficient. As a consequence, a speaker with developmental dysarthria may, in fact, slow the speech rate and not have to reduce significantly the number of syllables or words that he or she can produce comfortably on one expiration.

Practically every generalization that has been made regarding speech physiology problems associated with developmental dysarthria has required description of some exceptional cases, including these statements regarding speech rate. Some of these speakers tend to use a speech rate that is much slower than dictated by the physiology of their speech-producing systems. Those who attempt speech by using excessive generalized muscular efforts are examples. If use of the excessive effort for speech production can be modified, the rate of speech production may be increased without seriously degrading intelligibility.

Use of only drills designed solely to call the speaker's attention to speech rate and to have him or her modify the rate during the drill may not be optimally successful. It will be necessary to call attention to the speech rate in conjunction with other therapeutic activities. In the process of concentrating on an improved articulation, for example, the word or phrase to be produced may be demonstrated at a very slow rate, and the speaker may be told that he or she will produce that speech sample better if it is said slowly. As with clinical activities designed to instill use of short phrases as habitual speaking behavior, once it has been established that rate modification is a management goal, reinforcement of the desired rate should be consistent throughout all clinical activities.

management of articulatory errors

The results of the assessment of articulatory function should reveal at least an initial indication of groups of articulatory errors that seem to be the result of the manner in which the speaker has come to use the speech-producing system in the presence of the limitations of the speech-producing mechanisms. As has been emphasized, consideration should be given to simultaneous remediation of as many of these consonants and vowels as possible without confusing the speaker.

After the vowels and consonants have been selected for remediation at any particular stage in the management program, there may be a strong inclination to use the type of speech samples with which a speaker showed the best ability to produce the targeted consonants and vowels in the assessment procedures. For example, if those consonants and vowels can be spoken more precisely in CV syllables than in words, use of CV syllables for articulation work may seem indicated. That may initially draw the speaker's attention to production of the specific articulations that are desired. However, as soon as it is possible to do so, drill on the targeted consonants and vowels should be undertaken in words and phrases. If a child is working to improve the precision of the prevocalic /g/, for example, and that child can drive the vocal tract reasonably well over an utterance of four syllables in length and produce all other elements of the statement, "I want to go," the articulation drill for the prevocalic /g/ should utilize such statements.

It may be extremely difficult to devise speech samples of words and meaningful phrases for articulation work in which the speaker shows good potential for early improvement of both the consonant and vowel productions contained therein and that provide a variety of appropriate consonant-vowel combinations. Nevertheless, use of functional oral language as a routine component of articulation drills will (1) provide the opportunity to attend to appropriate use of the respiratory system and any other speech-producing behaviors that are subject to remediation such as establishing the most desirable speech rate, (2) provide a vehicle for attention to prosodic characteristics of the speech signal, and (3) enhance the chance that the speaker will be learning to produce speech skills that he or she will be using outside the clinical situation.

The more accurately the speaker can produce all of the speech samples, the better. Ideally, the samples should contain only phone-types whose production the speaker can improve at the time. If that criteria is held too rigidly, however, it may seriously restrict the repertoire. If phone-types that the speaker shows no capability for improving must be present in the drill materials, improved production of only those phone-types that have been identified for remediation should be emphasized.

With respect to work to improve production of vowels, it should be remembered that sustained vowels are relatively difficult to perceive accurately. Therefore, work to improve their production should proceed, at a minimum, through use of CV syllables. As is the case with consonants, however, concentration on vowel productions in words and phrases of functional language is preferable.

Confusion among a number of phone-types that are being simultaneously remediated may be circumvented to some extent by designing specific articulatory drills that emphasize only one, or a very few, consonants and/or vowels simultaneously. One phrase may be repeated, first with concentration on a consonant, then on a vowel, and finally on both. In cooperation with a classroom teacher, an oral reading assignment may be used, and over repeated readings concentration may be given to a specific phone-type each time.

With respect to the attention the speaker needs to give to monitoring the auditory signal of his or her speech accurately, the therapeutic regimen should include activities designed to maintain and improve that monitoring. Also, a review will be provided of methods that may be used to initiate articulatory movements and contacts that are not within the speaker's current speech-producing patterns. Those activities, such as the speakers observing his or her attempts at speech production in a mirror, may be used for ongoing monitoring during articulation drill where appropriate.

As alluded to earlier, as the program for articulation remediation reaches that stage where the physiological limits of the system are approached, repetitive, potentially laborious drill will be necessary. The initiative of even the most imaginative clinician will be taxed in designing stimulating activities that will keep children motivated.

A contingency system for rewarding appropriate articulatory performance is probably more applicable to articulation remediation than to other aspects of the therapeutic process. Those programs should be used, of course, for any set of speech-producing behaviors where possible.

Postvocalic Consonants. Consonants that are misarticulated in some way in the postvocalic position, but which are usually articulated well in the prevocalic position, may be among the easiest for the speaker to learn to produce correctly. Although his or her doing so may be dependent upon modification of use of the respiratory system, slowing the speech rate, attending to the need to maintain the effort required to complete syllables, and consistently drawing the speaker's attention to the desirability of completing syllables may result in the speaker's rather easily making all of the required adjustments to accomplish this task.

In stimulating the production of postvocalic consonants, the clinician should avoid exaggerating the productions. Such exaggerations may lead to inappropriate productions, such as aspiration of postvocalic voiceless stops. That type of inappropriate articulation should be avoided even in drill of CVC and VC syllables if such drill is used.

For these postvocalic consonants to be incorporated into speech habitually, continued attention to this aspect of the speech pattern may be needed. The inclination to omit postvocalic consonants in order to maintain a somewhat normal speech rate, to complete as much speech upon one expiration as possible, or to conserve the general physiological effort needed to produce speech may make it difficult for the speaker to overcome this articulatory pattern.

Articulatory Distortions. There has been frequent mention that imprecise articulation is a general characteristic of developmental dysarthria. This imprecision frequently can be described as distortions of consonants in which the articulatory gestures are inaccurate with respect to duration and extent of the articulatory gestures and misproduction of vowels. With respect to vowels, the inappropriate tongue positions may be said to lead to substitutions for the appropriate vowel. To me, that is a semantic differentiation not worth debating. The tongue's not reaching the appropriate vowel target position results in distortions of such desired vowels in that the acoustic signal falls within the perceptual class of other vowels.

The articulatory dynamics that lead to many of the vowel distortions (or substitutions) apply to a number of distortions of consonants. That is, the articulators at least move in the appropriate direction toward the target position. This group of articulatory errors is likely to have shown good potential for remediation during assessment procedures.

There may be a number of articulatory distortions, however, which the speaker demonstrates minimum ability to improve. These are most likely to be consonants for which precise posturing of the tongue is required (e.g., /s/). Remediation of such distortions may be more difficult.

Omissions and Substitutions. Although omissions of consonants also may result from incomplete articulatory gestures that the speaker shows capability of making, it is likely that these types of articulatory errors represent a greater degree of physiological restriction to the desired articulatory movement than is the case with distortions. In contrast to the usual assumption that omissions of consonant productions are easier to alleviate in cases of functional articulation problems, in the population who has developmental dysarthria, this type of articulatory error is likely to be more difficult to remediate. That is particularly so in the case of some omissions of voiceless consonants. If the particular pattern is due to velopharyngeal incompetence, it may be extremely difficult for the speaker to generate sufficient intraoral air pressures to produce those consonants in lieu of management of the incompetence.

Selected speakers may show substitution errors in which consonants that are inappropriate with respect to place of articulation are substituted for the appropriate consonant. Thus, the substitution of /d/ for /g/ may appear to be the result of inappropriate learning and only remotely related to the physiological problem. On the other hand, such errors may be the direct result of a physiological limitation to the appropriate articulation. In the example cited, the restricted mobility of the dorsum of the tongue may have prohibited the speaker from producing /g/, and in the presence of greater mobility of the anterior portion of the tongue, the speaker has come to substitute /d/. Remediation is likely to be difficult for those substitutions and omissions that result from such physiological limitations.

Initiating Desired Articulatory Movements. Consideration of a greater variety of management procedures may be needed for remediation of articulatory omissions and substitutions that involves extending the physiological capability of the articulatory mechanism. At a minimum the task will involve establishing a different or more extensive articulatory movement. One of the more difficult stages of articulation work may be that of establishing a desired pattern of movement. I have found no general rule of thumb in this regard that will be successful generally.

In those cases where the desired movements are within the capability of the speaker, drawing that speaker's attention to the auditory signal may be sufficient to stimulate him or her to produce the desired articulation. However, some desired articulatory gestures seem not to be within the speaker's repertoire of articulatory gestures, and initiation of the needed movements may seem almost impossible. That may be so even if the speaker can make comparable articulatory gestures to produce other phone-types.

Elicitation of these articulatory gestures may be facilitated by the clinician's demonstrating the desired articulations; having the speaker watch the clinician's mouth to observe the elevation of the tongue behind the teeth for production of a lingua-alveolar consonant may result in that speaker's being able to duplicate the movement and produce the consonant. Some speakers may respond favorably to instructions as to how to position the articulators for initiation of a given sound; for example, a specific child may respond best when attempting to produce /d/ to the instruction, "Now put your tongue up behind your teeth and say 'duh.' " Observing the movements of their oral structures in a mirror may be helpful to some.

Care should be taken, however, in using any form of instructions in which the cerebral palsied speaker's attention is drawn specifically to the structure or structures that are to be moved or positioned in specific ways. The reactions of those for whom such instructions may be inappropriate may suggest strongly that such attention creates more problems than it solves. Similarly, some cerebral palsied individuals seem to have even more difficulty accomplishing movements of the oral structures when they are concentrating on observing themselves in a mirror. What really is being said here is that all types of instructions and demonstrations for accomplishing articulatory movements should be attempted with the recognition that some will be more productive with specific speakers than others and that some seem contraindicated for reasons that have no ready explanation.

I have, however, become totally disenchanted with procedures that call for passive positioning or manipulation of a speaker's oral structures. I have personally spent significant amounts of time holding together the lips of a child whose upper lip was too hypertense to permit bilabial contact, asking the child to then phonate, and achieving a reasonable production of /m/ or /b/ as I allowed the lips to open. Whether the activity involved my manipulation of the jaw and/or lips in any manner with my hands, or positioning of the tongue with a tongue blade, I eventually came to the conclusion that such procedures are generally ineffective.

When repeated efforts at whatever type of procedure show no favorable result in assisting the speaker to produce a desired articulation, continued work on that particular production probably should be deferred. The word *deferred* is used purposefully. If the continuing speech habilitation program is successful in improving other deleterious speech-producing behaviors, it may be possible to return successfully to work on a specific articulatory act that previously seemed impossible for the speaker. No better example exists than results that are sometimes obtained from resolution of velopharyngeal incompetence; after successful management of that problem some dysarthric speakers may begin to show tongue mobility that previously did not seem to be present. I refuse to speculate as to the reasons for these changes in what seemed to be a physiological limit of the mechanism.

Voicing Errors. The tendency for speakers with developmental dysarthria to use voiced for voiceless consonants has been frequently mentioned.[3] This emphasis has been given to highlight the conceptualization of the speech-producing mechanism as an aerodynamic mechanical system and the advantages thereof to the understanding of the developmental dysarthric problem. It also has been given since it is my experience that the voiced-voiceless errors are relatively easy to remediate in a number of cases. As already implied, if the speaker can slow his or her speech rate while concentrating on producing the voiceless consonant, he or she may be able to do so relatively easily.

Such ease of remediation typically is not the case in the few instances in which the voiceless consonants are routinely produced for their voiced cognates. This pattern of voicing error, which is characteristic of hypofunction of the vocal folds, is found in a few of the more severely involved individuals who also manifest breathy vocal tones.

Management of Compensations. Some articulatory errors that are manifestations of compensation for physiological problems have been exemplified. The speech-language pathologist who works with the cerebral palsied population will be confronted with decisions as to whether such compensations should be allowed to persist. Firm generalizations cannot be made in that regard.

The clinician should keep in mind that working to eliminate such compensations where doing so proves physiologically impossible for the speaker may, in effect, work against that speaker's achieving some degree of speech intelligibility. An approximation of an intended phone-type may be less deleterious to intelligibility than eliminating the compensatory gesture with the result that there is an omission.

There have been arguments that compensations should not be permitted to develop or persist even when the compensatory articulation is acoustically acceptable. Compensatory movements may interfere with other needed gestures of the articulatory structures; they may preclude the possibility of ever developing normal articulation and in some cases, they may be aesthetically abnormal (e.g., /f/ for /θ/).

[3]Andrews, Platt, and their colleagues have provided a series of survey investigations of the oral communication characteristics of adult cerebral palsied individuals (e.g., Platt et al., 1980). In contrast to a number of findings that cerebral palsied dysarthric children misarticulate prevocalic voiceless consonants more frequently than voiced cognates, these adult subjects correctly articulated prevocalic voiced consonants proportionately more than voiceless cognates. The data were not presented in such a way as to delineate voicing errors, but the frequency of voiced for voiceless cognate errors found with children suggest that these adult subjects would have had to eliminate that problem in order to reduce the frequency of prevocalic voiceless consonant misarticulations. While the authors call for a replication to determine if such differences between adults and children will be a consistent finding, it may be that, in order to achieve better intelligibility, adults come to use the prevocalic voiceless consonants more frequently even though that use increases the aerodynamic inefficiency with which they produce speech.

As pointed out repeatedly, however, the goal of normal speech is frequently unrealistic, and a more pragmatic philosophy toward compensatory speech-production behaviors may be that they should be allowed to develop, persist, and actually encouraged if they contribute more to intelligibility than available alternatives. The best example that I can cite is a fourteen-year-old, mildly involved dyskinetic young man whose speech was usually intelligible despite rather severe restriction of mobility of the anterior portion of the tongue. He was producing lingua-alveolar stop consonants by moving the tongue mass forward against the alveolar ridge, but he could not retroflex the tongue to produce /l/. He had learned, however, to produce an acoustically acceptable prevocalic consonant /l/. Cinefluorographic films demonstrated that he was, in some way, accomplishing this feat by movement of the entire tongue mass in and out of the posterior oral cavity. Considerable clinic work made it apparent that he was going to be unable to produce /l/ with the tongue tip, and, moreover, the work began to result in a deterioration of the manner in which he had come to produce /l/. Even though with that compensatory gesture he produced prevocalic consonant /l/ clusters with an intervening neutral vowel (e.g., /bʌlæk/ for /blæk/), his degree of intelligibility would have been jeopardized by continuing to work toward a normal production of the consonant. This case exemplifies the need for giving due consideration to the potential deleterious effects of changing compensatory speech behaviors.

management of dysprosody

As a consequence of the rapid, subtle adjustments of musculatures throughout the entirety of the speech-producing system that are associated with prosody, development of normal prosodic patterns is unrealistic for many speakers with developmental dysarthria. That is particularly true of those whose neuromotor disorder is primarily spasticity. The usual topographical distribution of spasticity in which there is characteristically respiratory and laryngeal dysfunction, even though that latter dysfunction may result from hypertonicity of the neck musculatures, predisposes most of the cerebral palsied dysarthric speakers with spasticity to irreversible dysprosody. Those speakers who manifest primarily dyskinesia characteristically are dysprosodic, but a number of the mildly involved dyskinetic speakers may be able to improve their dysprosody.

Prosody, or the suprasegmentals of the speech signal, does convey meaning under certain circumstances, such as the rising inflection and strong stress to convey that a declarative statement is, in fact, a question. Therefore, dysprosody may interfere with efficient oral communication. Even so, dysprosodic speakers usually can convey their meaning if their production of phonology is sufficient that their speech is readily intelligible. Remediation of dysprosody, therefore, may not be crucial to enabling a speaker with developmental dysarthria to become a reasonably effective speaker.

Although using normal prosody is physiologically impossible for many individuals with developmental dysarthria, improving their dysprosody may be a highly desirable management goal. The dysprosodic characteristics of their speech are very distracting to listeners.

Even though some of these speakers will be unable to use reasonable ranges of fundamental frequency for inflection patterns and rapid intensity changes for stress contrasts, they may be able to use changes in durations of syllables and pause times between words. It may take considerable experimentation to determine the speaker's capability to vary these aspects of the speech signal along with limited pitch and loudness changes and to learn how they may be manipulated to produce a less distracting speech pattern.

It typically will be found that a prime contributor to the dysprosody will be lack of deemphasis. Multisyllable words are likely to be produced with comparable, relatively strong, levels of stress on each syllable, creating the impression that durations of syllables are relatively equal. Finally, there is usually an overriding characteristic of a tendency toward constant voicing even across word boundaries.

This equal stress of syllables, including durations of syllables, is not perceptually comparable to the dysprosodic pattern referred to as "scanning speech." That pattern, which is sometimes a component of acquired dysarthria, is characterized by a perceptual separation between syllables. In contrast to this "syllable-by-syllable" production of scanning speech, the dysprosody with equal stress on syllables in developmental dysarthria seems to include a lack of decrease in vocal effort to demark syllables. This latter characteristic might be described as a "droning" characteristic of the speech pattern.

Attempts to establish deemphasis of syllables may not be successful. It may be possible in such cases, however, to work with some success toward overemphasis of syllables that should be stressed. That is, since it probably will be desirable to slow the speaker's speech rate, it may be possible to reinforce even longer durations of syllables that are to be stressed and thus introduce some stress contrasts into the speech signal.

Bringing about substantial improvements in dysprosody may be an exceedingly slow process. The desired changes in the speech pattern may have to be directly emphasized as a somewhat separate component of the management program.

If the speaker begins to show improvement in other aspects of deleterious speech-producing behaviors, better prosody may be possible than would have been predicted early in the management program. For example, improvements in the precision of articulatory gestures may alleviate the dysprosody to some extent. That is particularly so if voiceless consonants and pause times also can be incorporated into a speech pattern that has been characterized by consistent voicing.

Even when improvement in dysprosody is not a management goal, consistent care must be taken to avoid reinforcing unnecessary dysprosody through the therapeutical process. In demonstrations of desired articulations, the clinician may lapse into stimulating the speaker by consistently strongly stressing syllables and accept such productions as appropriate responses. There should be constant attempts made to have the speaker use the best prosodic patterns that are possible.

○ MANAGEMENT OF CASES WITH MILD AND UNUSUAL PATTERNS OF INVOLVEMENT

Characteristics of the speech-production problem in the presence of mild involvement of the speech-producing musculatures result in somewhat dramatically different problems between the subgroups of cerebral palsied individuals with spasticity and dyskinesia. The major problem for the spastic subgroup is likely to be that of dysprosody. For the dyskinetic subgroup, the problems that are likely to be clinically significant are relatively mild articulation problems. These differences for the two diagnostic groups are, of course, due to the distribution of the neuromotor disorder throughout the speech producing musculatures.

As just reviewed in the discussion of management of dysprosody, the prognosis for dramatic improvement of this characteristic of mild dysarthria of the spastic group usually is guarded. If the distribution of the neuromotor problem extends to musculatures of the oral structures, and misarticulations are present, alleviating the articulation problems may be a realistic goal. Achieving that goal may depend on establishing optimum use of the respiratory mechanism since torso wall musculatures are routinely involved. Although relatively normal articulation skills may be a reasonable prognosis, "normal speech production" frequently cannot be expected due to the resistance of the dysprosody to remediation.

The mildly involved dyskinetic speaker may be able to alleviate his or her misarticulations, and reasonably normal-sounding speech may be a realistic management goal. If the respiratory musculatures do show some restricted mobility, extreme levels of vocal intensity may not be possible, and mild dysfunction of the laryngeal mechanism may result in a very mild dysprosody. Even that problem may be alleviated by using a somewhat slower rate of speech, which will permit different durations of syllables and hence stress contrasts.

These very mild cases of developmental dysarthria, as well as the very mildly involved child with whom there is little or no involvement of the speech mechanisms, are those that are likely to have types of speech problems other than dysarthria. Children whose speech possesses all of the characteristics of the dysfluent patterns of stuttering may be encountered, and articulation disorders that have no apparent physiological basis are sometimes seen. As has been mentioned, and as will be reviewed in the forthcoming chapter, it may be extremely difficult to convince parents and other professional persons that these speech-production problems are not the direct result of the child's having cerebral palsy or being "brain-damaged."

Within both of these diagnostic subgroups, however, there are a few speakers in which the neuromotor disorder in the extremities may be relatively mild, but involvement of selected musculatures of the oral structures may be quite severe. That situation could be expected for the dyskinetic subgroup, based on the earlier discussion of the topographical distribution of that type of neuromotor disorder. However, an occasional person with developmental dysarthria whose prime problem is spasticity will also show this unusual, somewhat isolated involvement of selected oral musculatures. The management goals and therapeutic activities should be based on the same considerations that have been discussed throughout this chapter. The prognosis for improvement of any aspect of speech production will depend on the muscle groups that manifest restricted function and the manner in which the speaker has come to use the totality of the speech-producing mechanism in the presence of that restricted function.

○ OUTCOME OF MANAGEMENT

Establishing realistic management goals for specific aspects of speech production will be aided greatly by thorough, early consideration of the long-term outcome of management. A speech signal that sounds normal is an unrealistic outcome for the great bulk of speakers with developmental dysarthria, even those with relatively mild involvement of some of the speech-producing musculatures.

Management goals should be established within that perspective. Maintaining a normal speaking rate may be counterproductive to improvement of selected aspects of the problem during early management, but there is the strong possibility that most of these speakers will never be able to use a normal rate of speech while maintaining a degree of intelligibility. To anticipate otherwise is to deny the reality of the problem.

For cerebral palsied speakers for whom a degree of functional oral communication seems to be a reasonable outcome of management, persistent attempts should continue to bring that outcome to fruition. For such speakers with relatively mild involvement of the speech-producing musculatures, efforts to assist them with specific articulation errors may show eventual promise of reducing the negative impact that their speech makes on their listeners. However, to continue doggedly working toward achievement of any specific management goal in the face of strong indicators that further progress is unrealistic is of questionable value to the client and to anyone who is closely associated with the client.

No firm generalizations are possible for anticipating the outcome of management. From my point of view, the speech-language pathologist should maintain contact with a number of individuals with developmental dysarthria through adolescence or the early adult years. The nature of that contact, however, will vary dramatically from individual to individual. Frequent, direct therapeutic intervention is called for until there is convincing evidence that progress is no longer being made. However, that evidence should signal the need for change in the frequency and type of contact. The use of alternatives to oral communication may be needed for specific aspects of the individual's daily living, as will be discussed in Chapter Ten. Even then, it may appear desirable to continue work to maintain or improve some aspect of the individual's oral communicative ability.

There will be persons for whom direct management has been terminated, and follow-up contacts will indicate the desirability for its resumption. A speaker with developmental dysarthria frequently will regress in the habitual use of optimum speech-producing behaviors, and a short therapy program may be indicated to alleviate that regression. As a child matures, he or she may become highly motivated to overcome what seemed earlier to be an insurmountable speech physiology problem. The eventual level of the person's aspirations and capability for employment and independence may dictate revisions in an earlier decision to terminate direct clinical work.

An attitude of guarded optimism should be maintained toward the outcome of management. Improvements in functional oral communication are realistic for a number of cerebral palsied individuals who have significant degrees of involvement of their speech-producing musculatures, and a much improved life style will result from that improved level of communicative ability.

A number of school-age children and adults who have cerebral palsy and obvious significant neuromotor involvement of their speech-producing musculatures frequently will be capable of improving the intelligibility of their speech. The assessment procedures should provide an indication of the changes that these speakers can make in their speech-producing behaviors that will contribute most to an improved speech signal that will enable the speaker to make further improvements.

In general, attempts should be made to achieve a set of short-term goals by (1) devoting attention to modifying those deleterious speech-producing behaviors that are not due to the physiological limitations of the speaker's speech physiology system and (2) incorporating into his or her speaking behavior a number of general changes that permit better speech-production within the limits of that system. Other changes, which may be thought of as long-term goals, are likely to be those that involve extending the physiological limits of the speech-producing system; those goals may be much more difficult to achieve.

The nature of the problem of developmental dysarthria dictates a number of general considerations throughout the management process. It is very desirable to maintain records of changes in the client's speech in order to retain objectivity since those changes are likely to be slow. Because of that slow progress and because developmental dysarthria usually presents a highly complex and interrelated set of clinical features, work should proceed simultaneously on as many therapeutic goals as possible. The nature of the neuromotor disorders that comprise cerebral palsy contraindicate asking the client to engage in acts that require maximum physiological efforts. Even though the developmental dysarthric problem is, by definition, one of motor performance, it is frequently necessary to work on the client's ability to carefully monitor his or her speech signal. Finally, attention must be given to a variety of means to assist the speaker to use those improved speech skills achieved in clinical settings in all other speaking situations.

Work on specific changes in speech-producing behaviors should be designed to assist the speaker in producing the best speech signal possible within the limits of his or her speech producing system. There are a number of such changes that frequently bring about very desirable general improvements. Two such changes are using the respiratory mechanism so that speech is produced over lung volume levels where the mechanism is capable of driving the vocal tract and producing relatively short phrases between inspirations in order to do so. Slowing the speech rate is frequently a requisite for speakers with developmental dysarthria since additional time is needed for their articulatory structures to complete articulatory gestures, and attention usually needs to be given to the speaker maintaining an appropriate level of physiological effort in generating the speech signal.

Although specific attention may be needed for those undesirable characteristics of the speech signal due to laryngeal dysfunction, changes in those characteristics are usually very difficult to achieve. However, deviations from normal laryngeal function seldom prevent accomplishing desirable changes in other aspects of speech production with speakers who are otherwise capable of improving their intelligibility.

In contrast, velopharyngeal incompetence may singly prevent significant progress. Moreover, many cases of velopharyngeal dysfunction associated with developmental dysarthria require either prosthetic or surgical management. The method of management should be chosen on the basis of the experience and skills of the persons who are to accomplish the needed procedures.

Remediation of articulatory errors will seldom be the only goal in work with developmental dysarthria. Rather, such work is most likely to be carried out appropriately along with attempts to achieve or maintain other goals. Special considerations relative to work on articulation skills include the need to concentrate heavily on those aspects of phonology that will contribute most in improving intelligibility.

Special consideration needs to be given to compensatory articulatory gestures that may or may not contribute to intelligibility. Dysprosody, which may be the most distinctive feature of developmental dysarthria, may be very resistive to management.

The same guidelines may be applied to the management of cases of developmental dysarthria in which the neuromotor disorder is relatively mild. Although it might be anticipated that progress with such cases will be good, their dysprosody may also be resistant to change. Special considerations will be needed for cases in which there is a very unusual distribution of the neuromotor involvement.

As is true for establishing a prognosis as a result of any set of assessment procedures, there should be strong efforts to maintain an objective perspective of the on-going results of the management program. Decisions regarding needed changes in the program or its continuation should be based upon such a perspective.

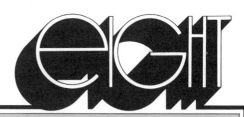

Associated disabilities, disorders, and problems

The fact that cerebral palsy results from an abnormality of the developing brain predisposes this population for consideration that its members may possess all of the various disabilities and disorders that have been demonstrated or inferred to result from brain dysfunction. As related previously, one of the obstacles to the understanding of the neuromotor disorders that constitute cerebral palsy was the natural tendency to assume that they should be comparable to disorders observed in adults who have sustained lesions to their brains. There also has been a strong tendency to explain a variety of atypical behaviors in children on the basis of alleged "brain damage" whenever similar behaviors have been noted to be sequelae of damage to adult brains.

There may be far less justification for such analogies relative to many other aspects of deviant behavior in children than for developmental neuromotor disorders since, of the functional neuronal organizations, the neuromotor systems are relatively resistant to change as a result of neural learning. It seems reasonable, then, that more plastic systems, such as those that come to mediate use of the language code, would be capable of considerable reorganization in the presence of an early lesion unless that lesion destroyed a large portion of the neural tissue that could become involved in those functions. It is likely, then, that a general decrement in brain function will result.

There is a tendency that stems from deeply imbedded historical ideas, however, to attribute specific dysfunctions in children to inferred damage to neurological systems. There seems to be the assumption that if a specific disability or disorder can be explained on the basis of some specific neurological abnormality, the indications for management and the prognosis will be clearer. Those are tenuous assumptions in many instances. Moreover, assuming that the basis for some specific deficit in a child's development is due to physiological factors in the absence of firm evidence to that effect frequently leads to a cessation of searches for other contributors to the problem. Many times those other contributors may have more predictable consequences than an assumed lesion to, or dysfunction of, some specific neurological system.

The conditions of cerebral palsy also are usually accompanied by a set of psychological-sociological problems that frequently deserve clinical attention, and those problems may impact directly on the responsibilities of the speech-language pathologist. In some cases these problems may deserve as much, or even more, consideration in clinical management of the population as the often strongly emphasized associated disabilities. In fact, examples will be cited in which a continuing search for other explanations of a clinical problem would have revealed that a sociological situation was a prime contributing factor that should have been given attention. This attention should not be given, however, with the assumption that these problems can be overcome easily because their roots may be in some behavioral domain, such as parent-child relationships. To the contrary, some of these associated problems may be extremely resistant to management.

○ ASSOCIATED DISABILITIES AND DISORDERS

Descriptions of "word deaf" and "word blind" children appeared in the literature prior to the turn of this century. Children were described who seemed to function normally otherwise and who seemed to see well, but who appeared to have specific problems learning to read. Others seemed to hear well but had difficulty understanding what was said to them. Great interest also had developed in the disabilities of adults who had sustained lesions to their brains, and it was being observed that some of these adults seemed to have specific deficits, such as reading or understanding what was said to them. Therefore, the "word deafness" and "word blindness" of selected children were being attributed to prenatal lesions of their brains.

By the 1930s a vernacular had been well developed to label such specific disordered behaviors of brain-damaged adults. Although that vernacular had been used much earlier, primarily by persons of the medical profession, it was beginning to be generally used by other professions that deal with children. The term agnosia, for example, had come to be used in reference to disorders in which a brain-damaged person seemed to be confused relative to characteristics of various sensory stimuli. Therefore, for example, the diagnostic label "visual agnosia" was applied to children with reading deficits, and damage to circumscribed areas of their brains was believed to be the basis of reading problems of numerous children who showed no other developmental problems.

This orientation was intuitively appealing. It seemed to offer answers to many questions that were being asked regarding atypical behaviors in children. By the post–World War II era, this orientation began to be accepted almost uncritically by large numbers of professional persons.

The concept of "congenital aphasia" was an outgrowth of this orientation in the field of speech-language pathology and audiology. Numerous descriptions of behaviors, in addition to delayed development of communication skills, appeared as lists of diagnostic criteria for the condition. Literally thousands of children throughout this nation were diagnosed as being "congenitally aphasic." The lists of diagnostic criteria were inconsistent, and many children were assumed to have some type of anatomical deviation of their brain primarily on the basis of a delay in development of speech and language skills.

Another orientation evolved during the post–World War II era for which the origin is more difficult to trace. Numerous brain-injured adults had been observed to be highly distractible to extraneous stimuli, and as already mentioned, they tended to show selective functional deficits. In addition, some children who had survived infections of their brains had been reported as being extremely active and distractible.

From the concentrated attention being given to mentally retarded children, there came the observation that some of these children could be also described as hyperactive and distractible and showing selective abilities to learn certain skills. The ideas of Strauss and Lehtinen (1947) had a tremendous impact on the thinking of their time. They postulated that the mental retardation of that subgroup of the intellectually handicapped was due, in fact, to brain damage. The remainder of the intellectually handicapped population was said to have the handicap due to genetic factors.

This concept of the "brain-damage syndrome," which was mentioned in the introductory comments of this book, was quickly generalized to include children who were not intellectually handicapped but who were believed to show the clusters of behaviors that had been set forth as indicators of the syndrome. Again, these formulations were looked to as providing answers to many problems facing educators of atypical children and persons from a variety of professions who were involved in assisting those children and their families.

Many of these earlier concepts have not fared well as a result of critical analysis and research. Signs that were alleged to signify brain abnormality and that were said to distinguish one disorder from another could be observed in other diagnostic groups of children. For example, characteristics that were said to distinguish children with congenital aphasia also could be observed in groups of children who had been demonstrated to be mentally retarded. The fact of brain damage could not be established in a sizable proportion of the children (1) who manifested serious delay in speech and language development and who were diagnosed as having congenital aphasia or (2) who possessed signs of the so-called brain-damaged syndrome.

With respect to the brain-damaged syndrome, the lack of direct correspondence between its signs and demonstrable central nervous system abnormality led to changes in the label. The terms "soft brain damage" and "minimal brain damage" began to be used. The so-called "soft signs" of brain abnormality thus evolved. In contrast, signs of the neuromotor disorders that led to the diagnosis of cerebral palsy were included among the "hard signs" of central nervous system abnormality in children.

As might be expected, when behaviors that resembled these soft signs were noted in selected children with cerebral palsy, who by definition possessed firm signs of brain abnormality, they were frequently attributed to the brain problem, and investigations attempted to demonstrate with cerebral palsied subjects the presence of these other disorders that were said to result from damage to the developing brain. These disorders, however, were not routinely present in cerebral palsied subjects, and their frequent absence in that population cast doubt on the assertions that soft signs uniformly resulted from early brain damage.

As sophistication in diagnostic techniques and understanding of other potential bases of developmental and educational problems of children advanced, other causes of the signs of alleged brain damage were found. Numerous children with reading problems were determined to have visual defects that did not interfere significantly with their daily living activities but did present significant obstacles to their academic performance, and it is now recognized that reading problems may result from a variety of causes. It also became recognized that children under stress for a variety of reasons frequently demonstrate learning problems and behaviors that were being ascribed to brain lesions. Problems of social maturation, academic performance, and parent-child relationships may cause children to react in these ways.

Other explanations were found for some of the disabilities that were being attributed to the brain lesions of selected cerebral palsied children. As mentioned previously, the subgroup of dyskinetic children known as the Rh athetoid subgroup routinely demonstrate bilateral high-frequency hearing impairments. Those children frequently exhibited what seemed to be bizarre patterns of language development, leading to conjectures that congenital aphasia was characteristic of the subgroup. As more was learned regarding the effects of bilateral high-frequency impairments on language development of children, it began to be demonstrated that it was the characteristic of the hearing impairment that led to the patterns of language development (e.g., Flower, Viehwig, and Ruzicka, 1966).

Numerous examples of clinical mismanagement can be cited that resulted from these early concepts. The application of the label "congenital aphasia" undoubtedly diverted attention away from the most efficacious management of the hearing impairment and language-related disability of a number of children with dyskinesia due to kernicterus. That concept, and the use of the label, also undoubtedly obscured the most responsible diagnosis in a number of badly neurologically devastated cerebral palsied children, namely mental retardation. With respect to use of the label of "brain-damaged syndrome," I can recall very well a mildly involved dyskinetic boy who was distractible, showed a short attention span, and experienced more problems academically than his overall capability seemed to predict throughout his elementary school years. He was labeled as having the "brain-damage syndrome," and the professional people who worked with him designed their programs accordingly, including counseling his parents regarding management of the problem. I later had contact with him as a young adult, and he related a long history of alcoholism in his home, with frequent abusive and violent episodes between his parents that often involved him as a young child. Yet, because of the presence of cerebral palsy and the assumptions surrounding the presence of "brain damage," the possibility that the home situation was a prime contributor to the child's general problems was completely overlooked.

The examples given above occurred in the somewhat distant past, and the concepts that led to their occurrence may no longer form the bases of decisions in many current clinical operations. Yet, history is difficult to disregard, and many of the questionable aspects of the earlier concepts remain a basis for clinical decisions. Terms such as "minimal brain damage" were replaced by "cerebral dysfunction," and that term continues to be used. Children who have problems in developing communication skills that are believed to be due to unconfirmed brain lesions now tend to be placed in one of two classifications, those who seem to have some type of auditory-receptive or processing problem and those who seem to have some type of motor-related difficulty in programing the neuromotor systems for speech production. The former group continues to be called congenitally aphasic by some, and the latter may be said to have developmental speech apraxia. Both of these entities still have problems of differential diagnostic criteria, but to the extent that these two classes of communication problems are being accepted as being related to developmental brain problems, their incidence is admittedly much lower than the previously advocated condition of "congenital aphasia."[1]

[1]One of the more extreme examples are the suggestions that "catastrophic reactions" occur in persons with cerebral palsy. That term has been used in reference to a physiological reaction in which brain-damaged persons become unresponsive, pale and show autonomic nervous systems signs such as perspiring excessively. In extreme cases, loss of bowel and bladder control are described. These reactions were sometimes suggested to be the result of the individual's being unable to tolerate consistent failure in a clinical situation. The possibility that even brain-damaged adults are subject to such reactions probably has been emphasized inappropriately in the literature dealing with aphasia. Throughout the numerous years in which I have been clinically involved with large numbers of both children and adults with communication disorders associated with nervous system dysfunction, I have never worked with any adult who has had a catastrophic reaction. Of numerous persons whose clinical experience in this area is as extensive, if not more so, than mine, I have been told of only one brain-damaged adult who had such a reaction. I have never witnessed nor heard of a child with cerebral palsy having a catastrophic reaction.

The literature adds to the problems of placing some of the earlier ideas in appropriate perspective. There are references to alleged possible disorders in a manner that provides no basis for critical evaluation as to their efficacy.

I take strong exception to statements in the literature on cerebral palsy that (1) propagate many questionable aspects of these earlier concepts and (2) imply that almost any type of problem that has been mentioned as a sequelae of brain damage can be found in the cerebral palsied population.[1] There are frequent reviews of the literature in which previous authors are said to have "delineated" or "elucidated" the presence of specific dysfunctions, and such reviews imply that the dysfunctions have been defined and demonstrated by data. In many instances, those "delineations" are no more than constructs that have been formulated on the basis of intuition relative to alleged results of brain dysfunction. This is a perplexing situation to the beginning clinical worker, and even experienced clinicians may be swayed in their perspectives of given cases.

The intent here should not be misconstrued. The evolution of many of the early concepts regarding the possible effects of a lesion to the developing brain have expanded knowledge regarding developmental and education problems in children. The current thinking relative to learning disabilities, for example, is a direct outgrowth of the early attention to selective differences of children's abilities to learn. Moreover, it cannot be denied that certain children manifest specific developmental problems that most reasonably can be explained on the basis of a lesion to and/or maldevelopment of their brains.

A prime intent here is to encourage clinical workers to analyze constantly and critically the bases for any suggestions that are made in the literature that may lead to repetition of historical difficulties in dealing with the variety of problems that (1) may or may not be associated with developmental brain abnormalities and (2) may or may not have implications for communication processes and disorders thereof. There currently is the suggestion, for example, that the cluster of developmental problems that are subsumed under the label "childhood autism" are due to "brain damage," and this idea is drawing both support and criticism. It would be unfortunate if children with cerebral palsy began to be labeled as having autistic tendencies simply because of their confirmed brain lesions.

Even the research literature relative to disabilities that are associated with cerebral palsy can be misleading. In order to assure that the neuromotor disorder does not confound the results of many studies, the subjects have had to be relatively mildly involved. In cases where the results show only a statistically nonsignificant tendency for the cerebral palsied subjects to demonstrate the problem under investigation, there has been the inclination to infer that the more severely involved portion of the population will have the problem to a greater degree. That is an unsatisfactory state of affairs.

Multiple measures from cerebral palsied subjects may show correlations that are significant statistically, but a statistically significant correlation says only that the demonstrated relationship occurs in the population due to other than chance factors. Whether the scores being used as criterion measures are shown to be significantly different in subgroups of the cerebral palsied population, or whether such measures are shown to be related within the population, there may be a conclusion offered that there is a cause-effect relationship.

Such conclusions may disregard that the differences or relationships may be due to the presence of a common variable, namely, the severity of the brain dysfunction. For example, levels of intellectual ability of cerebral palsied persons do vary, to some extent, with the severity of their neuromotor disorder. Severe spastic diplegic and quadriplegic individuals do tend to have reduced intellectual capabilities compared to those with paraplegia. The incidence of mental retardation in the former groups is greater than in the latter, and if reasonably good, comprehensive measures of physical ability could be devised, there is little doubt that a significant correlation could be shown between that measure and a measure of intellectual ability across these groups. As should be obvious, such findings could not be interpreted to mean that the intellectual level causes the neuromotor problem or vice versa.

The logic for the above statistical interpretation is obvious, and the clinical practitioner also recognizes that numerous severely involved spastic diplegic individuals have good intellectual ability, and some mildly involved spastic paraplegic individuals are severely mentally retarded. It is difficult to retain that perspective, however, in the face of elaborate statistical treatments of data that are reported regarding other variables. Interpretation of factorial analyses is difficult where multiple problems are present. A group of measures so analyzed may show a cluster of a few that seem related to some common factor. Yet, if a measure of some behavior that is not represented among the measures had been made, the results may have been dramatically different. Also, if a disproportionate number of measures in the group is related to one type of behavior, those measures will cluster in such an analysis.

There are different implications for the associated disabilities and disorders that are reviewed below. In some cases, the clinical implications may be minimal. The presence of some will dictate modification of the assessment procedures and/or the interpretations of the results of those procedures that are reviewed in Chapter Six, and of course, management procedures and the anticipated outcome also will be influenced. Since many of these associated disabilities and disorders will have a negative effect on the prognosis, it is imperative that determination of their presence is based, to the extent possible, on more than inference and a process of elimination. Establishing the presence of many of these associated disabilities and disorders is the role of other professional persons. Their significance many times must be determined through the interdisciplinary process discussed earlier that has, as a necessary component, critical evaluation of all assumptions.

intellectual status

During the era of accelerated interest in the conditions of cerebral palsy, it was becoming fully recognized that specification of levels of measured intelligence is dependent on assessing the ability of an examinee to respond to a variety of types of problem-solving activities with strict adherence to the administration for these behavioral tests. In recognition of all of the factors with the cerebral palsied population that preclude standardized administration of comprehensive intellectual batteries, a number of special tests were designed that could be administered with some confidence that different types of handicaps would not preclude standardized administration. For example, the vocabulary subtest of the Wechsler Intelligence Scale had been demonstrated to correlate most strongly of all the subtests with the total scores of those scales. It was only natural, then, to attempt to develop some type of vocabulary comprehension test that would circumvent poor oral communication ability, and the Ammons Full Range Picture Vocabulary Test was a result. Numerous suggestions were made as to how various psychometric materials of the two most well-developed comprehensive intellectual batteries (the Stanford-Binet and the Wechsler scales) could be modified to accommodate the physical handicaps and disabilities associated with cerebral palsy. There also was recognition of the facts that (1) a child with cerebral palsy frequently does not have the experiential background of a physically normal child, including experiences that lead to development of socialization, and (2) many of the items on psychometric scales reflect such aspects of normal child development.

Even though recognition was given to all of these factors that negate precise determination of intellectual status in the cerebral palsied population, the literature contained numerous reports of psychometric scores and intelligence quotients of group data gathered with this population. Those data, taken as a whole, suggested rather strongly that as much as 50 percent of the population probably should be classified as mentally retarded to some degree. There were those who argued, however, that such findings were inaccurate because of the inability to measure precisely the intellectual status of this population.

The reality of this aspect of the problem of cerebral palsy, nevertheless, began to be apparent. Whether, in fact, 40, 50, or 60 percent of the population can be said to fall at a subnormal level of measured intelligence, a very sizable proportion were recognized as functioning at that level of intellectual capability. It was also recognized that the psychologist carries enormous responsibility when assessing intellectual capability in the face of seemingly insurmountable difficulties. The usual approach to fulfilling this responsibility came to be use of as many subtests of the more comprehensive scales as could be administered with confidence, administration of a variety of the special tests that were being developed, observation of the child's performance in a variety of situations, and a synthesis of all the results, based on the examiner's experience.

Much more confidence is placed in the results of that method of intellectual assessment of multiply handicapped individuals now than was the case earlier. Even though, for example, methods of response for a specific test may have to be modified, a very low performance is accepted as highly suggestive of a problem. The meaning of various tests and their interrelations are better known. There is open recognition of the limitations of psychometric instruments as well as the need for comparison among a variety of test results in order to obtain evidence of intellectual capability. While the possible presence of confounding disabilities is recognized, there is a general tendency to require that those variables be demonstrated before they are assumed to influence the results of the assessment.

As a result, increasing numbers of children with cerebral palsy are being classified within general levels of intellectual ability at increasingly younger ages. Such classifications frequently carry numerous qualifications, but the broadened foundation of information upon which they are based usually gives substantial validity to the classification.

Of course, a reasonably accurate estimate of the intellectual capability of very young children with cerebral palsy may be impossible. The same may be said for some older children who have very severe neuromotor involvement and/or some associated disability, such as a hearing impairment. Deferring an estimate of intellectual capability may be appropriate, but ignoring the suggestive signs of mental retardation serves little positive purpose. Realistic planning for the habilitation of the child requires a comparable realistic estimate of his or her abilities.

Another very encouraging development which I perceive both in the literature that deals with psychological assessment of cerebral palsied individuals and in my contact with psychologists who are working clinically in that area is that there is a strong tendency to attempt to determine the reasons for unusual or deviant responses on psychometric instruments. There is recognition of the limits to which such responses should be attributed to ill-defined cerebral dysfunction, and the search for explanation of the responses frequently extends into investigation of all aspects of the child's behavior. The ramifications of various sociological factors are considered important as potential contributors to special learning problems. Even more important, there appears to be general recognition that the child's demonstrable handicaps will tend to create problems in the child's home, school, and society, and that these associated problems of adjustment in the presence of handicaps must be strongly considered in any management program.

The effects of mental retardation upon the development of speech and language skills are relatively well known, and once the presence of a significant intellectual handicap is established with a given cerebral palsied individual, the management program for remediation of speech and language skills must be adjusted accordingly. Of course, the outcome of the management of a dysarthria, which is also likely to be present, will be less favorable than if normal intellectual capability were present.

Depending on the level of the individual's retardation and other factors, continuing strong emphasis on remediation of speech-production skills may lead to a level of stress that jeopardizes the individual's ability to participate with optimal success in other aspects of educational and training programs. While it would be impractical to review even superficially the general characteristics of the intellectually handicapped, one characteristic of many such individuals is a disinclination to persist in developing a skill when doing so requires constant repetitive effort with minimum short-term success. The speech-language pathologist who has experience working with the mentally retarded population will recognize that it may be relatively difficult to convince parents, other lay persons, and individuals from other professions that continued work on speech production skills should be deemphasized. Nevertheless, the combination of limited ability to utilize language and difficulty in overcoming neuromotor involvement of the speech-generating mechanism to produce intelligible speech may indicate that some type of augmentative communication system should be used. That may be so even though functional oral communication might be possible for a child with a comparable degree of dysarthria who has normal intellectual capability.

The most realistic management goals and the most efficacious management planning calls for early recognition that the communication habilitation program should be designed with regard to the child's total needs. Therapeutic activities should be fully integrated with those programs that are being provided by other professional persons. Selected portions of the work by Lloyd (1976) deals specifically with communication problems of the intellectually handicapped, and some portions of the work also consider the confounding effects of a developmental dysarthria. Reference should be made to that material, or comparable material, in the design of a total communication remediation program for the individual who is mentally retarded and who has cerebral palsy.

Fortunately, the evolving favorable attitudes regarding the rights of all individuals, including the intellectually handicapped, make it much more feasible now than in the past to mount the long-range programs that are required to help the multiply handicapped reach their optimum potential. More important, efforts to program appropriately for the intellectually handicapped have demonstrated that much more can be accomplished than was thought possible as recently as ten years ago.

sensory disabilities and disorders

Both auditory and visual perceptual disorders have come to be mentioned routinely as associated disabilities to cerebral palsy. More recently, disorders of bodily sensation also are routinely mentioned. These sensory related disabilities are often discussed in a manner that implies they can be defined and identified precisely, with clear implications for the clinician. Yet, investigations of these disorders with the cerebral palsied populations do not consistently provide a justification for such discussions.

Lack of firm agreement as to what constitutes perceptual processes and the neurological organizations underlying those processes contributes to the ambiguities in this area. The literature reports a wide variety of different types of stimulus-response acts in investigations and tests of perceptual disorders. In some cases the tasks call for discrimination as to whether stimuli are alike or dissimilar. In other cases the response requires naming a stimulus that is perceived visually or repeating words that are heard. In a number of the latter cases memory processes, use of the language code, and cognitive abilities are involved in the experimental paradigms. Yet, there is the tendency to interpret the results of such studies as relating only to perceptual processes.

If a perceptual problem can be identified in an individual case and if it has clinical significance, the management goals and therapeutic activities should be designed accordingly. However, the possibility of relatively poorly defined perceptual problems should not be considered unless other related disabilities, including sensory impairments, have been determined not to be present.

Visual Impairments. Most reports of visual impairments in the cerebral palsied population date to the 1960s or earlier. Estimates from that relatively old literature indicate that as many as 25 to 50 percent of children with cerebral palsy have visual impairments that could significantly affect academic work and, of course, many of the activities that usually are used in speech remediation programs.

The most prevalent of the visual impairments in the population (strabismus and nystagmus) can be related to muscle imbalance and muscular control respectively. Strabismus is known to lead to suppression of use of one eye (amblyopia) in order to avoid the double image (diplopia) that results from the inappropriate rotation of the visual axis. Through this adaptation, binocular vision may be hindered or lost. The inappropriate movement of the eyes (nystagmus) may prevent maintaining the visual gaze as desired. It seems likely that if comprehensive, detailed visual examinations of cerebral palsied youngsters were routinely reported, the presence of other visual impairments would be documented to be present at least as frequently as in nonhandicapped populations.

Thorough screening for visual impairments is essential for members of this population. Precise assessment of the visual status of many cerebral palsied children will present some of the same problems to the ophthalmologist or optometrist as is presented to any professional person who attempts to assess their function. Ophthalmologists routinely have little experience with this population, and they may have difficulty in adapting their assessment procedures to the limited cooperation and response capabilities of many cerebral palsied children. Those professional persons who routinely occupy a place on the habilitation team should make their knowledge regarding individual cases available to either the optometrist or ophthalmologist who may initially provide screening of visual impairments. The speech-language pathologist should consider accompanying many of these children to the examination in order to assist in interpreting the child's responses.

Many physically normal children have the types of visual impairments that are suspected to be most prevalent with the cerebral palsied population, and they adapt to those impairments reasonably well. However, adaptation may be more difficult in the presence of reduced or uncontrolled head movements. Such visual impairments are not reported as being considered routinely in the studies of visual perceptual problems of the population, and most unfortunately, they are not considered routinely in some clinical programs.

Disorders of Visual Perception. Much of the work that has been interpreted as demonstrating some type of visual perception disorder to be characteristic of the cerebral palsied population has utilized stimulus-response paradigms that are of the type mentioned earlier and that involve more than visual processes. There have been indications that a few children with cerebral palsy may have some difficulty in depth perception, which would be a natural result of some of the visual impairments that are prevalent. Work done in conjunction with the visual-motor disorders that will be discussed later suggests that disorders in matching visual stimuli of geometric line figures usually are not present.

Compared to normal children, children with cerebral palsy may have difficulty on visual tasks that require responding to figures presented against backgrounds of different types. There are suggestions that these background-foreground perceptual problems contribute to distractibility and, hence, academic problems. However, errors on these types of tasks may be related more to intellectual ability than to other variables.

A variety of tests that may be given by a psychologist or other members of the habilitation team may suggest the presence of what may be called visual-perception problems. However, alternative reasons for the behavior should be thoroughly explored before it is assumed that it is related to visual processing of stimuli, and any potential clinical implications should be drawn on the basis of observed performance rather than inference.

Hearing Impairments. As is the case with reports of visual impairments, incidence of hearing impairments in the cerebral palsied population was reported in the 1950s and 1960s, and significant hearing impairments were found from somewhat above 8 percent to around 30 percent of this population. These reports suffered from inconsistencies in the definition of what constituted a significant hearing impairment and, undoubtedly, in audiometric conditions. Most important, there were variations in the proportions of the population samples from the different subtypes of cerebral palsy.

Where the subjects were identified as having kernicterus as the basis of their problem, hearing impairments classified as "moderately severe" were reported in as many as 80 percent of the cases. My experience suggests strongly that where kernicterus has been established as the etiology of the problem, some degree of hearing impairment will be present. The impairment may be a relatively mild bilateral high-frequency loss. More typically, a pure tone threshold will show a moderate to severe bilateral high-frequency impairment with pure tone thresholds in the normal range in the lower frequencies up to 500 to 1,000 Hz. The bilateral threshold may then drop as much as 30 to 50 dB over one octave. This is the type of hearing impairment that leads to the problems in learning speech-production and language skills of the kernicteric dyskinetic child that have been mentioned earlier.

With the reduction of incidence in the kernicteric problem, the overall incidence of hearing impairments within the total cerebral palsied population probably is lower than some of the earlier incidence figures suggest. Nevertheless, it is imperative that an audiologist begin working with all children who have cerebral palsy as soon as possible in order to begin estimating their hearing status. As soon as their maturation permits, a pure tone threshold should be established.

That type of attention to the possible presence of a hearing impairment may seem so reasonable that its emphasis may be questioned. Yet, even with the current sophistication of habilitation services, numerous cerebral palsied children may be found who have been receiving clinical attention for a number of years, whose hearing thresholds have not been established, but who have a significant hearing impairment. This situation seems to result from the inclination to attribute a speech and language problem to dysarthria and/or associated disabilities that have been said to result from early brain lesions. This inclination may be so pervasive that the substantial needed efforts to obtain the audiometric information will not be made. It is tragic to encounter an eleven-year-old spastic quadriplegic child whose hearing status had not been confirmed, who had been suggested to be mildly intellectually handicapped, but who is found to have a moderate to severe sensorineural hearing loss once he has been taught to respond reliably to pure tones in some special manner.

In addition to the increased probability of sensorineural hearing impairments, children with cerebral palsy are subject to the same conductive hearing impairments as normal children. In addition, through my concentration on work with dysarthric speakers who have velopharyngeal incompetence, I am of the impression that cerebral palsied children with that problem are prone to recurrent middle ear infections.

Obtaining reliable audiometric information may take considerable time. Nevertheless, it is essential to do so.

The presence of dysarthria may create significant problems in obtaining speech reception thresholds and discrimination scores once the presence of a hearing impairment is established. The speech-language pathologist should work quite closely with the audiologist in order to assist in diminishing those problems to the extent possible. The speech-language pathologist may assist in training the cerebral palsied child to respond to audiometric procedures of any type that seems indicated, including pure-tone audiometry.

Remediation procedures, including amplification for the language and educational programs for the hearing-impaired are applicable when a significant hearing impairment is present. Such multiply handicapped cerebral palsied children require the utmost in professional collaboration among the speech-language pathologist, the audiologist, and the child's classroom teacher, who should be trained in instructional procedures for the hearing-impaired and/or deaf child. Speech-language pathologists should not expect the audiologist and classroom teacher to appreciate totally the ramifications of the developmental neuromotor disorder on development of communication capability. In most cases, that involvement will preclude the use of sign in any total communication approach to the child's communication handicaps. Some system of augmentative communication, such as those discussed in Chapter Ten, should be considered where communicative ability is extremely limited.

Disorders of Auditory Perception. Despite the historical assumptions that auditory perceptual disorders are frequent sequelae of cerebral dysfunction in children, there is minimal evidence that well-defined auditory perceptual disorders are often associated with cerebral palsy. In fact, careful scrutiny of what evidence is available suggests a surprising lack of prevalence of these types of disorders.

Speech sound discrimination tests in which a child is asked to determine if two words (or CV syllables) are alike or unlike usually show no more problems in the cerebral palsied population than in normal children of comparable mental age. As reviewed by Lencione (1976), tests of speech perception in varying noise levels and tests that have been designed to determine the presence of what now are called central auditory processing disorders (e.g., comprehension of compressed speech) do not show results that can be interpreted as reflecting auditory perceptual disorders; moreover, use of the Illinois Test of Psycholinguistic Abilities with cerebral palsied subjects do not show systematically lower scores among the subtests that are designed to assess auditory processing.

I have been involved clinically with two children who were diagnosed as having cerebral palsy who showed extreme signs of such problems. Each of these children seemed to ignore most auditory stimuli, including oral communication, during their daily activities, and they had great difficulty in following oral instructions. Yet, they demonstrated pure tone thresholds within the normal or near normal range. They scored no better than at a chance level on picture vocabulary tests and psychometrics where instructions were given orally. On nonverbal psychometric scales where instructions may be provided by demonstration, their performance was substantially better, usually within the upper range of mental retardation or lower range of normal functioning.

Each of these children had mild neuromotor problems of the predominantly spastic type, and the involvement was more severe on one side. Their oral output was quite limited, and the signs of mild neuromotor involvement of their speech musculatures was insufficient to explain their almost total lack of articulatory gestures that characterized their speech attempts. Educational programing that would be appropriate for profoundly hearing-impaired children was provided for each child, and at my last contact they were showing signs of beginning to use nonoral communication and to learn reading skills. Unfortunately, I do not know what long-range progress they have made. It had appeared that these children could not differentiate the acoustic patterns of the speech signal well enough to learn speech-production skills, and efforts to assist them to learn those skills had been abandoned for lack of progress.

These types of rare cases may lead to the assumption that milder forms of this type of disability might be frequently associated with cerebral palsy, but there may be little basis for such an assumption. These two children both showed unusual signs of the neuromotor disorder. The history of one suggested strongly that the neural damage occurred during the second year of life; there was reason to believe that the other sustained brain damage postnatally, but the history was unreliable. There are reports of such relatively severe auditory-perceptual disorders in children that result from postnatal brain injury (e.g., Stein and Curry, 1968). Even so, that is no justification for assuming that such disorders can be frequently identified as isolated, specific disorders in populations of children with whom the brain insult occurred prenatally.

An initial step to considering the presence of any type of auditory-perceptual disorder is to rule out a hearing loss. Then, a variety of appropriate tests should be used before concluding that any type of auditory-perceptual disorder is present with a specific case. Where those test results definitely show a disorder to be present, procedures to improve the auditory discrimination of the child probably should be incorporated into the management program. However, if the disorder is, in fact, based on organic problems rather than mislearning, the prognosis for improvement may be rather negative.

Disorders of Somesthesia. Discussions of cerebral palsy now refer to the presence of disorders of bodily sensations. These references imply that tactile, proprioceptive, and kinesthetic problems are frequent associated disorders, and these disorders are related to speech problems in the population.

There is a tendency to use terms such as *proprioceptive, kinesthetic,* and *tactile* in a confusing manner throughout all literature that deals with somesthesia, and in some cases they are used interchangeably. Definitions of this terminology, as used here, are needed to avoid confusion.

The term *tactile* is used here to refer to the total array of neural patterns that result from excitation of receptors in superficial tissues, primarily the skin of the extremities, torso, neck, face, and head, along with the mucosa of the oral cavity. *Proprioception,* as used here, refers to neural patterns that arise from receptors in deeper tissues, including muscle spindles (which respond to stretch of muscle), and golgi tendons (which respond to load upon muscle). As reviewed in Chapter Four, both tactile and proprioceptive patterns may have relatively direct influence on activity of the final common pathway, and those patterns also may be transmitted directly to the cerebellum as one of the sources of afferent information to be integrated and utilized for coordination of normal, ongoing motor activity. Proprioceptive and tactile information may also be transmitted directly to neural mechanisms of the autonomic nervous system to provide information regarding the superficial and internal status of the organism, and portions of that information are also transmitted to the postcentral gyrus of the cerebral cortex, via the thalamus, that leads to somesthetic perceptions.

Figure 4–1 (Chapter Four) provides a listing of types of stimuli to which various receptors in tissues respond. This list grossly oversimplifies the variety of receptors that probably generate neural patterns that carry tactile and proprioceptive information, and a considerable amount of this information may not arise in discriminable sensations, or what is called somesthesia. For example, stretch information from the internal structures of the larynx may be transmitted to the cerebellum for coordination of intrinsic layrngeal muscle activity; however, we have no perception of the position of the vocal folds.

Somesthesia, then, refers to those discriminable sensations that are transmitted to the postcentral gyrus of the cerebral hemispheres, and those sensations can be differentiated as separate sensory capabilities. Deep touch (or touch-pressure) and light touch are two separate discriminations. *Kinesthesia,* as usually used, refers to the relation of body structures to each other during movement, and *position sense* refers to perceptions of the relations of body parts to each other, the head, and gravity during static, no-movement conditions. There is some evidence that separate discriminatory mechanisms exist for perception of vibratory sensations, and, of course, perceptions of temperature and pain are separable discriminations.

The extent to which various groups of receptors contribute to these specific sensations that comprise somesthesia is controversial. There is some debate as to the extent to which the muscle spindles contribute to position sense, and although kinesthesia usually is thought of as resulting from proprioceptive information, there are arguments that tactile information contributes to kinesthesia due to pressure differences in the skin during movement. Irrespective of such controversies, there are differences in the afferent information from tissues transmitted into the central nervous system that results in somesthesia as compared to that which may be used for other purposes.

It has been suggested that the integrity of motor speech processes depends on monitoring of oral structure movements by somesthesia. This idea that motor activity is dependent on such feedback in a "closed-loop" fashion, however, has a number of problems. Carried to its logical conclusion, it says that if such feedback is not present, the motor system will not function properly. This type of theory with respect to motor processes, in general, has a long history of controversy. For example, the effects of depriving the limbs of experimental animals of all bodily afferent information have been studied through sectioning of dorsal root nerve trunks. The results of those and other types of study, taken as a whole, are equivocal. They seem to suggest that as long as there is the opportunity for monitoring movement by some remaining sensory modality, the motor systems will be able to function quite well.

Yet, there have continued to be indications that persons who have oral asomesthesia may sometimes have speech-production problems, and the disrupted sensory process seems a viable explanation for the speech problem. Other speakers, however, with similar oral sensory problems may develop good speech skills. Two-point discrimination and ability to monitor tongue position have been tested in the oral cavities of groups of both normal and abnormal speakers; intraoral afferent cranial nerve anesthesia has been used to test the effects of reduction in speaking ability. Some of these studies seem to have had significant procedural problems. When that possibility is taken into account, a consistent cause-effect relation between reduced intraoral somesthesia and speech deficits still seems open to question.

The research relative to this issue with cerebral palsied speakers also has been only suggestive. Methodological problems make clear interpretations difficult. A considerable portion of this research has been conducted using three-dimensional forms that are placed in the mouth. The subject is asked to identify the form, which he or she can manipulate in the oral cavity, from among an array of such forms that are displayed for visual inspection.

This integration of somesthetic information for three-dimensional form discrimination, or *stereognosis*, seems to be an independent integration capability of the human brain. Deficits in the ability to perceive three-dimensional forms by feeling with the hand and fingers, or astereognosis, was first demonstrated with some brain-damaged adults, and there is reason to believe that the problem frequently is associated with lesions to the cerebral hemisphere that is not dominant for communication processes. Although stereognostic capability may be dependent on intact somesthetic mechanisms, astereognosis may be present even though there are no demonstrable indications of somesthetic deficits. There also are problems in interpreting stereognostic test results in the presence of a neuromotor disorder where exploration of the objects to be perceived depends on normal mobility of the exploring structures, such as the fingers for hand stereognosis and the tongue for intraoral stereognosis. Where somesthetic capability (e.g., two-point discrimination on the hand) and stereognostic ability (e.g., identification of objects in the hand) has been compared directly with cerebral palsied children, the relationship among the measures has not been strong.

Both somesthetic and stereognostic problems among the spastic hemiplegic group of cerebral palsied speakers have been demonstrated, and those deficits seem to exist even on the side that shows minimal effects of a neuromotor disorder. These problems also seem to be related to some extent to the group's speech problems. However, as discussed in Chapter Six, speech problems of spastic hemiplegic children usually do not seem to have a neuromotor disorder as their basis. Rather, these problems appear to be more like those associated with difficulty in learning articulation skills.

It may be that somesthesia has a prime role during the learning stages of speech production. During the formation of the neural organizations that eventually participate in skilled, automatic types of motor activity, the central nervous systems may use all available sensory information to assist in developing the ability to emit the appropriate motor patterns. However, once the underlying mechanisms for these skilled, automatic movements are formed, sensory feedback may have the prime role of providing information regarding after-the-fact information about the accuracy of these types of movements. Such relations would permit some children to learn speech production in the presence of disrupted intraoral somesthesia. Others, however, might find it difficult to do so.

As reviewed by Kent (1976), one of the more acceptable theories of motor speech processes suggests that the guidance system for speech production is a mechanism that provides internally generated targets for the speech-producing structures that have been formed as a result of learning and that is capable of anticipating the movements needed to produce the end product, namely, the acoustic speech signal. Also, it may be that if, indeed, a "closed-loop" servomechanism theory has applicability to speech motor processes, the afferent side of that system is composed of those mechanisms that transmit tactile and proprioceptive information relatively directly to the alpha motor neurons.

In response to the data and case reports suggesting that somesthetic problems are directly linked to speech-production deficits, some writers advocate assessment and management procedures that consider such problems as direct contributors to speech deficits. Due to the equivocal nature of the evidence, however, I am reluctant to do so. Moreover, reasonably precise assessment of intraoral somesthesia, such as measurement of two-point discrimination for touch-pressure over surfaces of the oral cavity and quantification of kinesthesis of the oral structures, is quite difficult. Although testing of intraoral stereognosis can be done rather quickly, as has been mentioned, the extent to which the results reflect somesthetic problems is open to serious question.

I have worked with a number of cases of acquired dysarthria in which intraoral asomesthesia could be determined by lack of the speakers' ability to determine reliably if a stylus was firmly touching some of the surface areas of their intraoral structures. For each case, however, the presence of a neuromotor disorder had been established, and it appeared that that aspect of the problem was the prime cause for restricted mobility of the oral structures. Even though I have been unable to satisfy myself that a significant intraoral somesthesia has been contributory to the speech-production problems of cerebral palsied children with whom I have worked, were I to do so I would establish a management program comparable to that which seemed most efficacious for those acquired cases. Those programs were based on the same general principles as outlined in Chapter Seven for management of articulatory errors.

sensory-motor disorders

There are reasons in addition to those given above for suspecting that measures of intraoral stereognosis with the cerebral palsied population may not accurately reflect their intraoral somesthetic ability. There is considerable evidence that a number of its members may have difficulty in perceiving a stimulus through one modality and matching that stimulus from among a number of choices that are perceived through another modality. Stereognostic testing usually entails that type of activity. When a form that is unseen is perceived by touch and feel in the hands, and a second form is presented visually, there is likely to be a problem in indicating whether that visually perceived form is like the one held in the hand. Yet, there may be no problem in correctly indicating if a second form held in the hand is the same or different from the first one that was held.

The ability to transfer accurately the percept of a perceived stimulus through one modality so that appropriate matching can be accomplished with stimuli perceived through another modality has been demonstrated to be a chronological phenomenon. Cerebral palsied individuals tend to be delayed in maturation of that type of capability (e.g., Birch, 1964).

There also is a high percentage of what has come to be known as visual-motor problems in the cerebral palsied population. These problems are those that are demonstrated in the types of activities called for in the Bender Gestalt Test of Visual Motor Performance. The acts call for reproducing line drawings of geometric forms, and it is well known that persons with brain lesions, including individuals with cerebral palsy, tend to have problems with these types of tasks. However, the exact clinical implications of these visual-motor deficits are not known. There is some evidence that the visual-motor problem results from difficulty in formulating an appropriate motor pattern in an attempt to duplicate the visually perceived pattern. There are other suggestions that the difficulty lies in some type of integration process in transferring the visual percept to formulation of the motor response.

It has been suggested that these visual-motor problems form a barrier to the learning of academic tasks, and that they might therefore contribute to the short attention spans and distractibility frequently said to be the manifestations of cerebral dysfunction. However, I know of no data that confirm those suggestions. Moreover, individuals with cerebral palsy who have significant visual-motor problems may achieve quite well academically.

The current assessment and management paradigms being advocated within the profession of occupational therapy under the term "sensory integration" assumes that difficulty in formulating a variety of responses to various sensory stimuli does have clinical implications. The underlying theories upon which the practice of sensory integration is based include a number of ideas that also contributed to formation of some of the systems of treatment for cerebral palsied individuals discussed in Chapter Two. Fay's ideas that learning should follow a natural maturational sequence (development of skills that are related to both phylogenetic and ontogenetic sequences) and the Bobath's attention to reflexlike behaviors are examples. Sensory integration assessment now involves use of sets of tests of children's responses to a variety of stimuli (Ayres, 1978). The tests include, for examples, reports of perceptions of tactile stimuli, replication of various body postures that are assumed by the examiner, assessment of accuracy of movement of the hands, and visual motor acts that call for copying line designs. These tests have been used with groups of children who have various disorders, and the resulting data have been subjected to elaborate statistical treatment. The results must be interpreted in view of the types of problems mentioned earlier in this chapter. Nevertheless, clusters of test performance have been indicated to be associated with certain types of problems such as learning disabilities.

Management paradigms have been developed that are based on the clusters of test scores for the groups of atypical children. The paradigms call for training responses to visual stimuli, inhibition of reflexlike behaviors, stimulating sensory mechanisms, and training to enhance appreciation of movement. Even though applications of these programs of sensory integration may be limited for children with cerebral palsy, since responses to the tests may be deviant as a result of the neuromotor disorder rather than processing of afferent information, the assessment and management techniques are being applied to children with developmental neuromotor disorders.

This sensory integration approach to various types of disabilities in children has become extremely controversial. A thorough and fair review of the issues would necessitate a considerable discussion of neurophysiological and statistical theory. Naturally enough, there is an intuitive skepticism regarding suggestions that disabilities such as reading disorders can be alleviated by some of the recommended management techniques that involve physiological mechanisms other than those involved with visual processing and memory. It is likely that most speech-language pathologists also will find problems with interpretations of some of this work that suggests that a lack of integration of neural information being transmitted between specific portions of the brain is the basis for delayed development of speech and language skills. Much research remains to be done to clarify many of the issues inherent in these concepts of assessment, the implications of the results, and the indications for management.

attention and seizure disorders

The earlier concentration on hyperactive and distractible behaviors has led to the recognition that a number of children (1) have difficulty attending to tasks for a reasonable length of time, (2) are impulsive, (3) seem easily diverted to nonproductive activities, and (4) have problems learning. This type of behavior problem is now believed to have a familial basis in a great number of cases, and the prime precipating factors are the psychological-social problems mentioned earlier. If the stress-related behaviors continue for a substantial period of time, they frequently lead to reduced self-esteem. Alteration in the biochemistry of the brain and metabolic problems are now thought to be additional contributors to this cluster of behaviors. The physical handicaps of children with cerebral palsy reduce their ability to compete in academic and social endeavors, and that fact certainly may contribute to development of these behaviors. However, the example of the mildly involved dyskinetic boy given earlier who was said to have the brain-damage syndrome exemplifies that the same variables that seem to precipitate many of these behaviors in physically normal children may be those that precipitate this cluster of behaviors in physically handicapped children.

Distractibility. A few children with cerebral palsy may be observed to be distractible in a different manner from that associated with the above described disorder. This form of distractibility is manifested by the child's attention being diverted to stimuli that seem to be of no consequence to most children. Examples of these stimuli would be (1) footsteps of someone walking by the door of a room in which there is relative quiet and (2) the intermittent movement of a shadow of a tree limb that is cast on the wall of the room from a window. Such children's attention seems almost uncontrollably drawn to such stimuli, and it would appear that their nervous systems are not inhibiting such stimuli from strongly impinging on their concentration.

The number of cerebral palsied children in which I have observed this type of distractible behavior are so few that I hesitate to mention the problem for concern that there may be an overreaction to it. When a child with cerebral palsy possesses this type of behavior, it will be unmistakable, and as soon as it is documented, it should be brought to the attention of the other professional staff who are working with the child and the child's physician.

One should not jump too quickly to the assumption that even this overt form of distractibility is linked to a lesion of the brain. Again, children under significant stress or who are preoccupied with sources of that stress may show similar behaviors. On the other hand, the possibility remains that some type of developmental central nervous system problem is a prime basis for such behaviors in selected children. Such behaviors in the cerebral palsied population provide what is probably an impossible clinical dilemma. A lesion to the developing brain has been confirmed; that lesion may or may not lead to certain behaviors of which a prime component is distractibility; those same behaviors also are known to be associated with stress in children; the presence of the physical disability and sociological problems associated with cerebral palsy does make the cerebral palsied child especially vulnerable to stress. The most reasonable clinical posture would seem to be that all possible reasons for these behaviors in the individual child with cerebral palsy should be explored, and if those behaviors have clinical significance, management programs should be designed according to the findings. However, if the decision as to the basis of the problem is prematurely assumed to be organic, a serious disservice to the child may result.

Seizure Disorders. It is well established that paroxysmal disorders do exist in the cerebral palsied population with sufficient incidence that the clinical worker should be alert to their possible presence. Although generalized, relatively severe seizures are easily recognized, the more frequently occurring type, which are sometimes referred to as petit mal seizures, may take a variety of forms and may go undetected. A child with cerebral palsy who has a reasonably good gait but who begins falling for no apparent reason may be doing so because of onset of seizures. The speech-language pathologist may notice that a child with whom he or she is working may seem to intermittently lose contact with the environment for a period of seconds; the child may suddenly stop in the middle of a response, stare as if preoccupied, and then return to the activity at hand. These behaviors suggest a relatively low level of abnormal firing of neurons of the brain, or a mild seizure disorder.

The speech-language pathologist should make certain that a physician is informed of such behaviors. The presence of seizure disorders can be confirmed or refuted in the bulk of cases by various procedures, including the use of electroencephalography (EEG). As mentioned in Chapter Two, there are limitations as to the extent that EEG can specify the presence of a lesion and/or dysfunction of brain tissue that is isolated to a small area of the cortex. However, it can be used with considerable reliability to confirm the presence of seizure disorders. It is inappropriate for a speech-language pathologist to specify that certain diagnostic procedures should be arranged by a physician. Nevertheless, since confirmation of most seizure problems is possible, attempts to obtain a thorough evaluation to rule out or confirm the presence of such disorders should be reasonably persistent.

Some children, for whom there are no other signs of any problem, suffer from mild seizure problems that do not significantly interfere with their function and may not require treatment. Nevertheless, there always is the possibility that such seizure problems interfere significantly with attention and other aspects of function of a child, and their level of severity and frequency should be documented, particularly in the cerebral palsied population, to determine whether or not they do merit treatment and whether they may become more intense over time.

Management. By the time it had become generally recognized that the behavior that was said to be associated with the brain-damage syndrome was not necessarily a firm demonstration of central nervous system problems, pharmacological treatment had been demonstrated to be successful in alleviating the undesirable behaviors in many of the so-called brain-damaged children. Medications are still prescribed rather routinely to assist the child in reducing those behaviors, but it is now generally recognized that only the symptoms are being treated when the underlying causes of the behavior are stress on the child. While some physicians tend to prescribe certain medications for these behaviors, trial-and-error periods with different medications frequently are needed before the most desirable effects are realized.

There will now sometimes be an attempt to make a differentiation between those types of attention disorders that are due to psychological-social factors and those where there are indications of some type of brain abnormality. Some physicians attempt to make that differentiation on the basis of the child's reactions to different medications. Where seizure disorders are determined to be present, a wide variety of possible medications are now available for their control where indicated.

developmental speech apraxia

The apraxias are a group of neurological disorders that were described early in the study of effects of lesions to adult brains. The behaviors of some brain-damaged adults suggested that these disorders resulted from disruption of neural mechanisms that participate in planning movement. Apraxic disorders are relatively poorly defined, and many contemporary researchers and clinicians who deal with neurology find it difficult to accept that such disorders exist. Nevertheless, the disordered speech behavior of some brain-damaged adults suggests strongly that there has been disruption of the operation of some type of programming mechanism that, in a sense, distributes plans for speech-producing movements to the neuromotor systems. Some argue that the entity that became known as Broca's aphasia represents that type of problem. These arguments have been so compelling that the concept of a speech apraxia is now accepted by many as an identifiable clinical entity that results from some central nervous system problems.

Despite the problems in drawing analogies between disorders that result from lesions to adult brains and alleged developmental disorders in children, the concept of developmental speech apraxia seems, at least at this time, to be an identifiable clinical entity. It is being given as an explanation for relatively severe articulatory disorders of *selected children.* Yoss and Darley (1974) have provided a reasonably comprehensive description of this type of developmental speech disorder. That description certainly provides a better basis for differentiating suspect developmental neurological problems than many of the earlier descriptions of alleged neurological bases of developmental disorders in children. Moreover, it is my impression that most speech-language pathologists who have had extensive clinical experience with children tend to agree that some clinical entity of this type may be observed in a few children with severe articulatory problems.

The description by Yoss and Darley may suffer from the implication that the disorder occurs more frequently in the population of articulatory defective children than, in fact, is the case. Also, I have been unable to differentiate the disorder on the basis of the specific patterns of misarticulations that they describe. Otherwise, Yoss and Darley's description corresponds to my experience that there is a select group of severely articulatory-defective children (1) who show problems in accomplishing nonspeech movements of their tongue and lips, (2) whose severe articulatory disorder is resistant to modification, and (3) who rather routinely show firm indications of mild neurological problems. With respect to that latter characteristic, all of the children with whom I have been involved, and to whom I would be willing to apply the label of developmental speech apraxia, have shown more than the so-called soft signs of brain abnormality. Those signs usually have included at least mild hyperreflexia. Moreover, those signs frequently have led to the diagnosis of mild cerebral palsy.

The principal concern for the present purpose, then, is the differentiating characteristics between this disorder and a developmental dysarthria, which are (1) the prosody of the speech patterns and (2) the performance of nonspeech movements of the oral structures on instruction. As mentioned in Chapter Six, the most common deviant characteristic of developmental dysarthria is dysprosody. The children I would be willing to label as having developmental speech apraxia typically use very adequate prosodic patterns in their attempts to communicate. The differences between the two groups with respect to nonspeech movements of the oral structures deserves a somewhat elaborate description in order to avoid confusion.

The discussion in Chapter Six of assessment procedures that are appropriate for developmental dysarthria deemphasize the historical use of movements of the speech articulatory structures during nonspeech acts. However, there also was the suggestion that observation of such movements would be helpful in differentiating between developmental dysarthria and speech apraxia. The two disorders probably cannot be differentiated so much on the basis of the rates of these movements, which are likely to be slow, as on the characteristics of these movements. The speaker with a developmental dysarthria is likely to show an appropriate direction of movement, such as responding to the instruction, "Stick out your tongue." The resulting movement may be slow and perhaps incomplete; nevertheless, it usually will be obvious that the appropriate motor act has been attempted. The child with developmental speech apraxia, in contrast, is likely to perform a reasonably rapid movement, with the tongue appearing to be appropriately mobile, but the gesture may be grossly inappropriate. Even when the child is asked to view his or her mouth in a mirror to aid in accomplishing the movement, the child may sit and seem to be somewhat puzzled as his or her tongue moves rather aimlessly in the mouth. In addition, children with developmental dysarthria routinely will show manifestations of the neuromotor involvement of their oral structures during eating, while children with the apraxiclike problem typically show no difficulty with eating skills.

I have not found it of value to speculate as to whether or not a child with developmental dysarthria has an apraxiclike component to his or her speech-production deficit. If the mobility of the speech articulators is reduced due to neuromotor involvement, differentiating signs of an apraxiclike problem would be obscured. Even though I have carefully attempted to assess the possible presence of this type of disorder in selected children whose speech production deficit seems somewhat more severe than the obvious signs of neuromotor involvement of their speech mechanisms would predict, I have usually been comfortable in managing the problem as a dysarthria.

language problems

A review of the descriptions of oral communication ability of very young children with cerebral palsy will show that, as a group, they are delayed in language usage on all dimensions. Reports of ages at which first words are used meaningfully, development of usable words as a function of age, and other uses reflect gross delay. Many of the early descriptions of the communicative ability of cerebral palsied children in the 1950s were merely descriptive of their oral language performance. These reports usually did not consider that the neuromotor disorder might limit not only the ability of numerous young children with cerebral palsy to produce oral language but also their ability to respond in ways that would reflect their comprehension of language. Moreover, there was a tendency to overlook the prevalence of mental retardation in the population and the inherent effect on the development of language. Rather, there were more frequent discussions of the presence of specific disorders, such as perceptual problems, which were alleged to account for the delay in language development.

The prevailing belief that lesions to the developing brain may lead to a variety of specific isolated disorders suggested to many individuals that the delayed development of language usage among young children with cerebral palsy should be attributed to aphasiclike disorders. As already mentioned, the subgroup of children whose nervous systems had been damaged by kernicterus were believed, in particular, to have that type of problem. These children routinely responded to low-level auditory stimuli of all types since, as already described, their thresholds were in the normal, or near normal, range for low frequencies. This responsiveness, in combination with their poor development of oral communication, which frequently did not seem to correspond to the severity of the neuromotor involvement of their speech mechanisms, led to the assumption that a special language problem was present. With such seemingly firm evidence that special language problems existed in this subgroup, and with the concentration on congenital aphasia as the basis of language disorders in large numbers of nonphysically handicapped children, it seemed quite reasonable that language problems associated with cerebral palsy were frequently due to a specific brain lesion that selectively involved neural language processes.

There is much more general recognition now that delay in oral language behavior and lack of appropriate responsiveness to spoken language may be due to the limits imposed on the young cerebral palsied child by the neuromotor disorder and the possible presence of mental retardation. There still is some tendency to attribute these problems to undefined and undocumented problems, such as perceptual disorders, central auditory processing problems, and other aphasiclike deficits. Even those who do not rely on such bases to explain a serious lag in use or appreciation of language by a young cerebral palsied child are many times cautious in attributing the problem to the neuromotor disorder and/or mental retardation. As will be discussed in the next chapter, that is an appropriate posture with respect to mental retardation. It is as unjustified to speculate that intellectual retardation is the basis of delayed language development without confirmatory evidence as it is to conjecture that some type of specific perceptual disorder, or other unconfirmed neurological deficit, is the basis of the problem. As also will be reviewed in the next chapter, there now is a strong tendency to rely on lack of experiential stimulation with young cerebral palsied children to explain delayed language development.

It is most unfortunate that children with cerebral palsy have not been more frequent subjects for the vast amount of research that has dealt with language development and its disorders over the last decade. There are issues that need resolution. For example, Myers (1965) reported differences in the performance of dyskinetic children as compared to children with spasticity on subtests of the Illinois Test for Psycholinguistic Abilities (ITPA). Myers controlled for the effects of intelligence, age, and socioeconomic status of her subjects by statistical manipulation of those variables, and her results led her to conclude that children with spasticity routinely perform better on ITPA subtests that represent automatic-sequential types of activities, while dyskinetic children perform better on activities that are said to reflect representational level of language processing. These differences were attributed to the sites of lesions that result in dyskinesia as compared to spasticity. This interpretation needs considerable review in that there is no body of information that specifically implicates the basal ganglia, or other subcortical structures, in selective operations that are represented by the automatic-sequential types of activities of the ITPA subtests.

On the other hand, there are indications that no common types of language disorders are associated with cerebral palsy compared to other groups of children when hearing status and intellectual level are normal. As already reviewed, the language disorders of the kernicteric group appear to be no different than physically normal children who have comparable hearing losses (e.g., Flower, Viehweg, and Ruzicka, 1966). Love (1964) closely matched the intellectual levels, mental ages, and chronological ages of cerebral palsied children with children who had no neurological impairments; there were no differences between the groups on a selected set of measures of language performance. As will be mentioned in Chapter Ten, special disorders in learning language have not been emphasized in the numerous reports of individuals with cerebral palsy who have been taught to use nonoral methods of communication. Certainly, there are a number of highly intelligent cerebral palsied individuals for whom the presence of a special language deficit has not even been considered. Therefore, it seems likely that the most prudent clinical orientation toward delay in language development and language disorders in children with cerebral palsy is that whenever there are indications of such problems with a specific child, assessment procedures should be used to determine the nature of the child's language competence without any preconception as to the nature of the problem.

In many respects, clinical assessment of the language development of children with cerebral palsy is analogous to study and determination of intellectual status of the population. The potential is always present that the neuromotor disorder is the variable that limits the extent to which a child with cerebral palsy can respond in a testing situation that requires standardized procedures for accurate interpretation. However, the assessment of language development and disorders in any population is even more difficult at this time than assessment of intelligence. Although there are many theoretical arguments as to what constitutes intelligence, the many years of work with and study of measurement procedures have resulted in an operational definition of intellectual status that permits its measurement and that predicts reasonably well learning and various cognitive abilities of a child. There is no comparable unifying conceptualization for measurement of all of the known dimensions of language.

Numerous tests of language proficiency are now available to the speech-language pathologist. These tests sample, on a limited basis, select aspects of language performance. Some are based on models of the manner in which the nervous system processes language. Other assessment procedures call for sampling the manner in which a child has learned to use the rules of language. Whether the assessment procedures are based on some theoretical model of processes of language, are designed to assess mastery of the rules of language, or are combinations of these two approaches, none permits a clinician to assess the language of a child with confidence that the child can be placed on some continuum of comprehensive language development. The available procedures can identify disorders of language learning in selected children, but again, it usually is difficult to determine if the disorder represesents the totality of a child's language deficit.

These statements may be hard to accept by a number of speech-language pathologists who have gained confidence in the clinical utilization of some of the numerous language assessment procedures that are now available. Nevertheless, a thorough review of what is now known regarding the complexities of language behavior should be convincing that procedures for assessment of language development and disorders sample only a selected portion of behaviors that constitute all potentially clinically significant language problems.

Many of the procedures that are used to assess language competence assume that neural language systems consist of input and output mechanisms with some intervening neural operations. The receptive side of the systems are believed to result in the formation of neural percepts from which meaning can be derived. Various terms such as association, integration, and information processing have been applied to the operations that result in that derivation of meaning. Such conceptualizations of language processes usually incorporate some type of storage mechanisms from which language can be retrieved for use, and that retrieval and use may be referred to as the decoding or expressive side of the language system.

Observation of the disordered communication behavior of brain-damaged adults prior to the turn of this century led to the beginning ideas that the brain processes communication by use of such three-stage (receptive-integration-expressive) systems. Those ideas have now been elaborated to include various levels of operations that are performed on incoming neural percepts. Thus, terms such as automatic-sequential processing and conceptual processing have come to have meaning to those who view language processes from this perspective.

The recognition that memory processes play a strong role in language behavior is one of the relatively recent refinements of ideas regarding language systems. Derivation of meaning is now believed to be dependent on memory searches as a part of the decoding process. Retrieval from memory also seems requisite to selection and use of appropriate language. This recognition has opened a vast area related to strategies of memory search and retrieval of language units.

Consideration of linguistic rules by which language is learned and used must be integrated into any model of language mechanisms. There seems to be considerable validity to the idea that those mechanisms operate on the basis of rules by which language is comprehended and used for expression. It has long been known that expression must conform to certain syntactical rules of a language, and it has now been demonstrated that certain syntactical constructions are easier to comprehend than others. Given all of the possible meanings associated with words and the morphological and syntactical variations with which those meanings can be used to formulate messages, it makes considerable sense that language competence is dependent on a system of rules that is learned and becomes organized within the brain. Otherwise, it would be difficult to understand how there can be comprehension of meanings of sentences, or use of sentences, containing word combinations that a listener has never heard, or a speaker has never spoken, before. Yet, such uniquely formed messages are a routine part of human communication.

Determination of the adequacy with which a speaker utilizes the rules of language and, in some cases, an analysis of that utilization within the framework of the models of language processes is beginning to be possible. Nevertheless, no set of assessment procedures incorporates all known variables that relate to language development and disorders. It also is not known, in some cases, how a number of the measures used relate to other dimensions assumed to be important aspects of language. For example, the ability to repeat a series of numbers may be used as an index of the adequacy of memory use in language processing. Yet, the relationship of a deficiency on that type of task to a number of other language-related operations, such as the ability to retrieve word units from memory, is not known.

It is not possible to review here all of the considerations that now must be applied in assessing language. Such reviews are available elsewhere (e.g., Siegel and Broen, 1976). Not only must issues such as test reliability be considered in selection of language tests, but theoretical issues such as those just reviewed should be used in selection of assessment procedures.

Despite the difficulties inherent in assessing the language competence of a child, the speech-language pathologist should be able to apply currently existing assessment practices to evaluation of the language of numerous children with cerebral palsy. It would be unfortunate if such an assessment were restricted to only selected tests that inevitably reflect the biases of the persons who developed the test and any theoretical model used in design of the test. Rather, in view of the confirmed presence of a developmental brain lesion, the prevalence of intellectual retardation associated with cerebral palsy, and the unknown effects of developmental dysarthria on a child's total development of communication skills, language assessments should be as comprehensive as possible.

Care should be taken in interpreting the results. If a child with cerebral palsy is highly suspect of being mentally retarded, it is likely that his or her vocabulary will be limited, not only with respect to the words that will be comprehended and/or used, but with respect to the number of meanings attributed to words. Such limited vocabulary probably should not be interpreted as being on the basis of some special language deficit. Similarly, a dysarthria might interfere with a child's production of bound morphemes, and if that child shows comprehension of tense and plurality that is marked by those morphemes, it probably is inappropriate to assume that he or she has a specific expressive language problem. If a seven-year-old cerebral palsied child uses morphological and syntactical structures that are typical of a much younger child or morphological and syntactical structures that deviate from the common rules of those structures, there may be reason to believe that the child is delayed in development of syntax, or has a disorder in that regard, just as may be the case with numerous children who do not have cerebral palsy.

A language remediation program should be undertaken as indicated by results of the language assessment, the child's level of intellectual ability, and the degree to which such a program merits integration into the child's total habilitation program. While language activities may be used to reinforce use of the speech-producing behaviors that may improve intelligibility, as discussed in Chapter Seven, it probably will be desirable to present a separate language program from that which is designed to improve the way in which the child utilizes his or her speech-producing mechanism to generate an improved speech signal.

The selection of the activities for the language program should be based on as broad a perspective of the dimensions of language as the assessment. Recommendations that language programs should be designed in accordance with the activities used in some language tests are probably too restrictive; moreover, to actually teach the skills that are reflected in test activities places too much credence on the possibility that the test design reflects the neural operations that encompass the totality of processes by which language is learned and used. Critical reviews of the implications of assessment of language for design of language remediation programs (e.g., again, Seigel and Broen, 1976) should be helpful.

○ ASSOCIATED PSYCHOLOGICAL-SOCIOLOGICAL PROBLEMS

The reactions of parents to having a child with cerebral palsy and the impact of those reactions on the child and the management program have drawn considerable interest over the years. The emphasis in the 1970s on the rights of handicapped children to appropriate special education programs and the federally mandated involvement of parents in that programing has lead to even more study of and emphasis on this area, and the literature on this topic is expansive.

There are a number of predictable effects on and reactions of parents as they are informed of the nature of the disability of their child and as they work through the process of raising that child. Occasionally, however, these reactions are extreme, and they must be viewed as pathological in selected instances. It is unfortunate that these latter types of situations have tended to be emphasized, since it should be helpful for speech-language pathologists to understand many of the problems faced by the majority of parents of the children that have cerebral palsy with whom they may work.

Unfortunately, the understanding is not so extensive regarding the attitudes and reactions of the individual who has cerebral palsy. From my point of view, some of these attitudes and reactions may be among the more significant obstacles facing the speech-language pathologist working with this population.

It may be exceedingly unwise for the speech-language pathologist to intervene directly as he or she becomes aware of some of the attitudes and reactions reviewed here. Such intervention frequently should be left to members of the professional team who are more appropriately trained for dealing with psychological reactions and problems. When such problems impact directly on the communication program of the client, however, the speech-language pathologist may be the person who has the knowledge and responsibility to attempt such intervention.

Even where the attitudes and interactions of parents with their child, or the general reactions of the child, are obviously hindering the habilitation program, there are a number of potentially detrimental consequences of direct intervention that must be weighed. In some cases an attitude and pattern of interaction that is obviously detrimental to the progress of a child may be a defensive mechanism that has evolved as a result of some untenable attitude on the part of a parent; when all aspects of the situation are considered, the most prudent decision may be to leave the situation as it is or to deal with it superficially. At the other end of the continuum, however, is the need to avoid overreacting to comments and behaviors of either the child with cerebral palsy or its parents as reflecting some serious problem that needs direct, professional attention of any type.

In numerous instances, however, the parents of a child with cerebral palsy will need to be told that their attitudes about and reactions to their child's communication problem are inappropriate and potentially detrimental to the child's improving his or her communication skills or adapting to the problem, and it will be necessary to offer recommendations for change. The information and recommendations can often be provided without reference to any general, underlying attitudinal problems, to which the parents may be quite sensitive or for which expectations for change may be unrealistic.

parent reactions

Most of the reactions of parents to their having a seriously handicapped child cannot be considered abnormal. Rather, they probably should be considered as very normal in view of their hard-core life problem. To the extent that the reactions are normal, a rather predictable pattern of behaviors results from having a child with cerebral palsy.

The Usual Reactions. Although management of the infant and very young child with cerebral palsy will be considered in the next chapter, the initial reactions of parents to having their newborn baby, infant, or very young child diagnosed as having cerebral palsy will be reviewed here. The predominating initial reaction has been described by such parents as grief and worry (or anxiety). There may be a certain degree of immobilization of their ability to deal with the situation, either because of those reactions or depression.

The early behaviors of many parents suggest strongly that a stage of denial develops very quickly. This reaction may be overtly manifest in the parents' "shopping around" for a more favorable professional opinion. Although there may be obvious signs of the handicap in the behavior of their baby, the parents may react to any normal-appearing behavior as an indication that the diagnosis is erroneous.

There may be a strong tendency to blame others for the situation. Depending on the quality of the marital relationship, one parent may begin to blame the other for the child's condition. The blame may be directed to physicians or other personnel who cared for the mother and baby or to an array of intangible factors that have been rationalized to have caused the problem.

Now that the diagnosis of cerebral palsy is made in the early months or shortly thereafter in a large number of cases, parental concerns over the long-range outcome of the situation may be one of the greatest causes of anxiety and problems in dealing realistically with their situation. Parents desperately want and need to know what they and their child are facing. Unfortunately, the fact that the long-range outcome of the problem cannot be specified during the early years probably enhances the difficulty that parents have in handling their initial reactions.

As the parents work through these early reactions, strong desires to do something to assist their child usually emerge, and denial may continue to be manifest in the strongly expressed beliefs that if they or professional people do enough, their child will be all right. As a result, the parents' drive to be of assistance may appear overzealous and inappropriate.

There are suggestions in the literature that these early reactions sub-side as others begin to evolve. Other reactions and attitudes may become more prevalent, and many parents of children with cerebral palsy come to manage their situation as well as, if not better, than might be expected. Even those parents, however, may occasionally show indications of denial through expressions of false hope, even though they have been repeated-ly counseled as to the reality of their situation, and they have demonstrat-ed every indication of having responded well to that counseling and to suggestions for management of their child. These seemingly well-adjusted parents occasionally may make a comment that they know that some way will be found to reduce their child's handicap, or they may suddenly react very unrealistically to hearing from some lay person or through the news media that a "cure" or miraculous new habilitation procedure has become available.

Whether the early reactions continue to be manifest in some way or whether they seem to subside, they probably have an effect on parents' long range adjustment. Either early in the sequence of events or later, a parent may develop the reaction of wanting to be out of the situation. "Why did this happen to me?" is a typical question. They may have to wrestle with feelings that they are, in fact, rejecting their child. Their feel-ings of resentment and hostility toward the child for the extra work re-quired in his or her care, embarrassment over the child's appearance, and lack of fulfillment of their aspirations for the child as a source of pride and extension of themselves may be impossible for them to accept. They may also develop guilt about these reactions.

It is the unusual individual who can grapple well with the practicalities of having a child with cerebral palsy and the resulting normal reactions without his or her life being dramatically affected. The extra demands for time and energy required for the child's care alone usually will have a tell-ing effect. The term "chronic sorrow" is used in the literature to describe a prevalent long-range effect of a handicapped child on its parents.

One of the more frequently mentioned patterns of parent-child inter-action with respect to the cerebral palsied population is the tendency for parents to be overprotective. The inclination of parents to protect their children is only natural, and whether or not such overprotectiveness is detrimental to the child's welfare and development of a sense of indepen-dence and self-esteem is quite relative. The physically handicapped child may, in fact, require more direct supervision than a physically normal child, and parents' concern in that regard may be quite justified.

Oversolicitousness is also frequently mentioned as a deleterious behav-ior pattern on the part of parents toward their cerebral palsied children. This characteristic may be a natural outgrowth of a tendency to want to provide for the child in ways that compensate him or her for the handi-cap. On the other hand, it is a fact that many children with cerebral palsy have to be cared for so closely that "doing everything" for the child is necessary, particularly during the child's early years. That behavior pattern on the part of the parents may become such a part of their interaction that they are unaware of the extent to which their child's motivation and ability to function is being thwarted later when the child can, in fact, do many of the things that the parents have been doing for him or her.

Extreme Reactions. The frequent mention of extreme examples of these parental reactions in the literature may convey a distorted view of the number of parents of cerebral palsied children who develop overtly extreme manifestations of them. It may be quite difficult to determine whether such manifestations are, in fact, well founded in reality or not.

A mother obviously is having real problems if she refuses to let her five-year-old cerebral palsied daughter from her sight and relates that she has never left the child alone with anyone else since the diagnosis was made. That is particularly so if the child is a five-year-old, mildly involved dyskinetic girl who is obviously bright, with good potential, and her mother demands that she be present in the child's classroom when the child begins school. The father who insists that the mother maintain such constant surveillance of their child also is having inordinate difficulty, as is the father who refuses to let the term cerebral palsy be mentioned in the presence of his ten-year-old, intelligent spastic diplegic son on the basis that "someday he will be all right." I have had direct experience with such cases.

Extreme oversolicitousness may be compensation for a parent's being unable to accept that he or she has, in fact, deep feelings of rejection toward the child. In general, it is likely that some rather serious psychological problem is present when any form of a parental attitude or reaction is extreme. As mentioned earlier, direct intervention usually should be provided by members of the professional team other than the speech-language pathologist; in some cases, it may be determined that no such intervention should be attempted.

There is one type of parental reaction, however, that I have come to believe must be modified if at all possible. Some parents tend to exert extreme pressure on their cerebral palsied child for improved performance to an extent that is unrealistic. This reaction may also result from parental rejection of the child. Such pressure may extend to all aspects of a child's activities, but when it is applied to speech-production skills, the speech-language pathologist should do what is possible to modify the parent's behavior. A number of examples come to mind, such as a seven-year-old girl with a relatively mild monoplegia that involved only her left foot and lower leg. The initial letter that requested an evaluation of the child at a speech and hearing clinic indicated that she had cerebral palsy and "a severe speech problem," and the parents had refused to allow the child's school records to be sent to the clinic. The child proved to be exceptionally bright and a very adequate child; other than her limp and inability to run, she manifested a relatively mild functional /w/ for /r/ substitution. The father had "given up" on obtaining the services of the speech-language pathologist in his daughter's school because "they said her problem was too mild, but I know they just don't know how to work with cerebral palsy." Upon being told at the clinic what he admittedly had been told by the school personnel, namely, that his daughter's "problem" had nothing to do with her neuromotor disorder and that it probably did not deserve clinical attention, he indicated that he would take his daughter to another clinic where "they would work with her." Throughout the evaluation the father had discussed his beliefs regarding his daughter's "problem" in her presence, and at one time he stated, "If it's not due to cerebral palsy, she is just talking lazy, and I can take care of that." This example may seem extreme, but comparable parental reactions may be encountered rather frequently.

Such parental reactions seem more likely in cases where the neuromotor disorder is relatively mild. However, parents of a child with a relatively severe neuromotor disorder may appear to be pressuring their child for improved performance to a degree that is unrealistic for his or her capabilities. For example, it may prove impossible to convince parents that demands should not be placed on their dysarthric child for dramatically improved articulation, and the speech-language pathologist may become convinced that the development of disfluencies in the child's speech pattern reflect, in fact, stuttering as it is observed in children who have no disorder of their neuromotor systems.

Effects on the Family. It should be readily apparent that the presence of a child with cerebral palsy can also have significant effects on a family constellation. As already indicated, if the situation evolves in which one parent blames the other for the child's condition, marital discord may be increased. One of the extreme reactions by one parent may present serious problems to the other. There are some indications that seriously disabled children are more frequently the subjects of parental abuse relative to their numbers in the general population.

Even in lieu of such extreme situations, strong disagreements sometimes ensue between the parents over what is the most desirable management for the child. The extra time, energy, and expense involved in caring for the handicapped child are likely to place a significant strain on the sound marital relationship.

Naturally enough, there is a strong possibility that the siblings of the cerebral palsied child also will be affected. The concentrated attention of the parents, which is realistically needed by the handicapped child, may lead to some neglect of both the psychological and material needs of the other children. Parents who involve siblings consistently in the care of the handicapped family member run the risk of the family's becoming oriented to the cerebral palsied child rather than to the needs of the total family. Reports are rather frequent of the evolution of behavior problems and feelings of deep resentment on the part of siblings of cerebral palsied persons.

working with parents

In view of the fact that the bulk of parental reactions to having a child with cerebral palsy must be viewed as normal, one of their greatest needs is to receive understanding support from professional people. Firm guidance as to the reality of their child's handicaps and what can and cannot be done to help the child overcome those handicaps is badly needed by most parents. Organizations of parents of disabled children may be a source of considerable assistance; learning directly from others who have had similar experiences and reactions may do more to convince parents that their reactions are common and normal than any discussions with professional persons.

The communication skills of children with cerebral palsy often have special significance to their parents. "If he could only talk, we would show you that he can learn," is a frequent comment of parents who have tended to maintain some denial relative to the status of their significantly intellectually handicapped and severely dysarthric children. On the other hand, some parents whose children are significantly dysarthric but not intellectually handicapped may need continual reinforcement that the speech-production problem is not an indication of mental retardation. There may be continued need for that reinforcement until ways have been developed whereby the child can demonstrate his or her learning capability. These tendencies to equate communication skills with intellectual ability may be the basis of many concerns expressed by parents to the speech-language pathologist.

In general, parents want to know the long-range outlook for their child's communicative abilities. Seldom is it disadvantageous to be honest and forthright. Parents may initially react negatively to a statement that the prognosis for speech development cannot be determined. Eventually, however, most parents will come to respect such honesty.

Certainly, admissions of not having good predictors are better than overly optimistic statements of the outcome. I have had to console far too many parents who have been told that their preschool-age dysarthric and mentally retarded child was going to develop speech on the basis that the child produced a variety of speech sounds at the age of eighteen months; on the other hand, I have heard a number of parents express appreciation for their child's being able to develop some oral communication skills some years after being told that he or she would never do so. Therefore, it may be better to err in the negative direction with stated prognoses.

It is not easy to tell parents that it is unlikely that their child will be able to develop oral communication. Fortunately, the systems of augmentative communication now available (see Chapter Ten) make options available, and the task is now easier than before those options existed. However, as a general rule, professional integrity and responsibility, as well as the long-range welfare of all concerned, dictates that, where appropriate, the reality of a poor prognosis be squarely faced.

Interactions that are judged to be detrimental to the child's progress in developing or improving communication skills probably are going to affect more than just the child's development of communication. As stated, intervention should be attempted by the most appropriate members of the professional team. Success in changing the parent interactions may or may not be possible.

There are a number of cases, however, in which parents simply do not recognize the significance of such interactions. A mother, for example, may have adopted the behavior of actually projecting what her five-year-old is trying to say. Intellectually she may be able to come to understand firmly that such behavior is contraindicated, but it may be some time before she is able to refrain from the behavior. Discussions of these problems should be conducted in a nonjudgmental way, and the examples of other parents who have adopted such interactions and the ways in which those other parents have accomplished the needed changes should be used wherever possible.

It is unfortunate that parents frequently are intimidated by professional persons, even in this day of relative sophistication on the part of parents and their involvement in programing for their handicapped children. Professional persons may tend to enhance that reaction by being directive and disregarding the parents' reactions to what they are being told. Parents have the need and the right to know what is being done to assist their child, why it is being done, and the expected outcome. They need to be educated, to the extent that is practical, in all aspects of the remediation program in order that they can comprehend its bases. Attempts to assist them in developing that understanding should be at their level of comprehension, and a great effort must be made to communicate with the parents rather than to them. Conversations with parents do need to be controlled to the extent that needed topics are covered, but the more the discussions can be made a sharing of impressions and exchange of ideas the better.

The extent to which parents should be expected to become directly involved in management should be based on factors inherent with each situation. The demands of time and energy and their effects on the parents and family members of the child with cerebral palsy should be kept in mind when offering any recommendations for home management. Home management regimens must be realistic, and none should be recommended that are impractical and that could lead to increased feelings of guilt on the part of the parent who lacks the ability to carry them out. Planning home management programs should be accomplished in an attitude of mutual cooperation.

The strong tendency to be judgmental of parents' inability or reluctance to carry out home management programs must be avoided. Many children, whether they are handicapped or not, do not respond favorably to structured, formal programs directed by their parents. No matter how good a parent's intellectual understanding of the problem may be, most are not trained to understand and to explore all of the options available to achieve a specific behavior in a child. They also are usually concerned that they may not be handling the recommended activities appropriately. If a home program is badly needed, it probably should be recommended in conjunction with extensive training of the parent.

No matter what parental role is judged appropriate in the professional program, a fundamental principle should be kept paramount: namely, no home therapeutic activity should be recommended that will jeopardize desirable parent-child relationships. Children do need parents. It may be far more conducive to development of a child's sense of worth and self-esteem, and to the eventual development of the desire to overcome his or her handicaps, for parents to spend constructive time in family-oriented activities that promote the child's belief that he or she is accepted and loved by the parents.

Neither should professional personnel place demands on the parents' life style that will further jeopardize their feelings of self-worth. Many parents become so preoccupied with their cerebral palsied child's physical handicap that they tend to neglect not only their child's psychological needs, but they tend to neglect their own needs for fulfillment in some way that is independent of the child. Professional recommendations for home management frequently have an unintended effect of reinforcing the parents' inclination to maintain a life style that is almost solely devoted to their handicapped child. Those recommendations should routinely consider the possibility that maintaining a sense of independent self-worth on the part of parents may have better long-range benefits to the handicapped child.

reactions to having cerebral palsy

A number of statements may be found that there are no common personality characteristics associated with cerebral palsy. Those statements result from early efforts to relate personality traits to the type of neuro-motor disorder and, hence, the general location of the brain lesion. It is also true that no common pathology of personality has been shown to be prevalent in this population. Rather, there seems to be general agreement that the varying degrees and complexities of the handicaps, the variety of parent-child interactions, and the different social situations encountered lead to great individual differences in personality development within the population. Also, most of the personality characteristics of individuals with cerebral palsy are those that would be expected to develop under the circumstances.

There is enough commonality of those circumstances that a number of general personality characteristics have been discussed on the basis of anticipated effects of being physically handicapped, known patterns of parent-child interactions and their potential effects on the child's personality, and empirical study of the personalities of individuals with cerebral palsy. The comments here are a brief synthesis of some of those characteristics that I believe should be helpful to speech-language pathologists in interacting with cerebral palsied clients and their families.

There is general agreement that parental concern over the child's physical handicap tends to lead to lack of recognition of their child's early needs for stimulation, exploration of the environment, and appropriate interpersonal interaction. Indeed, as will be discussed in the next chapter, providing the young physically handicapped child with such experiences may be exceedingly difficult. Parents may find it difficult to engage in activities with their handicapped baby or young child in a comfortable and spontaneous manner that will promote motivation to learn and there is the tendency for them to meet unquestionably all of the needs that they perceive the child to have. These factors may affect development of curiosity and interests on the part of the child.

The possibility that this type of situation may lead to delay in learning generally is a topic for the next chapter. However, it should be relatively easy to understand how this situation leads to an acceptance on the part of the child of his or her dependency. This acceptance may become so strong as to diminish the child's desire to accomplish what may be well within its capabilities, particularly if parents are extremely overprotective and solicitous.

This characteristic is, from my point of view, quite prevalent in children with cerebral palsy. This factor was mentioned in some of the earlier literature dealing with psychological testing as a variable that frequently works against determining the intellectual status of some cerebral palsied children, since they tend to put forth considerably less than optimum effort in any testing situation. It also may be one of the more significant obstacles to remediation of their speech-production deficits.

The speech-language pathologist may be able to develop a relationship with those cerebral palsied children who possess this characteristic that will motivate them to improvement of speech-production skills in the therapeutic situation. However, this tendency to be accepting of their status and to have minimal intrinsic motivation to improve it may be a strong contributing factor to the problems of carry-over that were mentioned in Chapter Six. It also may result in relatively lower aspirations for accomplishment than seem necessary for the degree of handicap.

This complex of the necessary provision of care and activities, limited ability to achieve, and acceptance of their dependency also results in immaturity in some cerebral palsied children, and they may come to expect that others should provide for them. This characteristic is particularly apparent in some parent-child interactions. Some children with cerebral palsy come to control their home situation. When the bases for ambivalence of parental reactions that have been reviewed are considered, it is little wonder that the children who adopt this immature, demanding posture within their families are successful. Like normal children who, for a variety of reasons, have become successful in substantially controlling their home environments, children with cerebral palsy may not show this tendency with professional people. Eventually, since the child does not receive appropriate direction and the usual constraints on his or her demands, the child may develop considerable insecurity and withdrawal tendencies.

Another dilemma presents itself with respect to many children with cerebral palsy. There are indications that some may develop guilt reactions for being unable to accomplish what is demanded of them in habilitation programs. Certainly, this same reaction has been noted for those whose parents express rejection through demands for unrealistic accomplishments. Hence, the child may not only lack an attitude that promotes his or her working toward improved performance, but the child is also faced with trying to meet unreasonable demands for performance.

As recognition grows of their inability to compete with siblings and peers and as the reality of their being "different" becomes apparent, many children with cerebral palsy may not only internalize their reactions as guilt, but they too may come to deny to a certain extent their situation. There also may have been ample opportunity for them to be able to deny their own contributions to their problems. They may have been allowed to behave in a number of unnecessary inappropriate ways, or not to work toward self-improvement, on the basis of their "being brain-damaged" or their "having cerebral palsy."

There are indications, however, that as individuals with cerebral palsy mature, a number come to be bitter and relatively hostile regarding the manner in which their parents reacted to and attempted to handle the problems surrounding their handicap. They may express strong feelings regarding their interpretations of parental comments and reactions as increasing their own guilt feelings by making it apparent that they required extra care and effort. Overprotectiveness on the part of parents frequently seems to come to be resented. Of course, many of the deep-seated feelings of parents regarding their situation are projected to their handicapped children in numerous, sometimes erroneous, ways, and many cerebral palsied individuals express hostility over those reactions.

Numerous persons with cerebral palsy also express resentment over their parents' refusal to discuss their problems openly with them. Not only does this problem seem to lead to resentment, but there are indications that the cerebral palsied individual may come to lose respect for his or her parents because they did not accept the reality of the situation.

I have encountered a number of young adults with cerebral palsy, many of whom are very mildly involved, for whom these types of reactions present real problems of adjustment. Just as parents have a difficult time accepting their reactions to having a cerebral palsied child, many of these young people have a difficult time handling their guilt relative to their feelings regarding their parents. These problems may be summarized by the comments of a university sophomore who had very mild dyskinesia. She had come to control her neuromotor problem so well that she would not be seen as handicapped unless she were suddenly forced into some type of rapid reaction. She was making close to an "A" average in her course work, but she had come to wonder, after reading a magazine article on the topic, if she were aphasic due to her "brain damage" since she sometimes could not perform up to her expectations on exams. Discussions with her revealed that she had numerous erroneous ideas regarding her condition. It took a considerable amount of time, including a visit with a physician, to convince this very pleasant young woman as to what constitutes "cerebral palsy." Her measured IQ was determined as 132, and I could not refrain from joking with her about what that finding indicated regarding her being aphasic. The young woman's reactions were summed up in a comment that she made as she seemed to be becoming convinced that she was a very adequate individual, "I suppose my mother was a good person, but I would have been so much happier if she would have talked to me about my problem."

This relatively common problem of lack of understanding of their condition among individuals who have cerebral palsy certainly can be offset with respect to their dysarthria. Older children with developmental dysarthria should be counseled by their speech-language pathologist as to the basis of their speech-production problem as a routine course of management. It is amazing how many teen-age and young adult individuals with developmental dysarthria have not been helped to understand that the neuromotor disorder that results in their physical disability and their communication handicap have the same basis. That understanding is particularly important for them because they, too, probably will have the same concerns about the relationship between their communication ability and their level of learning ability as was mentioned above in regard to parental concerns.

The numerous practical problems of those with cerebral palsy inherent in competing in society for eventual economic and functional independence, as well as the psychological problems of being handicapped, have not been discussed. Even without coverage of these topics, this brief review of the psychological-sociological problems associated with cerebral palsy may give the impression that there is little likelihood that families who have children with cerebral palsy will become as well adjusted to their problems as can be expected. There are a number of families, however, who succeed admirably in what seems to be a "no-win situation," and the favorable adjustment of their handicapped children attests to their having done so.

The speech-language pathologist should concentrate considerable attention, as is appropriate, on this aspect of the management program. In many cases, the resulting long-range dividends to the cerebral palsied individual are crucial to achieving the degree of functional oral communication that his or her speech physiology problems and associated disabilities permit.

In addition to the neuromotor disorder a special set of associated problems are inherent in the cerebral palsy situation. One or a combination of these problems are frequently as important, if not more so, in the remediation of the communication problems of an individual with cerebral palsy as is the developmental dysarthria. These problems range from mental retardation to the psychological-sociological problems that surround the individual with cerebral palsy.

There has been a historical inclination to attribute specific developmental problems in children to sometimes undetectable damage to their brains. This has been so for many children who appear to be otherwise physiologically normal. Therefore, it is not surprising that brain dysfunction in the cerebral palsied population has made its members a prime target for this type of thinking. Moreover, this perspective has remained with this population even though many of the suppositions in that regard have been found wanting with respect to children for whom the fact of brain damage cannot be established. This tendency to attribute what appears to be specific developmental problems to brain damage in the cerebral palsied group carries the same dangers as with other groups of children. It frequently results in obscuring what may be the actual bases of their problems since an explanation on the basis of brain damage tends to stop the search for alternatives and sometimes more viable explanations. Particularly with the cerebral palsied population, this type of thinking tends to overshadow the fact that the same types of variables that affect the development of physically normal children also affects that of children with cerebral palsy.

Due to the fact of brain damage in cerebral palsy, the probability of a higher incidence of developmental problems in addition to the neuromotor disorders in this population is dramatically increased. However, the tendency to assume without verification that there exists many of the specific problems found in adults subsequent to their brains being damaged is unwarranted. The tendency to assume a cause-effect relationship between sets of problems and dysfunctions that may be found in any multiply-handicapped population is many times indefensible.

Visual and hearing impairments, seizure and attention problems, and visual-motor deficits are found in the cerebral palsied population with greater frequency than the physically normal population. Visual perception, auditory perception, and somesthetic problems also may be found in individual cases. However, the exact character and significance of these latter problems has not been established. It is unfortunate that they may be assumed to be the bases of poor development of a variety of skills when the cause may be the most prevalent associated disorder of the cerebral palsied group, namely mental retardation.

The speech-language pathologist must form a defensible position regarding how these and other associated disorders relate to the clinical problem. That position must encompass the developmental language problems that are encountered. Again, the fact of brain damage in this population has been assumed to predispose its members to special types of developmental language disorders, but the evidence in that regard is equivocal. As with other associated disorders, it is unfortunate that special language problems are assumed to exist in individual cases without firm verification or due consideration of the effects of the dysarthria upon language development.

The set of almost inevitable interactions within a family who has a member with cerebral palsy will also need the attention of the speech-language pathologist. Many of these interactions must be considered as undesirable to optimum development of a child with cerebral palsy and the function of his or her family unit. However, it must be recognized that most of the patterns of parent-child relationships and family living that form the basis of these concerns are the result of people facing a hard-core life problem, namely rearing a child whose development is significantly impaired in some way.

Although a number of the commonly seen undesirable family interactions and the reactions to those interactions by the family member with cerebral palsy are most frequently normal reactions to the situation, efforts to modify them should be a part of the management program where appropriate. However, great care should be taken relative to intervention in this area. Those instances in which patterns of parental interaction seem extreme must be approached even more carefully.

It is easy to assume that this problem area of parental and family interactions can be changed through appropriate professional attention. It is equally easy to assume that the undesirable perceptions and attitudes that may be developed by the individual with cerebral palsy can be changed when they appear to be counterproductive to the individual's developing optimum functioning. Unfortunately, those assumptions are not valid in a number of cases.

A comprehensive, objective view of the total ramifications of the cerebral palsy problem might suggest that none who have the condition to a significant degree or their family members can be expected to carry on with a productive life style with reasonable self-esteem. Contrary to such an expectation, many of these individuals succeed most admirably. The speech-language pathologist who enters into this area of professional endeavor has the awesome responsibility of assisting them to achieve that success.

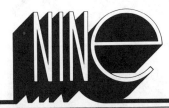

NINE

The infant
and young child

Discussions in previous chapters have emphasized the importance of the earliest possible interdisciplinary professional involvement with infants and very young children who have cerebral palsy. Reserving this discussion, which is specifically devoted to that aspect of management of cerebral palsy, until near the end of this book is not meant to undermine that emphasis. Rather, many of the guidelines for management of the general case of cerebral palsy are needed to set the stage for a discussion of management for the infant and very young child. These guidelines should provide a background of what the speech-language pathologist who works with cerebral palsied infants and young children should anticipate as his or her clients become older. In many cases early management may serve to diminish some of those problems.

Irrespective of the severity of the disorders of the infant or very young child, parents are very likely to need support, guidance, and assistance from professional personnel at the time some neurological abnormality is suspected and particularly, after the diagnosis of cerebral palsy is confirmed. In some cases, continued close monitoring by a physician is called for to rule out conditions other than a nonprogressive lesion of the brain. Initial management programs by an interdisciplinary professional team may be required for some aspect of the child's disability, and during the course of those programs, or through observation of the developing child, estimations may be made of his or her need for long-range programing. Firm prognoses are difficult to establish within the first two or three years of life, but establishing some idea of the outcome of long-range programing may be a goal of this early professional involvement.

As has been discussed, there is rather widespread belief that early management of the neuromotor disorder may result in a lessening of its manifestations as compared to results that may be realized if management is deferred until later in a child's life. The philosophies and techniques of this early therapy for developmental neuromotor disorders frequently entail components of some of the earlier systems of treatment that were mentioned in Chapter Two. There seems to be more general acceptance of these procedures as they are now used with the infant and very young child who has cerebral palsy than when they were advocated so strongly for general application throughout the population.

Among these philosophies and techniques of management is that which

is now referred to as the neurodevelopmental approach to habilitation of
the young cerebral palsied child. The assessment and treatment regimens
of that approach rely heavily on many of the ideas that were formulated
by the Bobaths, as described in Chapter Two. The revisions of those earlier ideas (Bobath, 1980; Bobath and Bobath, 1972) should be reviewed by
those professional persons who become involved in management of very
young children with cerebral palsy. Those persons also should take special
training relative to this approach to that management.

Recognition of these needs for early programing has led to development of a number of interdisciplinary programs designed specifically for
the cerebral palsied infant and very young child. There also has evolved
the belief on the part of some that such early programing results in (1) diminishing some aspects of the problems that would present more serious
obstacles to later habilitation efforts had they not received such early attention and (2) accelerating abilities of the child that might otherwise be
delayed more significantly. Concentrated attention may be given to assisting the infant and young child to develop physical abilities, functional
skills, communication, and socialization. Counseling, education, and instruction of parents are fundamental components of many of these programs, as is providing the infant and young child with a variety of
experiences that are designed to enhance learning of all types.

Lencione (1976) gives a review of some of these interdisciplinary programs, which vary with respect to the model of service delivery and the
theories on which they are based. However, most seem to embody some
common features that can serve as guidelines for services to this portion
of the cerebral palsied population.

○ ROLE OF THE SPEECH-LANGUAGE PATHOLOGIST

Prior to a discussion of what seems to be some of the more salient
features of these programs for the cerebral palsied infant and young
child, it seems worthwhile to review the role of the speech-language pathologist in provision of these services. The role which I believe to be
most appropriate differs from the current thinking of some, and each
speech-language pathologist who is involved with assessment and programing of these infants and young children will have to consider the
present points of view along with those of others that suggest other emphases.

The sustained interest in the abnormal reflex behaviors and postural
reactions that are a component of developmental neuromotor disorders
has led to identification of oral and pharyngeal behaviors in cerebral palsied speakers that are believed by some to interfere specifically with the
development of motor speech skills. There also has been a renewed interest in the chewing and swallowing difficulties experienced by many per-

sons with cerebral palsy and, as reviewed by Love, Hagerman, and Taimi (1980), programs for management of these mastication and deglutition difficulties by speech-language pathologists are now relatively common with young cerebral palsied children. Moreover, these programs are designed with the belief that they either (1) assist with development of oral reflexlike behaviors that may be diminished or (2) inhibit those that may be exaggerated. Frequently, the underlying rationale of these programs is that the development of more normal patterns of mastication and deglutition will lessen the severity of the dysarthria that is likely to emerge as the child matures.

As should be anticipated from the discussions in Chapter Five, I seriously question the idea that management of mastication and deglutition patterns will have direct influence on development of motor speech behavior. My rationale for strong reservations in this regard was reviewed in that chapter, and what I consider to be appropriate clinical utilization of observations of irregularities of motor patterns of the oral structures during nonspeech acts of persons with developmental dysarthria were reviewed in Chapters Six, Seven, and Eight.

Many of the comments made at the beginning of Chapter Eight regarding the problems of interpreting data that are gathered with the cerebral palsied population also apply to this discussion. There is no doubt that numerous infants and young children with cerebral palsy have problems in chewing and swallowing; there also may be observed in the group oral behaviors that appear to be reflexlike; a relatively large percentage of these infants and young children will have problems in developing speech-production skills for reasons that have been reviewed throughout this book. Moreover, these three areas of dysfunction will tend to occur commonly among those who have sustained more extensive damage to their neuromotor systems. That does not necessarily mean, however, that alleviation of one set of manifestations of the neurotomotor disorder will automatically lead to changes in the others. For that position to be held strongly, there would have to be demonstrated a very strong relationship among the sets of behaviors. The observations of Love et al. (1980) showed no such strong relationship between the prevalence of the abnormal oral-pharyngeal behaviors they identified, mastication and deglutition problems, and the speech status of their cerebral palsied subjects. A number of their subjects who had good speech had chewing and swallowing problems, and some who had poor speech showed few or none of those problems.

There is no doubt that some very young cerebral palsied children manifest these oral-pharyngeal behaviors when they attempt vocalization; similar behaviors may be observed to be associated with their eating. For others, these behaviors may be associated with vocalization attempts but not eating, and vice versa. To the extent that these reflexlike behaviors can be observed in normal infants, there also is no doubt that they can be observed in some cerebral palsied children to be exaggerated or retained past the age when they usually become inhibited. Any general management program of the developmental neuromotor disorder that can be shown to reduce the influence of such reflexlike behaviors on motor function during performance of any act may be helpful. However, the idea that improving chewing and swallowing behaviors is contributing to development of the neuronal nets that distribute neural patterns to the final common pathways of the efferent cranial nerves for the synchronous muscular activity for speech production has, from my point of view, minimal justification.

This type of issue, unfortunately, is not likely to be easily resolved. The clinician is forced to make choices on the basis of what seems most reasonable. Practical obstacles make clear resolution through research very difficult.

Irrespective of the efficacy of concentration on nonspeech oral behavior of infants and young children as a component of their speech remediation programs, such concentration is unfortunate if it detracts unduly from other contributions of the speech-language pathologist. Those other contributions may, in fact, relate more directly to development of speech-production skills of these infants and young children. As stated, I grant fully that, to the extent that procedures embodied with the neurodevelopmental approach or other approaches to management of developmental neuromotor disorders in these children results in diminishing the abnormal movement patterns associated with any functional act of the oral structures, those procedures should be applied. It also may be that the meager vocal output of more severely involved cerebral palsied infants may limit the extent to which the speech-language pathologist can design programs that deal directly with those children's development of speech-production skills. I also realize that whenever others of the interdisciplinary team that deal with young cerebral palsied children are uncomfortable with management of the mastication and deglutition problems, the speech-language pathologist may be in a reasonably good position to impact on those problems. However, the possibility should be seriously considered that the attention of the speech-language pathologist should be directed more to procedures that will minimize oral reflexlike behaviors and overflow of muscular activity into the speech-producing musculatures from postural reactions during vocalizations than during eating.

The speech-language pathologist should, without doubt, concentrate on determining ways in which these children's vocal output can be elicited. There is minimal information regarding stimulation and reinforcement paradigms that are known to increase and modify vocal behavior of cerebral palsied infants and young children. There is not sufficient information regarding those variables that will shape the vocal output of normal infants and young children as they develop speech skills to serve as a foundation for such programs. It is generally agreed that the vocal output of infants comes to conform to the phonology of the language through some array of reinforcement of their vocal output, or that reinforcement becomes self-perpetuating through internalized rewards. However, the lack of knowledge about the specific reinforcers that will optimally promote vocal-output and shape its acoustic characteristics in infants and very young children does not permit design of clinical techniques that consist of much more than general stimulation programs.

Even in the face of lack of such knowledge, the speech-language pathologist may be well advised to devote considerable attention to specific and systematic stimulation and reinforcement activities that will promote the vocal output and reinforce desired characteristics of that output in infants and young children with developmental neuromotor disorders. It is to be expected that the neuromotor involvement of the speech-producing musculatures may limit the degree to which many of these young children will be able to respond to such activities. Unfortunately, the limits of function imposed on the vocal behavior of cerebral palsied infants and young children for speech production by the neuromotor disorder probably should be considered as a reality of the situation.

In addition to the prime role of promoting speech production in the cerebral palsied infant and young child, the speech-language pathologist should attend to all of those variables that are believed to contribute to the development of language comprehension and its use. As already reviewed, the speech-language pathologist also has the responsibility for assisting parents of these infants and young children to adapt to and assist with remediation of their child's communication problem.

Even though the desirability of close and cooperative interdisciplinary management of the problems associated with cerebral palsy has been stressed to this point, such programing seems even more essential for optimum results with cerebral palsied infants and young children. The speech-language pathologist also has the role, then, of interacting with a variety of professional persons who are also involved with this type of service in order to maintain an optimally efficacious program. Sharing observations and information with the psychologist should lead to more sound conclusions regarding a child's intellectual status, potential for language development, and so on. Impressions regarding parental problems should be shared with the social worker and/or psychologist, and mutually agreed-upon plans for intervention should be designed with comparable cooperation from all others of the interdisciplinary team. From my point of view, an occupational therapist should assume prime responsibility for programs related to feeding problems, but as mentioned, the speech-language pathologist may have considerable input relative to the child's oral behavior. Interaction with the physical therapist may be essential; for example, a program related to gait training with a given child may elicit postural reactions that result in extensive abnormal muscular activity throughout the speech-producing musculatures. This one example is not, of course, the only type of potentially counterproductive management goal that must be resolved among members of the interdisciplinary team.

○ THE PROGRAM

the neuromotor disorder

Most programs for cerebral palsied infants and young children include analysis of the presence of abnormal reflex behaviors, patterns of abnormal muscle tone, and reactions to movement and posture. There seems to be considerable variation, however, in the methods of management of these behaviors, patterns, and reactions.

A method of management of the basic underlying neuromotor problem that has relatively wide use incorporates the principles of positioning in the manner in which the infant or young child is handled for all activities. That is, as the infant or child is assisted and cared for, care is taken in the handling to avoid postures or movements that bring about increases in abnormal, undesirable changes in the manifestation of the neuromotor disorder. In a number of programs, this type of handling may be coupled with a positioning program like that described earlier. The use of specially constructed seating devices, for example, may be an integral part of the management.

In some programs there may be initiation of therapeutic activities designed to facilitate those normal patterns and reactions that are believed to be diminished and to inhibit those that appear exaggerated or abnormal. This "normalization" of these behaviors, patterns, and reactions may be anticipated to result in long-range diminution of the overall manifestations of the developmental neuromotor disorder. In contrast to earlier claims, however, there seems to be a prevailing recognition that the objective is to reduce the influence of these behaviors and reactions and that to anticipate eventual normal motor activity is unrealistic.

interaction and stimulation

The fact that the restricted mobility of many cerebral palsied infants and young children leads to a general deprivation of opportunities for personal interaction and learning experiences has resulted in strong advocacy that appropriate programing should place heavy emphasis on these areas. The belief that optimum development of cognition and language is dependent on such experiences and that the amount and quality of interactions between the young child and the parents or other care providers will influence that learning is uniformally taken for granted. Many management programs include heavy emphasis on structuring the young child's daily activities in a manner that is designed to offset, to the extent possible, the child's limited ability to (1) explore the environment and (2) motivate those adults responsible for his or her care to engage in the usual type of interactions, which are judged to be fundamental to child development.

Unfortunately, enthusiasm for these early stimulation programs may lead to unrealistic expectations. Reliance on the logical assumption that experiential deprivation of the young physically impaired child contributes very significantly to delay in development of cognitive and language abilities can be misleading. There is ample evidence that environmental enrichment may enhance the learning performance of physically normal children who possess the innate capability to utilize that enrichment. However, there is equally compelling evidence that such enrichment can assist children who are intellectually retarded but who have no significant physical impairment only to a limited degree in the development of cognition and language. Finally, normal development of communication skills is characteristic of children with physical impairments who have normal intellectual ability and no anatomical or physiological problems of their speech-producing mechanism. Therefore, although it is important to recognize the benefits of environmental enrichment in programs of very young children with cerebral palsy, it is perhaps even more important to recognize the limitations of such programing for those of the population who have limited intellectual potential.

It would be equally unfortunate, however, if the need to be realistic about the effects of early stimulation programs resulted in overlooking the potential of those infants and very young children whose lack of responsiveness is due primarily to their neuromotor problem. Infants and young children who are developing receptive skills quite well will show sometimes subtle, but usually observable, differences to stimulation activities as compared to those who are not.

development of speech-production skills

The results of the speech-language pathologist's observation of the child's responsiveness and vocal behavior should impact strongly on the design of the activities that are recommended to meet the child's learning and psychological needs. When activities designed to promote vocal behavior should be initiated may depend on the severity of the neuromotor disorder and also on the general responsiveness of the child. It probably makes little sense to expect a six-month-old severely hypotonic infant to respond with abundant vocalizations in response to a stimulation program.

The speech-language pathologist should systematically observe all behaviors of the speech-producing musculatures to begin formulating impressions of the extent to which significant neuromotor involvement may be present. As with older children and adults who have developmental dysarthria, however, the best indicator of future dysarthria with cerebral palsied infants and young children will be the characteristics of the acoustic output of their vocal tracts. An abnormal vocal tone, restricted variations in pitch and loudness, limited emergence of different vowellike sounds, and, of course, a lack of development of appropriate articulatory gestures that produce consonantlike sounds in the child's vocal behavior all are indications of possible restricted mobility of the speech-producing musculatures. Observations of the movements of the speech-producing structures during vocalizations where possible will assist in confirming impressions of such restriction.

It is unlikely that specific dysfunctions of the various speech-producing structures can be identified until the child begins to attempt to produce words. At that time it may be possible to begin forming impressions of the physiological limits of the child's speech-producing mechanism.

Attention has been given to respiratory behaviors of cerebral palsied infants and very young children. Tidal breathing may be observed to be relatively rapid, and some specific procedures for changing these rates have been recommended. For example, using the hands to slowly compress the infant's abdomen to induce prolonged expirations and then releasing the pressure suddenly, which should result in rapid inspiration, has been considered to be an exercise that promotes the rapid inspiratory-prolonged expiration pattern associated with speech breathing patterns. I have seen procedures of this type used, but I have not been convinced that they are worthwhile, other than when they are used in conjunction with conditioning that has led to the child's phonating, or otherwise vocalizing, in conjunction with the induced, forced expirations. I also am not convinced, however, that this type of procedure eventually contributes to changes in the respiratory patterns so much as it provides an activity in which a young child may be conditioned, and come to appreciate, its ability to vocalize.

Most cerebral palsied infants will come to produce vocal behaviors of some type, particularly if procedures can be used that will minimize strong postural reactions and resulting overflow into the speech-producing musculatures of those who are more severely involved. As indicated previously, the speech-language pathologist should systematically explore a variety of stimulation activities to produce an increase in vocal output and modifications of that output. Use of facial expressions, tone of the voice, and other behaviors of the adult who is providing this stimulation should be comparable to those that are usually associated with parent-infant vocal play and interchange.

That particular point needs emphasis, since the bulk of this type of activity with cerebral palsied infants and very young children probably will have to be done by parents. As was pointed out at the end of the last chapter, the lack of responsiveness, the abnormal neuromotor behaviors, and the parental concerns over interacting appropriately with their handicapped infant or young child frequently diminishes what otherwise would be natural, spontaneous types of interaction. Even professional personnel may lapse into a mechanistic, unemotional type of vocal interaction with relatively unresponsive infants and young children.

Another major difference in vocal stimulation that deserves consideration with these infants and young children is the rapidity and amount of such stimulation. The presence of the neuromotor disorder will frequently result in a delay in the infant or young child's ability to respond. If the adult continues a relatively rapid patter of unceasing vocal stimulation, the child may be so inundated due to its limited ability to respond that its attempts to do so will be reduced. Indeed, careful observation of the effects of such overstimulation may lead to the conclusion that some of these young children actually seem to withdraw from participating in the activity.

During these stimulation activities designed to increase even the amount of vocal activity, it may be well to consider the potential long-range effects of a dysarthria on the child's eventual ability to produce speech. The rate of speech acts with which the child is stimulated probably might be slower than normal, and the duration of syllables may be slightly prolonged. It makes little sense to anticipate that the child can incorporate into its responses phone-types that he or she has shown no physiological capability to produce. Therefore, stimulation and reinforcement should emphasize those phone-types that the child is expected to be able to eventually produce.

As oral language begins to develop, the productions of identifiable words should be rewarded as strongly as possible, regardless of the extent to which they are well articulated. The child's need to develop and use expressive language dictates that attempts to modify specific misarticulations be very indirect, as is the case with shaping the articulatory skills of a normally developing child. The child's demonstrated ability to produce specific phone-types in CV syllables that may be elicited in vocal play can be used as a guide for realistic expectations of articulation in word productions. As the child develops oral communication skills, those procedures described in Chapter Seven will begin to be applicable.

It is likely that the speech-language pathologist will find it desirable to initiate language programs with most young children with developmental dysarthria. In many cases, such programs will consist of enhancing and reinforcing many aspects of the spontaneous language stimulation that is being provided by the child's parents.

Although there are no data relative to the next point to be made, I am under the strong impression that young dysarthric children tend to take as many linguistic shortcuts in oral expression as possible. Unnecessary words are frequently omitted, and as a result, the speech-language pathologist may wish to alter that behavior to the extent possible in order that the child's language usage will be optimally communicative. Care should be taken in this regard. Too much emphasis on grammatically correct and elaborate language may inhibit any young child's spontaneous attempts to communicate.

the task of the parents

As just mentioned, the bulk of the activities designed to promote learning, language development, and speech production skills of the cerebral palsied infant or young child usually will be provided by the parents. Due consideration must be given to the inherent problems faced by these parents, as reviewed in Chapter Eight, in recommending any program of activities and in instructing parents as to how to carry out the activities. It is unlikely that any set of instructions given orally or through reading material will enable a parent to interact comfortably with his or her cerebral palsied infant and young child in accomplishing the desired tasks. Not only should the recommended activities be demonstrated, but the parents should become involved in participating in those activities under the direct supervision of the professional team.

As mentioned in the discussion of management of the general case of developmental dysarthria, program planning for the speech-production deficits of the young cerebral palsied child is exceedingly difficult. There is the need to elicit from the child specific speech-production behaviors that will offset potential development of unnecessarily deleterious motor speech patterns and to attempt continually to improve the capability of the child's speech-producing mechanism. The difficulty in designing particular types of activities that will accomplish these purposes is compounded by the fact that most of the activities will have to be conducted by parents.

Whether parents are to assist in programs of physical activity, feeding, or vocal responses, the likelihood that the spontaneous parent-child interaction will be lacking cannot be emphasized enough. That is certainly true with respect to vocal interactions. Not only is it difficult to maintain continually an appropriate emotional climate, it is extremely difficult for an adult to provide vocal stimulation to a relatively unresponsive infant over any substantial period of time. No speech-language pathologist should recommend that a mother provide such stimulation to her relatively unresponsive six-month-old cerebral palsied infant until the speech-language pathologist has personally had that type of an experience.

Not only is reduced vocal behavior of an infant or young child not reinforcing to an adult to continue the vocal interchange, but without such responses, the adult is unable to judge what may be an expansive reinforcer to the child's response. A normally developing fourteen-month-old may exclaim "bow wow" when it sees a dog, and its mother may spontaneously respond, "Yes, dog's go bow wow." The relatively nonvocal cerebral palsied child may provide minimal opportunity for this type of parental interchange that is conducive to both speech and language development.

These difficulties, which result from normal reactions to their circumstance, should be explained to and discussed with parents. Possible ways to deal with them should be reviewed openly and frankly.

For parents whose child started receiving services very early in its life, the appropriate procedures for handling the child with a developmental neuromotor disorder should be accomplished as a matter of routine within a few months. The manner in which most babies are held, for example, with their head supported and their extremities well controlled in the adult's arm is likely to be a posture that minimizes exaggerated postural reactions. Most parents will continue to be comfortable with that type of handling as their baby becomes older.

The parent of a reasonably large thirteen-month-old who has just started a management program, however, may find it disconcerting to hold his or her child like a newborn infant. Such parents must come to understand, however, that many young cerebral palsied children cannot be expected to engage in vocal activity optimally unless they are secure in their position. Unfortunately, bouncing on daddy's knee with abundant vocal play between the child and father is contraindicated in many cases. For another example, even though some young children with reasonably severe involvement may learn to sit unsupported, and their parents will delight in their achieving that developmental milestone, they also must be made to realize that the child's relative insecurity against gravity may result in such generalized hypertonus throughout its musculature that vocalizations while he or she is sitting unsupported should not be expected.

The speech-language pathologist must constantly keep in mind all of the potential concerns and reactions of parents as the cooperative program with them is planned for their very young cerebral palsied child. Other than for those whose reactions to their situation are extreme, parents should be helped to recognize that their concerns and reactions are normal under the circumstances. Moreover, they should be assisted in recognizing and appreciating their own attributes in their attempts to help their child. With due cognizance of the practical and psychological problems they are facing, it usually is possible to design and carry out mutually satisfactory remediation programs with parents for their young cerebral palsied child's speech-production problem.

○ THE PROGNOSIS

The greatest difficulty experienced by those who work with the cerebral palsied infant and very young child may be determining a prognosis for their management program. Certainly, it is very likely the greatest difficulty for the speech-language pathologist. The professional responsibility for and desirability of being as objective as possible regarding the outcome of management with cerebral palsied individuals has been stressed throughout these discussions.

As was the case in discussion of the outcome of management for the speech-production problems of older speakers with cerebral palsy, the comments here are made in the context of infants and very young children whose prime basis for the speech-production deficit is a developmental dysarthria. To the extent that associated disabilities, disorders, and problems are determined to be present, the suggested program and anticipated outcome will have to be adjusted.

It is likely that the long-range effect of reasonably mild involvement of a young cerebral palsied child's speech-producing musculatures cannot be determined until the school-age years. It frequently will be possible, however, to make a judgment much earlier that functional oral communication is an unlikely possibility for many of the more severely involved young children.

Yet, predictors are so poor as to the eventual capability of many of these young children to learn to produce functional communication that even the most objective speech-language pathologist may be reluctant to offer a negative prognosis. That reluctance may be well-founded. There are numerous instances where negative prognoses for developing communication skills have been given for young cerebral palsied children and have proven to be erroneous.

As mentioned earlier, if a prognosis must be offered, it may be best to err in a somewhat negative direction. Maintaining false hopes too strongly probably is to no advantage to the parents or the professional persons involved. However, with these young children the professional endeavors should continue with the same effort until the prognostic indicators are so firm that they cannot be denied.

Fortunately, the options now available for augmentative communication systems make it possible for a young child who has little likelihood of developing functional speech, but who otherwise has ability to develop communication skills, to begin showing that ability relatively early. Moreover, as will be discussed in the next chapter, these systems may be considered to augment the limited ability of even less severely dysarthric young children to begin communicating.

There now are strong indications that interdisciplinary programs for infants and very young children with cerebral palsy have considerable value. Early counseling, instruction in care, and education relative to the problem for parents may do a great deal to offset numerous unnecessary concerns and inappropriate ideas and attitudes that parents tend to adopt during the early years with their cerebral palsied child.

The support provided to the parents during these initial stages by professional programs would justify their existence. However, there is the growing belief that direct work with the very young child with cerebral palsy is needed for the child's optimum development. This belief frequently includes the rationale that this early work will diminish some aspects of the child's disorders and accelerate others that otherwise might be delayed more significantly. These direct intervention programs frequently include working to reduce the manifestations of the neuromotor disorder generally and attempts to offset problems of experiential deprivation and motivation for learning through interaction and stimulation programs. It is unfortunate that there are sometimes overzealous claims made for the results of these programs, but there is little doubt that many young cerebral palsied children benefit from them.

The role of the speech-language pathologist is a fundamental component of such early programs. That role includes impacting upon the design of the program so that it includes activities to promote optimum development of speech and language. In some cases it is believed that this role should include a heavy emphasis upon reduction of exaggerated oral reflexlike behaviors and facilitation of more appropriate oral motor behaviors through feeding programs, but a more important role is likely to be concentration upon programs to stimulate and shape vocalizations as well as enhance language development.

Although prognoses are difficult to determine in the early years, these early management programs should make efforts in that regard. At a mininum, early planning can be accomplished relative to the needed long-term programs for many aspects of the child's needs.

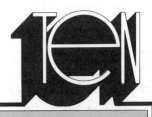

○ GENERAL CONSIDERATIONS

○ THE TECHNOLOGY

    expense
    ease of use
    positioning
    adaptations

○ CHARACTERISTICS OF THE
   NONSPEAKER

    physical abilities
    language development and integrity
    intellectual level
    other disabilities and disorders
    motivation

○ CHARACTERISTICS OF RECIPIENTS
   OF MESSAGES

○ COUNSELING

○ THE OUTCOME

○ SUMMARY

The severely involved:
Augmentative
communication systems

When the Nonoral Communication Project described by Vicker (1974) was being planned in the early 1960s, requests were made to potential funding agencies for the financial assistance that was anticipated to be needed to support the program. The requests were denied, and the uniform reason for the denial was that use of nonoral communication systems with severely dysarthric cerebral palsied children would reduce their motivation to continue to attempt development of oral communication skills. That philosophy of the era should not be criticized too severely. It represented the prevalent belief of the time: that efforts to promote oral communication with dysarthric cerebral palsied children should continue even when their speech physiology problems were extremely severe.

There is now much more acceptance of the reality of a negative prognosis for numerous severely involved children to develop functional oral communication. That acceptance has resulted in relatively widespread use of nonoral systems of communication with these children. Moreover, most speech-language pathologists who recommend and use such systems in the management of the communication disorders of speakers with cerebral palsy recognize the great psychological benefits that the nonoral child derives from developing the ability to communicate. Indeed, some of these professional persons take the position that such communication systems and devices may be used to assist in motivating children to improve their oral communicative ability.

This acceptance of these communication systems and devices for persons who cannot speak is only one aspect of the surge in use of assistive devices for physically impaired persons. Such devices are now being designed to improve their potential for independence and ambulation, daily living activities, vocational endeavors, participation in recreation, and control of the environment in which they live and work. Electronic, computer, and mechanical engineering technology is being applied to development and production of the needed equipment. Persons from the professional disciplines that work with the physically impaired are, in some programs, bringing interdisciplinary efforts to bear on analysis of the individual's capabilities and needs in conjunction with evaluation of commercially available equipment, modifications of that equipment, or specially designed equipment that can meet the individual's requirements.

A variety of terms has been used to designate these devices that are designed to assist nonspeakers to communicate. Nonoral communication devices, communication prostheses, and speech aides are but three of these terms. Special symbol sets (e.g., Blissymbols) are being used in conjunction with these devices to permit communication by those nonspeakers who cannot use orthography or manually coded communication systems (Sign English, Signing Exact English, etc.).

The use of these devices and systems has become so prevalent, and the professional expertise that is needed for their design and application has become so sophisticated that the American Speech-Language-Hearing Association (ASHA, 1980) has recently issued a position paper regarding the training, professional ethics, and guidelines for service delivery that are judged to be appropriate for the speech-language pathologist who becomes involved in this type of service to communicatively handicapped persons. This statement also recommends standardization of the terms used in this type of professional work, and the term augmentative communication system is recommended for reference to systems that involve assistive devices, symbol sets, and manually coded communication that may be designed and provided for nonspeaking persons. This position paper attests to what has become apparent to those who have been involved in providing those systems over the last few years; that is, an area of specialty of speech-language pathology has evolved that requires a professional expertise regarding technology, language systems, and needs of nonspeakers whose capabilities permit utilization of augmentative communication systems.

As a result of the evolution of this area, an extensive literature has been generated within recent years. There will be no attempt here to provide a comprehensive review of the specific systems that are now used or guidelines for this type of management. Rather, an attempt will be made to highlight what appears to be some of the more important issues that need consideration for entering a child with cerebral palsy into use of an augmentative communication system.[1]

○ GENERAL CONSIDERATIONS

The early concerns that augmentative communication systems will serve to diminish the motivation of severely dysarthric cerebral palsied children to attempt oral communication now appears ill-founded. There are relatively consistent reports that these systems may, in fact, serve to increase that motivation. This increase in motivation may result from the augmentative communication system's providing opportunity to partici-

[1]The bulk of cerebral palsied individuals for whom augmentative communication systems are appropriate have such severe impairments of hand usage that they cannot use manually coded systems of communication. Therefore, the term *augmentative communication systems* as used in this discussion refers to the use of nonstandard symbol systems, pictures, orthography, and/or recorded speech in conjunction with some assistive device by which messages may be constructed.

pate in verbal society at a better level than had previously been possible, but, because of some of the inherent practical problems with any augmentative system, these nonspeakers may become motivated to overcome those limitations through use of oral communication to the extent possible. The use of a communication system also may cause the nonspeaker to develop an appreciation for being able to communicate, and he or she may then become more motivated to enter into communicative interchange. Finally, having the augmentative system as an available method may reduce the anxieties associated with not being able to communicate; the child may then be able to enter into the process of improving his or her speech-production skills with fewer anxieties and concerns over being able to succeed.

Augmentative communication systems may also be used to great advantage in assessment of the capabilities of a child with cerebral palsy. As should have become quite clear from the material throughout this book, there are numerous, relatively severely involved children whose potential for developing communication skills is difficult to assess. A planned program of increasing the complexity of the language to be used with an augmentative system may clearly reveal a child's limitations with respect to comprehension of and ability to use language. The limitations that may be so demonstrated must, however, be viewed realistically. There is no justification for assuming that the use of an augmentative communication system will increase the basic capabilities of the child.

The inherent limitations of augmentative communication systems are a prime general consideration. The tremendous enthusiasm over the evolution of these systems may leave the impression that they may serve as a reasonably adequate substitute for oral communication. A more reasonable view is that these systems enable a nonspeaker to participate to some extent in our verbal society, but none will permit such a speaker to be an adequate, competitive communicator. Augmentative communication systems inevitably impose a number of practical problems relative to portability and flexibility of use. They also reduce efficiency of communication relative to the precision of language and time required for communication, and their use poses numerous problems to the recipient of the nonspeaker's messages.

The most important of these limitations of augmentative communication systems may be the restrictions that most place on the nonspeaker's ability to use expansive, flexible, and hence, precise language. Lexicon, syntactical structures, and flexibility of discourse are usually limited, even with the more sophisticated and elaborate assistive communication devices. As a result the nonspeaker's messages may be ambiguous. The unique language constructions that are a part of everyday communication are usually unavailable, and it is that almost infinite expansiveness and flexibility of oral language that contributes to our precision of communication through construction of unique messages. In general, those augmentative communication systems that have a more limited language corpus result in greater ambiguity of messages and, hence, increased opportunities for miscommunication.

There is an inherent trade-off between practicality of many augmentative communication systems and the expansiveness of expressive language that is available. Those systems that permit more expansive and precise language usually present greater practical problems, either with respect to size, portability, or expense. Those that are more practical and less expensive frequently impose the greater limitations on language usage. Exceptions are those augmentative communication devices for which printed orthography is the output medium (e.g., electric typewriters). These devices, however, routinely require relatively good arm, hand, and finger dexterity. As a result, their applicability across the nonspeaking cerebral palsied population is somewhat limited.

These problems of restricted lexicon, syntax, and so on are compounded by the fact that suprasegmentals (or prosody) are routinely unavailable to the nonspeaker. All these restrictions on expansiveness of language dictate that nonspeakers be trained to recognize that their communication attempts may be highly ambiguous and miscommunication may be frequent, and that they be rigorously trained as to how their particular system can best be used to offset that problem. Extensive training in vocabulary use and grammatical structures is called for, and the more that the nonspeaker can anticipate the reasons as to why a particular message may be misinterpreted, the more he or she will be in a position to overcome the problems.

These limitations on the efficiency and precision of messages should be a prime consideration in planning any nonspeaker's use of an augmentative communication system. That is particularly so, however, when the nonspeaker is a child. For cerebral palsied children who have quite severe dysarthria and good intellectual capability and who, as a result, show good potential for use of a system, plans for use of these systems should be designed with consideration of the type that will best meet these children's needs later in life. That is, it may be necessary to begin a child with a more restrictive system initially due to the child's abilities. However, the assumption that his or her needs as a child can be met by that more limited system may be in error. It may be better to begin a planned program of introducing the child to more elaborate systems as soon as possible. By doing so, the child may have the opportunity to be more communicative during the developing years, and may also be better able to learn to use the even more elaborate systems that may be introduced later in life.

○ THE TECHNOLOGY

The types of assistive devices that have been used successfully as components of augmentative communication systems with nonspeaking cerebral palsied individuals range from very simple devices, by which a nonspeaker who may be mentally retarded selects from a number of limited responses that usually include yes and no by either pointing to a display of the messages or pushing buttons to turn on lights on the display, to highly sophisticated devices that permit access to and retrieval of a language corpus with a storage capacity of hundreds of lexical and syntactical units through a microcomputer. The expense associated with these devices ranges from very little cost for those that may be constructed by drawing and/or writing symbols, letters, pictures, and orthographic units on a display board to which the nonspeaker points to thousands of dollars for construction and/or purchase of the more sophisticated electronic devices.

The number of devices and potential adaptations that can be used as assistive communication devices currently seems limited only by the imaginations of those involved in designing them. Anyone who becomes involved in providing services related to these systems is well advised to review as much of the literature in this area as possible. The above mentioned work of Vicker (1974) and the work of Vanderheiden and associates (Vanderheiden and Grilley, 1975; and Vanderheiden, 1978) provide early, relatively comprehensive reviews of some basic systems and potential adaptations that may serve as a basis for formulating decisions as to an appropriate system and modifications.

The literal explosion of use of augmentative communication systems will make any list or discussion of specific systems obsolete in a relatively short time. A major difficulty in this area is simply keeping abreast of the commercially available devices as they are marketed, ideas from knowledge of devices constructed by professional persons, and adaptations of all such devices. The speech-language pathologist may obtain current and updated information by requesting mailings from a number of sources.[2] This expanding technology is tremendously exciting, and its continuing expansion undoubtedly will resolve many of the inherent limitations of augmentative communication systems. The natural fascination with the technology, however, can lead to some serious, unnecessary problems.

[2]Information relative to augmentative communicative systems may be obtained from a variety of sources, including commercial firms who manufacture or market assistive communication devices. The relatively few sources given here should be included among those contacted, and the information that will be received will list most others, including commercial firms. The publication *Communication Outlook* (available by subscription from *Communication Outlook*, Artificial Language Laboratory, Computer Science Department, Michigan State University, East Lansing, Mich. 48824) provides current articles and announcements regarding augmentative communication systems; the National Rehabilitation Information Center (NARIC, The Catholic University of America, 4407 8th Street NE, Washington, D.C. 20064) is a rehabilitation research library funded by the National Institute of Handicapped Research, U.S. Department of Education, and it provides information from a computerized data base that contains bibliographic data and abstracts regarding all types of assistive devices; *The Resource Guide, Rehabilitation Engineering*

The strong tendency to review the number of devices and adaptations that are available, select the one that seems most appropriate, and then literally require the nonspeaker to adapt to that particular system or device must be avoided. The capabilities and needs of the nonspeaker must be the paramount consideration.

Many times that consideration will lead to the selection of a device or system that is among the less complex and expensive ones available. It is most unfortunate when some elaborate, sophisticated, and very expensive assistive device has been purchased and hours of professional time have been spent in training the nonspeaker to utilize that device, only to find that within a relatively short period of time the nonspeaker ceases to utilize it because it does not meet his or her needs. In many cases, relatively simple and inexpensive devices will, in fact, prove to be more optimally useful for a given nonspeaker.

expense

One of the major issues that needs resolution relative to services for handicapped individuals is making available funds to support their utilization of assistive devices. A very practical limitation imposed on the choice of an augmentative communication system may be the cost. In some cases, third-party payers may bear this expense. In other cases, special education programs in schools may be able to do so, but there is considerable debate as to whether or not educational programs should bear this kind of fiscal responsibility.

Initial selection and long-range plans for future acquisition of devices for an augmentative communication system must be made in view of availability of funding. There is little utility in teaching a ten-year-old cerebral palsied child the beginning skills requisite to using some assistive device that may be unavailable later due to lack of available funding. This factor alone should motivate the speech-language pathologist to review as comprehensively as possible all available options for less expensive systems. As indicated above, some of the more economical options may, in fact, meet the needs of the nonspeaker better than the more expensive alternatives.

---

and Product Information, (Publication No. E-80-2205, September 1980) may be obtained from the U.S. Department of Education, Office of Special Education and Rehabilitation Services, Office for Handicapped Individuals, Washington, D.C. 20202. This guide lists nationwide sources of information relative to assistive devices, among which is The Trace Research and Development Center for the Severely Communicatively Handicapped, University of Wisconsin, Madison, Wis. 53706; Accent on Information (Post Office Box 700, Bloomington, Ill. 61701) is an information sharing system operated on a nonprofit basis. It utilizes computer searches and retrieval of information relative to a wide array of assistive devices for persons with disabilities.

ease of use

Despite the advantages that the nonspeaker may realize from being able to communicate, if the device used with his or her augmentative communication system imposes too many difficulties, the nonspeaker may become disinclined to use it. In general, of course, the smaller the size and the greater the portability of the device, the better. The severely physically impaired nonspeaker may be disinclined to use larger and more bulky devices due to their appearance of accentuating his or her handicap or out of reluctance to having to ask those who care for him or her to make the device consistently available. The environments in which relatively large devices can be used will be restricted. Those caring for the nonspeaker may simply not wish to bother making more cumbersome devices available to the nonspeaker. As far as size and portability is concerned, of course, the ideal assistive device is one that can be unobtrusively transported with the nonspeaker at all times.

Concern regarding ease of use of an augmentative communication system applies not only to the user of the device but, perhaps even more importantly, to the recipient of the nonspeaker's messages. A device whose access and/or output takes a considerable amount of time may make many recipients disinclined to participate in conversation with the nonspeaker. For that matter, any augmentative communication system that entails prolonged completion of a message may create memory problems both for the nonspeaker and recipient, and details of the initial part of a message may be forgotten before its completion.

The ease with which messages can be received is an equally important consideration, and the problem of time of message construction that is presented to the recipient has already been mentioned. The position that must be assumed by the recipient in relation to the nonspeaker and the device is also important. Most recipients will have much more patience if they have freedom of position when listening to messages generated through some device that uses recorded speech for output in contrast to having to stand behind the nonspeaker in order to see the series of characters to which the nonspeaker is pointing. The sophisticated nature of devices that display orthographic messages on an oscilloscope may be intriguing, but they require the recipient to be able to view the scope face; a small paper writer that generates a hard copy of the message, which the recipient can simply hold and read, may be preferable.

positioning

It is generally accepted that positioning of the physically impaired nonspeaker so that he or she can physically operate the device with ease is essential. A prime requirement with cerebral palsied individuals is that they be posturally secure during use of their system so that there will be minimum influence of postural reactions and manifestations of their neuromotor disorder. A child with dyskinesia who has considerable problems using a typewriter when he is required to lean forward to reach a keyboard is an example. A desirable management in such a case would be to (1) assure that the child is positioned adequately in his chair so that there is optimal postural security and (2) mount the keyboard, perhaps to the positioning chair, in such a way that it is within easy reach of the child and the keyboard can be maintained within his range of vision with a minimum of head and body movement.

adaptations

Very frequently simple adaptations to assistive devices, when used in conjunction with positioning devices, dramatically increase the ease with which an augmentative communication system can be used. For example, a given nonspeaker may be limited to use of one or two switches; the access to the assistive communication device may be a visual scanner on which lights are illuminated in a serial order; pushing a button when a given light is illuminated directs access to a specific mode of operation of the device. Ease of use of such a device may be increased dramatically by simply mounting the visual scanner on some type of rod that is attached to the positioning device and that holds the scanner at face level. In many cases imaginative but very simple adaptations of the basic assistive communicative devices can enhance their utilization significantly.

○ CHARACTERISTICS OF THE NONSPEAKER

Whenever it has been determined that a developmental dysarthria is so severe that a child will not be able to develop functional oral communication that will meet his or her minimal communicative needs, some type of augmentative communication system may be considered. In addition, the presence of an intellectual handicap along with a developmental dysarthria of less severity may suggest that some type of augmentative communication system with the use of a nonstandard symbol system may be advisable (McDonald, 1980).

The degree of involvement of the individual's extremities usually will limit the selection of the types of access to assistive communication devices and, as already mentioned, the nature of that access may be a prime determiner of the basic characteristics of the augmentative communication system. In addition, however, numerous other variables may dictate the characteristics and success of the system. A child's level of language development and/or integrity of the language system must enter strongly into the choice of the communicative device to be used initially and a determination of the amount of training that will be needed to bring the child to some level of communicative competence. Optimal planning for an augmentative communication system also, of course, must consider the child's intellectual level. The presence of a significant visual impairment or visual perception problem may limit the type of system that can be used. Another prime consideration is the extent to which the child is likely to be motivated to use an augmentative communication system. The attitudes and reactions of those with whom the child uses the system may be deciding factors in the child's maintaining appropriate motivation to use the system.

physical abilities

In most cases an occupational therapist, and many times a physical therapist, should participate in the selection and design of an assistive communicative device. Not only will determination of range, control, and force of movement be needed, but in many cases it will also be desirable to design an augmentative communicative system as an integral part of a child's general positioning program. The child's ability to control switching devices may be totally dependent on adequate positioning with a concomitant reduction in postural reactions and manifestations of the neuromotor disorder. The characteristics of the assistive communicative device to be used may dictate the design of posturing devices and vice versa. In addition, assistive devices to promote function for other than communication may be indicated, and the total design of positioning and assistive devices programs must be an integrated process.

The need to coordinate the planning of an augmentative communication system for children with cerebral palsy with an occupational therapist usually is taken for granted since use of the upper extremities probably will be a prime determinant in the type of assistive communication device that can be used. Coleman, Cook, and Myers (1980) review some of the specific evaluations of upper extremity and hand dexterity that may be needed. In addition, the occupational therapist may be able to estimate the extent to which the function of a cerebral palsied child's upper extremities can be expected to improve. If such improvement seems likely, the initial system may be designed in anticipation of later changes that the improved function will permit.

When upper extremity function is so limited that the use of the hands for the assistive communication device is not a viable consideration, use of head movements may be an alternative. Pointing sticks mounted to a head band are frequently used with good success, and switches controlled by head movements are also sometimes possible, as is use of the feet and toes with rare dyskinetic nonspeakers who have lesser involvement of the lower extremities.

language development and integrity

The level of language development of children, of course, will dictate many of the characteristics of the initial augmentative communication system that is to be used, and the prognosis for continued language development must be considered in long-range planning for increasing the capability of the system. Since most of the systems that are appropriate for use by young children require language concepts to be associated with some type of drawn or printed characters, use of a nonstandard symbol system such as Blissymbolics (McDonald, 1980) may have applicability, or use of pictures in combination with orthography, as in the type of systems described by Vicker (1974), may be considered. When it appears that the child has normal intellectual capability, my preference is for the latter.

The level of the child's language development will dictate the level of the language corpus and constructions to be used initially with the system. However, an augmentative communication system can be a powerful tool in teaching language skills. Strong emphasis should be placed on using appropriate syntactical structures in the construction of messages. As mentioned in the discussion of language in Chapter Eight, conformance to syntactical rules is known to enhance comprehension of oral language, and the same can be said for messages generated with an augmentative communication system. As a result, a child may be taught such rules through use of his or her system. Expansion of vocabulary also is a frequent outgrowth of the use of these systems.

Descriptions of use of augmentative communication systems frequently mention the need to use a variety of tests to determine the language integrity of a potential user. As mentioned earlier, the lack of reference to specific language disorders in this literature create doubt on the prevalence of such disorders in cerebral palsy.

intellectual level

Not only will reduced intellectual capability of a nonspeaking child with cerebral palsy limit the level of language that can be incorporated into an augmentative communication system, but it also may impose limits on the complexity of the operation of the system, to include use of a nonstandard symbol system. The nonspeaking dysarthric and mentally retarded child may show gross limitations to his or her ability to comprehend or appreciate the need for relatively simple grammatical constructions and lexicon that may be incorporated into even a beginning augmentative communication system. It may be much more feasible to limit the number of responses and to have those responses be formed messages rather than to expect the child to formulate messages from smaller linguistic units. In addition, intellectual retardation may reduce a child's appreciation of the advantages of participating verbally in his or her educational and daily living activities.

other disabilities and disorders

A number of cerebral palsied children may be unable to perform a set of basic tasks that are requisite to use of an augmentative communication system. These problems may range from having poor ability to discriminate symbols visually to being unable to attend to the task to formulate messages for sufficient lengths of time.

Although relatively significant visual impairments can be circumvented in a program of management of speech-production skills, such an impairment may be a significant obstacle to use of an augmentative communication system. Ability to discriminate among visual stimuli and to use memory to attach consistent linguistic significance to those stimuli are requisite to use of many systems. Testing for visual perception problems has been recommended as prerequisite to determine the candidacy of cerebral palsied children for use of augmentative communication systems, and determining digit span recall are among the assessments that are used. As mentioned in Chapter Eight, however, it may be exceedingly difficult to determine the basis of erroneous responses to various types of visual discrimination tests, and the precise implications of tests for memory for communication processes is not known.

Although such tests may be helpful, their results may not predict the extent to which the child can learn to perform the various tasks associated with use of an augmentative communication system. In training a child to use Blissymbols, for example, initial difficulty may be encountered with an intellectually handicapped cerebral palsied child, and that difficulty may seem to be on the basis of poor ability to discriminate the symbols. As training in the use of this nonstandard symbol system proceeds, however, the child may show increasing capability to make the necessary visual discriminations.

Problems of attention also have been mentioned as limiting the extent to which a child can use these systems. If training activities can be made sufficiently stimulating, a child's inclination and ability to attend to the tasks may improve.

motivation

Children may initially be quite fascinated with the somewhat unique tasks associated with learning to use an augmentative communication system. However, as soon as the initial fascination subsides, the enthusiasm may wane, and it may be surprisingly difficult to motivate them to continue to participate optimally in the training programs. One basis of

this difficulty may be the general attitude of being accepting of their de-
pendence and not being willing to put forth effort to improve their communicative ability. Also, the tasks that are involved may simply be quite
difficult for the child, and care should be taken to maintain an appropriate level of difficulty. There is also the possibility that lack of motivation
results from the child's not perceiving the functional significance of the
system. Early practical use of the system is indicated, no matter how limited that use may be. Drill that generates messages with little applicability to
the child's daily activities should be used only to the extent that it does not
diminish a child's desire to use the system. Actually using the system to
communicate with his or her therapists, teacher, and parents may be a
strong motivating vehicle for the child.

○ CHARACTERISTICS OF RECIPIENTS OF MESSAGES

A prime deterrent to the child's motivation to utilize an augmentative communication system and perceive the advantages in doing so may
be the reactions and attitude of the adults with whom he or she attempts
to use the system. As mentioned, none of these systems are as efficient as
oral communication. Adults with whom a child attempts to communicate
may not take the time to allow the child to formulate messages; they may
prematurely and erroneously misinterpret the message; they may not be
willing to interact with the child in a manner that will assist with appropriate elaboration of a message so that it can be interpreted reasonably well;
or they may project an attitude of impatience and discontent as a result of
the time-consuming and relatively inefficient communication process.

Potential recipients of the child's augmentative communication attempts should be trained to avoid these reactions. In particular, the child's
parents should be optimally supportive of and enthusiastic about their
child's use of the system. If they are not, that variable alone may result in
poor or unsuccessful usage of the system. Whether or not the system that
is planned for a given child is the type of language display with which
messages are generated by pointing to displays of language units, the discussions of use of those systems with cerebral palsied children in Vicker
(1974) review very well some of these contributors to success, or lack
thereof, that are associated with adult reactions to a cerebral palsied
child's use of augmentative communication.

○ COUNSELING

In some cases an augmentative communication system may be introduced into the cerebral palsied child's program of habilitation and

used with minimal problems. Despite the limitations and difficulties with these systems, the child may enter into the use of his or her system enthusiastically; the parents may simply accept the limitations and intuitively work to adjust to them.

More frequently, however, there will be need to counsel both the user and frequent recipients as to the ramifications of using an augmentative communication system. Frank and open discussions of the problems are usually indicated. Even young children may be able to understand and to respond amazingly well to such discussions. However, the speech-language pathologist should not take for granted that the opportunity for the child to communicate will motivate the child to work through all of the possible frustrations that he or she will encounter. Such frustrations may be overwhelming relative to the rewards received.

Such frustrations may become defeating even for those children who have accepted and learned to use their system quite successfully. Such a child may become a proficient user of the system in the environment of his or her home and school. Within those environments, the more important persons to the child may have learned to interact very appropriately. They may make significant attempts to interpret messages accurately; they may repeat their interpretations of a message so that the child may correct any misinterpretations; and they may ask questions that will permit the child to elaborate the messages with optimum efficiency. Children may come to expect equally appropriate interaction from most adults with whom they use the system. When that interaction fails to occur, a child may experience significant frustrations and become disinclined to attempt to use his or her system with persons other than those he or she knows will interact appropriately. Again, frank discussions of the child's feelings to this type of circumstance may be amazingly helpful, as will reviews with the child of practical ways to overcome the problems.

The speech-language pathologist also should not take for granted that parents will welcome the recommendation of a nonoral system of communication for their severely dysarthric cerebral palsied child. Even though the system may give their child the opportunity to communicate, and even though, intellectually, they may be able to accept the potential benefits to their child, parents frequently react negatively to this type of recommendation. It may represent concrete, final evidence that their child is not going to be able to communicate orally. Parents who otherwise have shown very realistic acceptance of their situation may suddenly display unrealistic expectations. A few may totally reject the recommendation or be unable to cooperate optimally in the needed counseling and training programs with their child. As a consequence, the initial recommendations to parents for augmentative communication systems should be approached cautiously and with considerable understanding.

○ THE OUTCOME

There is little doubt that optimum use of augmentative communication systems will lead to an improved life style for many cerebral palsied nonspeakers. Significantly intellectually handicapped and severely involved individuals who have cerebral palsy may be able to communicate basic needs and thereby receive better care and more appropriate responses from caretakers. The intelligent severely dysarthric individual with cerebral palsy may be able to use an elaborate, complicated assistive communication device to express ideas and to communicate relatively well to selected individuals.

Persons with the latter characteristics may face more significant obstacles in optimal utilization of their augmentative communication systems than do those with the former characteristics. The most significant obstacle for those whose basic capabilities permit good communicative ability may be the cluster of factors that were just reviewed relative to reactions of recipients to their communication attempts. For that matter, cerebral palsied speakers who are dysarthric but who develop functional oral communication face the same set of obstacles to being able to communicate, and thus interact, appropriately within society. When a person possesses as obvious a communication disorder as do most dysarthric individuals with cerebral palsy they routinely encounter reactions from nonhandicapped individuals that diminish appropriate interaction. A moderately severe dysarthric young man with spasticity may be easily intelligible with relatively careful listening. Yet, a nonhandicapped listener may initially react to his dysprosody, and his general appearance, as if he is not worth listening to. His slow rate of speech may create considerable impatience on the part of other listeners. Others may become very uncomfortable as they make a concentrated effort to understand his speech or to attempt to understand fully a message of a cerebral palsied nonspeaker using an augmentative communication system.

In contrast, these reactions are not likely to be as extreme or obvious to the quadriplegic spinal cord injury victim who has normal communicative skills. The numerous reports by individuals with cerebral palsy of the reactions of persons in society generally to their effort to communicate reflect the previously described inclination to associate communicative ability with intellect, and probably personal worth of the communicatively handicapped person. When this handicap is associated with a significant physical disability, these inclinations to degrade the capabilities of the disabled individual probably are intensified. Therefore, whether the individual with cerebral palsy must use an augmentative communication device or uses obviously abnormal oral communication, the most significant obstacle to optimum fruition of the speech-language pathologist's efforts to assist these communicatively persons may be society's reaction to their modes of communication. While tremendous advances have been made in the general public's understanding of needs and abilities of disabled persons, much more needs to be accomplished to achieve their acceptance as human beings, and this need is especially great for the individual who has a communicative disorder as a result of having cerebral palsy.

SUMMARY

The rapidly expanding technology of assistive devices for persons with handicaps is now enabling those persons to achieve higher levels of functional independence. Augmentative communication systems are now accepted as a means to provide persons who are unable to speak with the ability to communicate. As a consequence, these systems are now being used with many severely dysarthric nonspeakers who have cerebral palsy.

The design, construction, and issues related to the use of these augmentative communication systems requires special expertise, and a specialty area of speech-language pathology is evolving to provide it. Not only does the use of these devices permit numerous nonspeaking persons with cerebral palsy to dramatically improve their life style, but they may be used to assess a number of aspects of the abilities of nonspeaking children with cerebral palsy and to stimulate some to improve their oral communication abilities.

The enthusiasm that has been generated for these systems must not cloud a number of problems inherent in their utilization. Most importantly, they are not a wholly satisfactory substitute for oral communication. These systems usually curtail the efficiency of communication in a number of ways. The language corpus that is available to the nonspeaker is limited. As a result, the ability to form unique, precise messages is curtailed. The communication process places numerous demands on both the nonspeaker and the recipient of his or her communications due to the frequent ambiguity of the messages and the time it takes to construct them. Some type of device usually must be made accessible to the nonspeaker, and the recipient of the messages usually must terminate his or her other activities to participate in the communication. Moreover, the recipient frequently must actively participate in order to make the messages reasonably precise.

It is easy to assume that both the nonspeaker and his or her associates, particularly parents of nonspeaking children, will be enthusiastic over the communicative potential that is offered by augmentative communication systems. However, some of the above problems may make it difficult for the nonspeaker to maintain his or her level of motivation to use them. Parents may even reject their use due to their reluctance to accept the fact that their child will not be able to develop oral communication.

A number of the augmentative communication devices that will best meet the needs of some nonspeaking persons with cerebral palsy are extremely expensive.

Obtaining the necessary monies for their purchase is one of the significant problems in this area of professional work.

The program of the speech-language pathologist for these systems should rely heavily upon interaction with the other professional persons who are involved with a specific client, and it should be designed to diminish as many of the above problems as possible. It is likely that the value of these programs is just beginning to be realized, and continued advances in technology is likely to make them even more successful. As increased knowledge is gained relative to matching a nonspeaker's language skills, physical abilities, intellectual level, and communication needs with the system that will best meet those needs, further emphasis on this aspect of management of cerebral palsy will result.

This concentration upon assisting the nonspeaking person with cerebral palsy is long overdue. It represents a significant advance to enable an increased number of those persons to participate in society at a level that is more commensurate with their potential, and it presents another stimulating and challenging area to the speech-language pathologist who works with them.

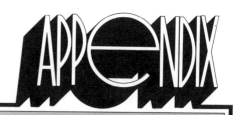

○ A   TERMS AND CONCEPTS RELATIVE
TO NEUROMOTOR DISORDERS

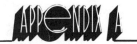

APPENDIX A

This synthesis of the manner in which terms are used relative to disorders of the motor (and neuromuscular) systems is not exhaustive. Rather, the more frequently used terms, their definitions, related concepts, and their implications for conditions associated with cerebral palsy are presented.

○ LOWER MOTOR NEURON DISORDERS

The term *lower motor neuron disorder,* or *lesion,* refers to dysfunction of the alpha motor neurons (or final common pathway). Lesions to the neuromotor systems of the developing brain that result in conditions of cerebral palsy typically are above the level of even the efferent cranial nerves. Therefore, lower motor neuron disorders are not typically associated with cerebral palsy. However, there may be occasions when terms that are related to lower motor neuron problems may be found in records of individuals who do have cerebral palsy, and it is helpful to understand that in most instances those terms probably have been used erroneously.

The term *segmental disorder,* or *lesion,* also may be used in reference to a lower motor neuron problem that is confined to a segment (or vertebral level) of the spinal cord that affects functions of the alpha motor neuron that emerge from that vertebral, or segmental, level. The term *bulb* is used to refer generally to the brain stem, and the term *bulbar palsy* may be used in reference to lower motor neuron disorders, or final common pathway problems, that result from dysfunction of the efferent cranial nerves since the cell bodies of the alpha motor neurons that make up those nerve trunks reside in the brain stem.

fasciculation

The term *fasciculation* refers to an abnormal, random discharge of the alpha motor neurons. Such a single discharge results in contraction of the muscle fibers innervated by the telodendria of a single alpha motor neuron (or motor unit). That contraction produces a twitch within the muscle that may be perceived by the individual and may be observable.

Fasciculations are a normal occurrence under conditions of fatigue (e.g., twitching within muscles of the eye lid). Fasciculations may occur at any time when the alpha motor neuron is irritated (e.g., as a result of some disease state prior to the alpha cells dying due to that disease).

fibrillation

Fibrillations are random contractions of individual muscle fibers that begin to occur after those fibers are denervated, and they may persist for a period of months. Thus, fibrillations may result from a variety of conditions of the myoneural junction. Since these contractions are non-synchronous even within the motor units, they may produce no observable contraction of muscle tissue, and their presence usually must be confirmed by intramuscular electromyography.

neuromuscular disorder

The term *neuromuscular disorder* usually is reserved for disorders of the myoneural junction and of muscle tissue. Since fibrillations are the result of such disorders, the term usually should be used in reference to the state of the total neuromotor-neuromuscular systems where random firing of muscle fibers is present. That term also is used in reference to some abnormal conditions of alpha neurons that result in fasciculations. The term neuromuscular disorder, therefore, probably should not be used in reference to the motor problems associated with cerebral palsy. (The term *neuromotor disorders* is now used commonly in reference to disorders of muscle tone, movement, and coordination that result from dysfunction of neural motor systems above the level of the final common pathway.)

hypotonia

When a number of motor units of a muscle become dysfunctional, due to some lower motor neuron or neuromuscular problem, resistance of the muscle to stretch will be diminished, and the muscle will be weak. The term *hypotonia* is applicable to this condition, but, as will be discussed below, this term also is used in reference to neuromotor disorders in which there is insufficient influence on the alpha motor neurons by those neuromotor systems that contribute to maintenance of normal muscle tone.

flaccidity

When there is denervation of essentially all fibers of a muscle, the resulting lack of muscle tone and contractibility is referred to as *flaccidity*. Flaccid muscle is a different phenomenon than the extreme forms of hypotonia that may be seen in some cerebral palsied infants and that will be discussed below.

atrophy

A lower motor neuron disorder that results in denervation of muscle fibers also results in a wasting of the tissue of those fibers. Muscle *atrophy* also results from disuse of muscle, and if atrophy exists in conditions of cerebral palsy, it would be because of disuse rather than denervation. However, the muscles of an essentially immobile arm of someone with spasticity are being "used" in the sense that there is contraction of those muscles. Therefore, disuse atrophy usually is not considered to be present in cerebral palsy.

○ UPPER MOTOR NEURON DISORDER

If the term *upper motor neuron disorder* were used in a manner semantically parallel to the term lower motor neuron disorder, it would be used in reference to motor problems that result from dysfunction of any of those descending neuromotor systems that influence activity of the final common pathway. Such use would make it applicable to all conditions of cerebral palsy. However, the term is routinely used only in reference to spasticity.

The term *suprasegmental disorder,* or *lesion,* is used in reference to an upper motor neuron disorder (spasticity) since it implies that the lesion to the neuromotor systems is above the level of the vertebral segments of the spinal cord and, hence, the cells of the motor units throughout the cord. It is conceivable then, that damage to an adult's brain stem may result in (1) *bulbar palsy,* or a lower motor neuron problem, of the efferent cranial nerves as a result of damage to the alpha cells of those nerves, and (2) an upper motor neuron disorder of the musculatures innervated by spinal nerves as a result of the *suprasegmental* lesion that results in the spasticity in those musculatures. The term *pseudobulbar palsy* is used in reference to an upper motor neuron disorder of the efferent cranial nerves; it implies an upper motor neuron disorder of the efferent cranial nerve system that is not due to damage within the level of the brain stem, and, hence, to the cell bodies of those neurons. This term, also, is routinely used only in reference to spasticity. Unfortunately, even though the term *suprasegmental lesion,* or *disorder,* implies dysfunction of spinal efferent nerves, it also is used in reference to conditions of spasticity regardless of the site of lesion, and therefore the individual who may be said to have a suprasegmental lesion also may have pseudobulbar palsy, or dysarthria, resulting from a lesion above the level of the brain stem. Except for bulbar palsy, all of these terms may be used in reference to individuals with cerebral palsy for whom the predominant neuromotor disorder is spasticity.

○ DISORDERS OF MUSCLE TONE

Muscle tone is routinely defined on the basis of a muscle's ability to resist stretch and/or the normal, constant contraction of muscle fibers that are associated with normal muscle function. A reduction or absence of that normal state of contraction and/or a muscle's resistance to stretch is referred to as *hypotonia,* and an increase in that normal state of contraction or a muscle's being overly resistive to stretch is referred to as *hypertonia.*

hypotonia

The term *hypotonia* is probably one of the less specific terms used in reference to neuromotor disorders since it can result from a variety of conditions that may lead to diminution of the normal tone-generating activity of motor units. Hypotonia is most frequently mentioned in reference to (1) lower motor neuron disorders as mentioned above and (2) damage to cerebellar mechanisms, which strongly influence maintenance of muscle tone for normal function. As has also been indicated above, the former is not typically seen in conditions associated with cerebral palsy. Neither is hypotonia usually mentioned as being present in the relatively infrequent cases of cerebral palsy that may be due to cerebellar damage and for which the prime neuromotor problems is incoordination.

Even though it is not routinely mentioned, indications of hypotonia can be found with numerous individuals who have sustained brain lesions and who have predominant signs of other types of neuromotor disorders. It is generally assumed that these cases of hypotonia result from damage to some excitatory mechanism or mechanisms within the neuromotor systems. Similarly, indications of hypotonia may be found in persons with cerebral palsy for whom the prime problem is some other type of neuromotor disorder.

Hypotonia is frequently an initial prime manifestation of cerebral palsy in infants, and it may be so severe as to draw the term *atonia.* That term probably is misapplied, since some muscle tone frequently is present. This form of hypotonia evidently results from a generalized lack of excitatory influence to the alpha motor neurons. As the damaged neuromotor systems of these infants mature, some of the more prevalent forms of the neuromotor disorders associated with cerebral palsy (i.e., spasticity or dyskinesia) probably will evolve. The site of the lesions and disruption of the neural mechanisms that result in this form of hypotonia have not been specified.

hypertonias

Two forms of hypertonia, namely, spasticity and rigidity, are frequently reviewed in discussions of neuromotor disorders acquired by adults. The third form, tension, is usually confined to discussions of developmental neuromotor disorders. Of these three hypertonias, spasticity is the most frequent predominant neuromotor disorder in both acquired and developmental disorders of the neuromotor systems. Even though there is considerable knowledge regarding the physiological basis of spasticity, a number of questions remain unanswered as to the exact central nervous system operations that result in its manifestation. While it is generally assumed that spasticity results from damage to the pyramidal motor system (i.e., corticobulbar and/or corticospinal tracts) in combination with some extrapyramidal system, the specific mechanisms that, when damaged, may result in rigidity or tension are unknown.

Spasticity. There is general agreement that *spasticity* results from hypersensitivity of the gamma system of those musculatures below the level of the lesion to the pyramidal system, and it appears that hyperactivity of the gamma efferent neurons is the basis for that abnormally high response to stretch of muscle spindles. The associated diminution of influence of corticobulbar and/or corticospinal tract influence on the alpha motor neurons results, then, in hypertonia through the gamma alpha loop and an exaggerated response of muscle to stretch. Spasticity also has been classically defined as affecting antigravity muscles of the extremities to a greater degree than muscles that work with gravity when the individual is in an upright position. Therefore, the flexors of the elbow joint that lift the lower arm against gravity are more severely involved than the extensors, and the muscles that extend the knee and push the foot downward are more involved than their antagonists. As a consequence, the individual with spasticity is likely to show routinely the posture of a flexed arm and stiffly extended leg while walking up on the ball of the foot.

The hyperstretch phenomena may be manifested by what is known as the "*clasp knife phenomenon*"; when the elbow or knee is passively flexed rapidly, the joint may initially close with minimal resistance; after flexion of a few degrees a firm resistance will be encountered as a result of the abnormally high discharge of muscle spindles in the extensors of the joints that are being stretched by the passive movements; if the passively induced force for joint flexion continues to be applied, this strong resistance may subside and the joint may be moved through its range of motion. *Deep tendon reflexes* also *are hyperactive* as a result, again, of exaggerated reaction of the muscle spindles in the muscle that has been stretched by a sudden force being applied to its attached tendons. Where spastic muscle can be stretched by applying an elastic force, a phenomenon known as *clonus* may be elicited. When an examiner pushes the foot upward toward the knee, the stretch reaction may result in the foot's being moved downward against the examiner's hand; when the angle of the ankle joint is thus increased to the point where stretch on the muscles of the calf of the leg is diminished, the foot then may be pushed back upward toward the knee; if the force continues to be applied, a reverberating action (ankle clonus) may result in which the foot literally vibrates against the examiner's hand. Some cutaneous reflexes also may be hyperactive and/or have an extended zone over which they can be elicited, and a prime diagnostic indication of spasticity is a Babinski response, or upward movement of the big toe and a curling of the other four toes in response to stroking the distal portion of the foot longitudinally toward the ball of the foot.

The consistent presence of hypertonia may result in slow and/or diminished movement of the limb of someone with spasticity. It is generally assumed, however, that attempts at rapid movement will be further restricted due to the increased reaction to stretch of the antagonistic muscles.

Rigidity. Although the sites of lesions that result in *rigidity* are infrequently specified, it usually is assumed that some inhibitory system that serves to diminish and/or control activity of excitatory neuromotor systems is damaged. Although descriptions of subtypes of cerebral palsy continue to refer to rigidity as being seen in developmental neuromotor disorders, most diagnosticians seldom, if ever, differentiate rigidity as a predominant problem in cerebral palsy.

Rigidity usually is said to be differentiated from spasticity by relatively equal hypertonia in all muscle groups and equal resistance to flexion of joints throughout their range of motion. One exception is what is referred to as a *"cogwheel" phenomenon,* in which there is an intermittent strong resistance to passive flexion of joints. These types of differentiation between rigidity and spasticity are somewhat unsatisfactory. It has been suggested that some cases of rigidity are, in fact, due to hyperactivity of the gamma system and that others are due to overexcitation of alpha neurons due to damage to some inhibitory neuromotor system.

Tension. The hypertonia referred to as *tension* in discussions of cerebral palsy is seldom mentioned in reviews of neuromotor disorders that result from lesions to mature brains. Its prime characteristics are that it (1) may be "shaken away" and (2) may vary in severity as a function of

the individual's affective state. Vigorous shaking of an arm whose musculatures manifest this type of hypertonia will result in a dramatic reduction
in the hypertonus; within a few minutes the tension will return. This form
of hypertonia will also increase in severity when the individual becomes
excited, angry, or otherwise emotionally stimulated, and it tends to diminish dramatically when the individual is relaxed or asleep.

When tension is present in individuals with cerebral palsy, it usually is
in conjunction with signs of dyskinesia. Although it is assumed that some
type of inhibitory neuromotor mechanism has been damaged, the site of
the lesion that produces tension and its neuroanatomical basis is unknown.

O DISORDERS OF MOVEMENT

Disorders of muscle tone result, of course, in an impairment of
movement capability. However, some neuromotor disorders are manifested by either excessive movement (hyperkinesia) or diminished ability to
move (hypokinesia).

hyperkinesias (involuntary movement)

Classical descriptions of the hyperkinesias have attempted to differentiate subtypes on the basis of the character of the movement (e.g., either rapid or slow involuntary motions). However, the poor reliability
with which some of these forms of movement can be differentiated on
that basis has led to suggestions that in some cases these so-called types of
involuntary motion disorders are simply variations of a common problem. Nevertheless, most reviews of this group of disorders continue to
specify distinct characteristics of subtypes of hyperkinesias as given below.

Dyskinesia (Extrapyramidal Signs). The term *dyskinesia* is beginning to be used with increasing frequency to refer to what classically has
been defined as a set of different disorders. Other terms that have been
used to designate these disorders are *athetosis, chorea,* and *choreoathetosis.*

Athetosis has classically been said to be characterized by slow, writhing
involuntary motions of the extremities. The movements have been described as "wormlike" when they are superimposed on voluntary movements. There also may be finger movements that are opposite to the
intended movement (e.g., a fanning and extending of the fingers prior to
their closing on an object to be grasped). Rapid, jerking, and flailing involuntary movements of the extremities have been designated as chorea,
or choreoform movements. The term *choreoathetosis* has been used in reference to involuntary motions in which the rapid choreoform movements
appear to be superimposed on the slow, writhing athetotic movements.

Although these three terms are still found in the literature, there now appears to be a growing belief that these involuntary movements are variations of a common disorder. The term *extrapyramidal signs* is frequently used in reference to some of these manifestations of damage to the neuromotor systems of adults. *Dyskinesia* or *athetosis* are the terms that are most frequently used in reference to the large proportion of individuals who have cerebral palsy and for whom involuntary motions are the prime neuromotor disorder.

Dystonia. Some reviews of acquired neuromotor disorders describe dystonia as an extreme form of athetosis in which the posturing of hands and/or feet are pulled and held into abnormal positions. These types of phenomena probably would be said to be the result of tension in developmental neuromotor disorders.

Dystonia is more typically described as involuntary contractions of the muscles of the torso, neck, and face. These contractions increase relatively slowly in intensity, and they may result in grotesque postures due to the extremely forceful contractions of the involved muscles before relaxation. The basal ganglia and other extrapyramidal mechanisms are usually indicated as potential sites of causal lesions.

Ballismus. Lesions to a relatively small nucleus below the thalamus (subthalamic nucleus of Luys) is known to result in rapid, violent, flailing movements of the extremities on the contralateral side. This usual, but not consistent, involvement of only one side has lead to a frequent designation of this condition as *hemiballismus.*

Of the hyperkinesias, ballismus is the only form that seems to result from a site of lesion that can be specified. Even so, there are suggestions that some of the rapid, flailing movements of the dyskinetic group of disorders are a form of ballismus. There have also been suggestions that ballismus may be seen in selected individuals with cerebral palsy. However, neither of these suggestions seem to be generally accepted.

tremors

Tremors are routinely defined as a back and forth, pendular movement of the extremities and/or head. Tremors may be included in discussions of forms of hyperkinesias, or they may be discussed as a separate group of disorders. In general, tremors seem to result from damage to some type of inhibitory mechanism that permits oscillatory patterns of excitation to influence the final common pathways. Two types of tremor are usually described: tremor at rest and action tremor. As the label implies, the former occurs during rest, and it usually is attributed to some type of lesion or disorder of the basal ganglia and associated nuclei; tremor at rest is usually mentioned as one of the characteristics of Parkinson's

disease. Action tremor is manifested during movements, and it is a frequent sequelae of damage to cerebellar mechanisms.

There are discussions of other types of tremors. These discussions,
however, routinely do not review the tremors that may be observed in individuals who have sustained damage to their brains from a variety of
causes or who are aged. Also, in spite of some suggestions to the contrary,
tremors should not be expected to be seen with individuals who have developmental neuromotor disorders.

myoclonus and spasmodic disorders

As in the case of tremors, discussions of hyperkinesias may also
include myoclonus and a variety of conditions in which there are rapid,
twitching contractions of muscles or musculatures. However, they also are
discussed separately. The term *myoclonus* is used in reference to what
probably is a variety of disorders in which some inhibitory mechanism
among the extrapyramidal mechanisms has been damaged such that
surges of excitatory activity reaches the final common pathways and result
in very rapid, spasmodic muscle contractions. Such rapid contractions result in movement, including contortions of the face, depending on the
muscles that are involved. Palatal myoclonus is characterized by a rhyth-
mic, continual elevation of the palate. Palatal myoclonus is probably a distinct type of disorder that differs considerably from the myoclonus that
results in rapid, abrupt contractions of, for example, a muscle within or
muscles of the arm. This variety of disorders is not seen in conditions of
cerebral palsy.

hypokinesia

A characteristic referred to as paucity of movement has been recognized for some time as a component of the cluster of neuromotor disorders that constitute Parkinson's disease. Its manifestations include delay in
initiating movement, slowness of movement, and diminution of what
might be referred to as associated movements such as the swinging of the
arms while walking. These characteristics have been attributed to other
forms of neuromotor disorders (e.g., rigidity) as observed in Parkinson patients. These manifestations of a neuromotor problem are now being referred to as *hypokinesia,* and in some cases this disorder is now believed to be
the basis of what were formerly thought to be different disorders in Parkinson's disease such as rigidity and/or spasticity.

There appears to be a growing tendency to identify hypokinesia as a
separate entity that may also result from other etiologies, such as trauma
to the brain. Again, to the extent that it is recognized as a separate neuromotor disorder, hypokinesia has been attributed to dysfunction of the

basal ganglia and associated mechanisms, but it is not recognized as being present in developmental neuromotor disorders.

O DISORDERS OF COORDINATION (ATAXIA)

Lesions to cerebellar mechanisms may result in an individual's being unable to perform smoothly coordinated movements, often displaying disturbances of gait and balance. The basis of this incoordination is believed to be a disruption of the cerebellum's ability to compare incoming afferent information from somesthetic, vestibular, visual, and perhaps, auditory mechanisms to intended movements and targets of the motor systems. As a result, there is abnormal cerebellar influence into the neuromotor systems that ordinarily assist in relatively minute adjustments needed to accomplish coordinated movements. This incoordination, or *ataxia,* is believed now to occur only rarely as a subtype of cerebral palsy.

O PROBLEMS WITH LABELS

In reviewing lists and descriptions of neuromotor disorders such as the above, there is a strong inclination to assume that the various labels represent discrete, well-defined, and readily identifiable disorders. As exemplified by the above discussion of the dyskinesias, there may be reasons to question the extent to which a number of the neuromotor disorders as routinely labeled are distinct and result from unique sites of lesions. On the other hand, as is exemplified in the above discussion of hypotonia, one label may be applied to disorders of obviously different origins.

Such lists and brief descriptions also may lead to the misconception that most individuals who have some disorder of the neuromotor systems manifest signs of only one type of these disorders. Definite indications of combinations of disorders may be present. For example, an individual who has sustained brain damage as a result of an accident may show a generalized involvement of some form of hypertonia and exaggerated deep tendon reflexes in three extremities but with a violent action tremor in one arm. Such extreme variations are not likely to be seen in developmental neuromotor disorders.

Such lists of labels and descriptions of neuromotor disorders often imply that, for both acquired and developmental neuromotor disorders, the identifying characteristics are consistently present. Whether an individual with predominant spasticity of a lower limb is a recent car accident victim or a child with cerebral palsy, a Babinski response may or may not be elicited consistently. The variety of influences to the final common pathways of the musculatures of the lower leg and foot may inhibit the response at any moment in time. This example of the dynamic nature of the nervous system points out the problems of conceptualizing that system as consistently producing the behaviors that are described as manifestations of neuromotor disorders.

○ CONTRACTURES

Muscle tissue tends to adopt, anatomically, the length in which it is routinely held. When an arm, for example, that has been broken is removed from a cast that has held the elbow at 90 degrees for a period of weeks, it may be impossible for the elbow to be straightened completely. Disuse atrophy of the triceps may be present to some degree, but a likely reason for the inability to extend the elbow completely is that the bicep will be somewhat shorter than before the casting. Exercise will not only relieve what disuse atrophy may be present, but will also reverse the contracture of the bicep, and the muscle will lengthen as it begins to be stretched as the arm is exercised and the elbow joint extended.

While contracture is not a neuromotor disorder per se, it is a phenomenon that affects musculatures of many individuals with neuromotor disorders. When there is imbalance among hypertonic muscles, for example, that results in one of those muscles routinely being maintained in a less than normal length, contractures are likely to develop. That is particularly so with spastic muscle; moreover, such contractures in the presence of a neuromotor disorder may be irreversible.

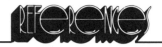

ASHA Ad Hoc Committee on Communication Processes and Nonspeaking Persons, "Nonspeech Communication: A Position Paper," *Asha,* 22, no. 4 (April 1980), 267–272.

AYRES, A. JEAN, *Southern California Sensory Integration Tests* (Manual), (6th ed.). Los Angeles, Ca.: Western Psychological Service, 1978.

BIRCH, HERBERT G., (ed.), *Brain Damage in Children—The Biological and Social Aspects.* Baltimore, Md.: The Williams and Wilkins Co., 1964.

BOBATH, KAREL, *A Neurophysiological Basis for the Treatment of Cerebral Palsy* (2nd ed.), Philadelphia, Pa.: J. B. Lippincott Co., 1980.

BOBATH, KAREL, and BERTA BOBATH, "The Facilitation of Normal Postural Reactions and Movements in the Treatment of Cerebral Palsy," *Physiotherapy,* August 1964.

BOBATH, KAREL, and BERTA BOBATH, "Cerebral Palsy," Chapter 3 in *Physical Therapy Services in the Developmental Disabilities,* ed. Paul H. Pearson and Carol Ethun Williams. Springfield, Ill.: Charles C Thomas, 1972.

BYRNE, MARGARET C., "Speech and Language Development of Athetoid and Spastic Children," *Journal of Speech and Hearing Disorders,* 24, no. 3 (August 1959), 231–240.

COLEMAN, COLETTE L., ALBERT M. COOK, and LAWRENCE S. MYERS, "Assessing Non-Oral Clients for Assistive Communication Devices," *Journal of Speech and Hearing Disorders,* 45, no. 4 (November 1980), 515–526.

CROTHERS, BRONSON, and RICHMOND S. PAINE, *The Natural History of Cerebral Palsy.* Cambridge, Mass.: Harvard University Press, 1959.

FLOWER, RICHARD M., RICHARD VIEHWEG, and WILLIAM R. RUZICKA, "The Communicative Disorders of Children with Kernicteric Athetosis: II. Problems in Language Comprehension and Use," *Journal of Speech and Hearing Disorders,* 31, no. 1, (February 1966), 60–68.

FREUD, SIGMUND, *Infantile Cerebral Paralysis* (1st ed.), trans. Lester A. Russin. Coral Gables, Fla.: University of Miami Press, 1968.

GILLETTE, HARRIET E., *Systems of Therapy in Cerebral Palsy.* Springfield, Ill.: Charles C Thomas, 1969.

HARDY, JAMES C., "Lung Function of Athetoid and Spastic Quadriplegic Children," *Developmental Medicine and Child Neurology,* 6, no. 4 (August 1964), 378–388.

HARDY, JAMES C., "Suggestions for Physiological Research in Dysarthria," *Cortex,* 3 (1967), 128–156.

HARDY, JAMES C., RAYMOND R. REMBOLT, DUANE C. SPRIESTERSBACH, and B. JAYAPATHY, "Surgical Management of Palatal Paresis and Speech Problems in Cerebral Palsy: A Preliminary Report," *Journal of Speech and Hearing Disorders*, 26, no. 4 (November 1961), 320–325.

HARDY, JAMES C., and H. J. ARKEBAUER, "Development of a Test for Velopharyngeal Competence During Speech," *Cleft Palate Journal*, 3 (1966), 6–21.

HARDY, JAMES C., and T. D. EDMONDS, "Electronic Integrator for Measurement of Partitions of the Lung Volume," *Journal of Speech and Hearing Research*, 11, no. 4 (December 1968), 777–786.

HARDY, JAMES C., RONALD NETSELL, JAMES W. SCHWEIGER, and HUGHLETT L. MORRIS, "Management of Velopharyngeal Dysfunction in Cerebral Palsy," *Journal of Speech and Hearing Disorders*, 34, no. 2 (May 1969), 123–137.

HIXON, THOMAS J., "Some New Techniques for Measuring the Biomechanical Events of Speech Production: One Laboratory's Experiences," *Asha Reports*, 7 (July 1972), 68–103.

HIXON, THOMAS J., "Respiratory Function in Speech," Chapter 3 in *Normal Aspects of Speech, Hearing, and Language*, ed. Fred D. Minifie, Thomas J. Hixon, and Frederick Williams. Englewood Cliffs, N.J.: Prentice-Hall, 1973.

HIXON, THOMAS J., and JAMES C. HARDY, "Restricted Motility of the Speech Articulators in Cerebral Palsy," *Journal of Speech and Hearing Disorders*, 29, no. 3 (August 1964), 293–306.

HIXON, THOMAS J., JERE MEAD, and MICHAEL D. GOLDMAN, "Dynamics of the Chest Wall During Speech Production: Function of the Thorax, Rib Cage, Diaphragm, and Abdomen," *Journal of Speech and Hearing Research*, 19, no. 2 (June 1976), 297–356.

JOHNS, DONNELL F., and KENNETH E. SALYER, "Surgical and Prosthetic Management of Neurogenic Speech Disorders," Chapter 7 in *Clinical Management of Neurogenic Communicative Disorders*, ed. Donnell F. Johns. Boston, Mass.: Little, Brown & Company, 1978.

KENT, RAYMOND D., "Models of Speech Production," Chapter 3 in *Contemporary Issues in Experimental Phonetics*, ed. Norman J. Lass. New York: Academic Press, 1976.

KENT, RAYMOND D., and RONALD NETSELL, "Articulatory Abnormalities in Athetoid Cerebral Palsy," *Journal of Speech and Hearing Disorders*, 43, no. 3 (August 1978), 353–373.

LAVELLE, WILLIAM E., and JAMES C. HARDY, "Palatal Lift Prostheses for Treatment of Palatopharyngeal Incompetence," *Journal of Prosthetic Dentistry*, 42, no. 3 (September 1979), 308–315.

LENCIONE, RUTH M., "Speech and Language Problems in Cerebral Palsy," Chapter 5 in *Cerebral Palsy, Its Individual and Community Problems* (2nd ed.), ed. William K. Cruickshank. Syracuse, N.Y.: Syracuse University Press, 1966.

LENCIONE, RUTH M., "The Development of Communication Skills," Chapter 6 in *Cerebral Palsy: A Developmental Disability* (3rd ed.), ed. William M. Cruickshank. Syracuse, N.Y.: Syracuse University Press, 1976.

LITTLE, W. J., "Course of Lectures on Deformation of the Human Frame," Lecture No. 8, *Lancet*, 1 (1843), 318.

LITTLE, W. J., "On the Influence of Abnormal Parturition, Difficult Labor, Premature Birth, and Asphyxia Neonatorum, on the Mental and Physical Condition of the Child, Especially in Relation to Deformities," *Lancet*, 2 (October 1861), 378–380.

LLOYD, LYLE L., **(ed.)**, *Communication Assessment and Intervention Strategies.* Baltimore, Md.: University Park Press, 1976.

LOVE, RUSSELL J., "Oral Language Behavior of Older Cerebral Palsied Children," *Journal of Speech and Hearing Research,* 7, no. 4 (December 1964), 349–359.

LOVE, RUSSELL J., **EVELYN L. HAGERMAN**, **and ELAINE G. TAIMI**, "Speech Performance, Dysphagia and Oral Reflexes in Cerebral Palsy," *Journal of Speech and Hearing Disorders,* 45, no. 1 (February 1980), 59–75.

McDONALD, EUGENE T., *Teaching and Using Blissymbolics.* Toronto: Blissymbolics Communication Institute, 1980.

McDONALD, EUGENE T., **and BURTON CHANCE, JR.**, *Cerebral Palsy,* ed. Charles Van Riper. Foundations of Speech Pathology Series. Englewood Cliffs, N.J.: Prentice-Hall, 1964.

MINEAR, W. L., "A Classification of Cerebral Palsy," *Pediatrics,* 18 (1956), 841–852.

MYERS, PATRICIA, "A Study of Language Disabilities in Cerebral Palsied Children," *Journal of Speech and Hearing Research,* 8, no. 2 (June 1965), 129–136.

NETSELL, RONALD, "Evaluation of Velopharyngeal Function in Dysarthria," *Journal of Speech and Hearing Disorders,* 34, no. 2 (May 1969), 113–122. (a)

NETSELL, RONALD, "Changes in Oropharyngeal Cavity Size of Dysarthric Children," *Journal of Speech and Hearing Research,* 12, no. 3 (September 1969), 646–649. (b)

PAILLARD, JACQUES, "The Patterning of Skilled Movements," Chapter 67 in *Handbook of Physiology, Section 1: Neurophysiology Volume III*, ed. John Field. Baltimore, Md.: Williams & Wilkins, 1960.

PAYTON, OTTO D., **SUSANNE HIRT**, **and ROBERTA A. NEWTON** (eds.), *Scientific Bases for Neurophysiologic Approaches to Therapeutic Exercise, An Anthology.* Philadelphia, Pa.: F. A. Davis Company, 1977.

PHELPS, WINTHROP M., "Classification of Athetosis with Special Reference to the Motor Classification," *American Journal of Physical Medicine,* 35 (1956), 24–31.

PLATT, J. F., **GAVIN ANDREWS**, **MARGRETTE YOUNG**, **and PETER T. QUINN**, "Dysarthria of Adult Cerebral Palsy: I. Intelligibility and Articulatory Impairment," *Journal of Speech and Hearing Research,* 23, no. 1 (March 1980), 28–38.

SACHS, B., "Little's Disease; Shall We Retain the Name?" *Journal of Nervous and Mental Disease,* December 1897, pp. 3–15.

SIEGEL, GERALD M., **and PATRICIA A. BROEN**, "Language Assessment," Chapter 3 in *Communication Assessment and Intervention Strategies,* ed. Lyle L. Lloyd. Baltimore, Md.: University Park Press, 1976.

STEIN, LASZLO K., **and FREDERIC K. W. CURRY**, "Childhood Auditory Agnosia," *Journal of Speech and Hearing Disorders,* 33, no. 4 (November 1968), 361–370.

STRAUSS, A., **and L. LEHTINEN**, *Psychopathology and Education of the Brain-Injured Child.* New York, N.Y.: Grune & Stratton, 1947.

VANDERHEIDEN, G. C., **(ed.)**, *Non-Vocal Communication Resource Book.* Baltimore, Md.: University Park Press, 1978.

VANDERHEIDEN, G. C., and K. GRILLEY (eds.) *Non-Vocal Communication Techniques and Aids for the Severely Physically Handicapped.* Madison, Wis.: Trace Center, University of Wisconsin, 1975.

VICKER, B., (ed.) *Nonoral Communication System Project: 1964/1973.* Iowa City: University of Iowa, 1974.

WESTLAKE, HAROLD, and DAVID RUTHERFORD, *Speech Therapy for the Cerebral Palsied.* Chicago: National Society for Crippled Children and Adults, 1961.

YOSS, KATHE ALLEN, and FREDERIC L. DARLEY, "Developmental Apraxia of Speech in Children with Defective Articulation," *Journal of Speech and Hearing Research,* 17, no. 3 (September 1974), 399–416.